Nutrition and Biochemistry for Nurses

Nutrition and Biochemistry for Nurses

Second Edition

Jacob Anthikad
MA (Psy) BEd MA (Chem) DTech (Biochem)

Retired Wing Commander
Indian Air Force (IAF)
Bengaluru, Karnataka, India

Visiting Professor
Kempegowda College of Nursing
MS Ramaiah College of Nursing
St John's College of Nursing
St Philomena's College of Nursing
Bengaluru, Karnataka, India

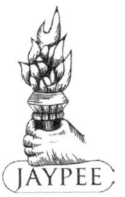

JAYPEE BROTHERS MEDICAL PUBLISHERS (P) LTD
New Delhi • London • Philadelphia • Panama

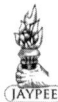 **Jaypee Brothers Medical Publishers (P) Ltd**

Headquarters

Jaypee Brothers Medical Publishers (P) Ltd
4838/24, Ansari Road, Daryaganj
New Delhi 110 002, India
Phone: +91-11-43574357
Fax: +91-11-43574314
Email: jaypee@jaypeebrothers.com

Overseas Offices

J.P. Medical Ltd
83, Victoria Street, London
SW1H 0HW (UK)
Phone: +44-2031708910
Fax: +44(0)2030086180
Email: info@jpmedpub.com

Jaypee Medical Inc
The Bourse
111 South Independence Mall East
Suite 835, Philadelphia, PA 19106, USA
Phone: +1 267-519-9789
Email: jpmed.us@gmail.com

Jaypee-Highlights Medical Publishers Inc.
City of Knowledge, Bld. 237, Clayton
Panama City, Panama
Phone: +1 507-301-0496
Fax: +1 507-301-0499
Email: cservice@jphmedical.com

Jaypee Brothers Medical Publishers (P) Ltd
17/1-B Babar Road, Block-B, Shaymali
Mohammadpur, Dhaka-1207
Bangladesh
Mobile: +08801912003485
Email: jaypeedhaka@gmail.com

Jaypee Brothers Medical Publishers (P) Ltd
Bhotahity, Kathmandu, Nepal
Phone: +977-9741283608
Email: kathmandu@jaypeebrothers.com

Website: www.jaypeebrothers.com
Website: www.jaypeedigital.com

© 2014, Jaypee Brothers Medical Publishers

The views and opinions expressed in this book are solely those of the original contributor(s)/author(s) and do not necessarily represent those of editor(s) of the book.

All rights reserved. No part of this publication may be reproduced, stored or transmitted in any form or by any means, electronic, mechanical, photocopying, recording or otherwise, without the prior permission in writing of the publishers.

All brand names and product names used in this book are trade names, service marks, trademarks or registered trademarks of their respective owners. The publisher and author are not associated with any product or vendor mentioned in this book.

Medical knowledge and practice change constantly. This book is designed to provide accurate, authoritative information about the subject matter in question. However, readers are advised to check the most current information available on procedures included and check information from the manufacturer of each product to be administered, to verify the recommended dose, formula, method and duration of administration, adverse effects and contraindications. It is the responsibility of the practitioner to take all appropriate safety precautions. Neither the publisher nor the author(s)/editor(s) assume any liability for any injury and/or damage to persons or property arising from or related to use of material in this book.

This book is sold on the understanding that the publisher is not engaged in providing professional medical services. If such advice or services are required, the services of a competent medical professional should be sought.

Every effort has been made where necessary to contact holders of copyright to obtain permission to reproduce copyright material. If any have been inadvertently overlooked, the publisher will be pleased to make the necessary arrangements at the first opportunity.

Inquiries for bulk sales may be solicited at: jaypee@jaypeebrothers.com

Nutrition and Biochemistry for Nurses
First Edition: **2009**
Second Edition: **2014**
ISBN 978-93-5090-946-1
Printed at: Sterling Graphics Pvt. Ltd.

***Dedicated to**
Student Nurses
around the country
whose questions and comments
continue to inspire the fine-tuning
of this textbook*

Preface
to the Second Edition

The suggestions and comments received from the student community and teaching fraternity have been incorporated in this second edition. The findings of the UNICEF-2012 and Nutrition Survey-2011 have been highlighted in India's nutritional problems. Due importance has been accorded to the 'weaning section'.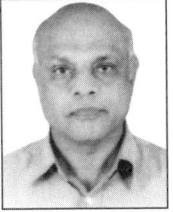

The question bank has been thoroughly overhauled by removing the question papers pertaining to the earlier syllabus and by adding new questions. Hope this student-friendly second edition meets all the requirements of the students and will be well received as usual by the students and their teachers. Wishing you all the best and best of all!

Jacob Anthikad

Preface
to the First Edition

This textbook has been carefully prepared as per the latest basic BSc (Nursing) Syllabus of the Nursing Council (revised: 2004) where nutrition has been combined with biochemistry. Nutrition is a relatively new science, which evolved from biochemistry and physiology. It is often treated as a branch of chemical science or biochemistry.

The separation of biochemistry in the syllabus is sometimes arbitrary. As an author, I have tried to separate some more principles of biochemistry from nutrition aspects and group them with the biochemistry portion of the prescribed syllabus. Blood chemistry and urinalysis have been included in Biochemistry as chapters 16 and 17 and will be essential for Pathology to be studied later in the basic BSc (Nursing) course. MCQs and plenty of study questions have been added to make the text still more student-friendly. Readers' constructive suggestions are most welcome and will be implemented in the subsequent editions.

I am grateful to Shri Jitendar P Vij (Chairman and Managing Director) and Mr Tarun Duneja (Director-Publishing) of M/s Jaypee Brothers Medical Publishers (P) Ltd, New Delhi, for their constant support and encouragement.

Jacob Anthikad

Acknowledgments

The first edition of 'Nutrition and Biochemistry' was published in 2009. It was very well received by the students and their teachers necessitating many reprints. With their constructive feedbacks, the book is now thoroughly revised for the second edition.

My task was made more pleasant by the cooperation and non-complaining attitude of my family members. I acknowledge their patience and also thank each and every one of them for their loving care.

I take this opportunity also to thank Shri Jitendar P Vij (Group Chairman), Mr Ankit Vij (Managing Director), Mr Tarun Duneja (Director-Publishing) and Mr Venugopal V (Regional Manager, Bengaluru Branch) of M/s Jaypee Brothers Medical Publishers (P) Ltd, New Delhi, India for encouraging and enabling me to meet the deadlines. I also thank Ms Sajini SV and others of M/s Jaypee Brothers Medical Publishers, Bengaluru branch for their assistance in completing the entire project.

Contents

Part 1: Biochemistry

1. Biochemical Perspective to Medicine   3
    Scope of Biochemistry   3
    Structure, Composition and Functions of a Cell   5
    Prokaryotes and Eukaryotes   9
    Microscopy   9
    Autoradiography   10
    Fluid Mosaic Model of Cell Membrane   11
    Transport Mechanisms Across the Cell Membrane   12

2. Chemistry of Carbohydrates   16
    Biological Importance   16
    Characteristics of Carbohydrates   18
    Reactions of Carbohydrates   22
    Classification   25

3. Chemistry of Lipids   36
    Occurrence   36
    Biological Significance of Fats   36
    Classification of Lipids   37
    Chemical Composition of Fats   38
    Essential Fatty Acids (Polyunsaturated
      Fatty Acids)   38
    Properties of Fats   39
    Characteristics of Fats   41
    Structural Lipids or Membrane Lipids   42
    Functions of Cholesterol   46
    Lipoproteins   47
    Estimation of Plasma Lipids   49

4. Amino Acids 52

Utilization or Metabolism of Proteins 52
Absorption of Proteins (Amino Acids) 54
Classification and Structure of Amino Acids 54
Functions of Amino Acids 55
Occurrence of Amino Acids 55
Properties of Amino Acids 55

5. Chemistry of Proteins 64

Biological Importance 64
Composition of Proteins 64
Biomedical Importance of Proteins 65
Structure of Proteins 66
Denaturation of Proteins 68
Classification of Proteins 68
Properties of Proteins 70
Color Reactions (Tests) of Proteins 73

6. Vitamins 77

Definition 77
Classification 77
Vitamins Not Acting as Coenzymes or
 Fat-soluble Vitamins 78
Water-soluble Vitamins 84

7. Nucleic Acids and Nucleotides 99

Nucleic Acids 99
Nucleosides (Nitrogen base + Sugar) 101
Nucleotides (Nitrogen base + Sugar
 + Phosphate) 101
Nucleotides of Biological Importance 104

8. Enzymology 112

General Properties of Enzymes 112
Classification of Enzymes 113
Enzyme Specificity 114
Mechanism of Enzyme Action 115
Coenzymes 120
Diagnostic Value of Plasma Enzymes 121

9. Digestion and Absorption 127

Digestive Fluids 127
Digestion of Carbohydrates 130
Digestion of Fats 131

Digestion of Proteins	131	
Absorption of Carbohydrates	132	
Absorption of Lipids	134	
Absorption of Proteins	135	
Absorption of Vitamins	135	
Bile Pigments: Biliverdin and Bilirubin	136	

10. Basic Concepts of Metabolism — 140

- Definition of Metabolism — 140
- Source of Energy — 140
- Biological Oxidation — 141
- Biomedical Importance of Metabolism — 145

11. Metabolism of Carbohydrates — 149

- Fate of Glucose after Absorption — 149
- Intermediary Metabolism of Carbohydrates — 149
- Glycolysis — 151
- Tricarboxylic Acid Cycle (Krebs Cycle/Citric Acid Cycle) — 153
- Eight Steps in Citric Acid Cycle — 156
- Energetics — 157
- Blood Sugar Level and its Clinical Significance — 159
- Regulation (Homeostasis) of Blood Glucose Level — 163
- Role of Hormones in the Homeostasis of Blood Sugar Level — 165

12. Metabolism of Lipids — 173

- Plasma Lipids — 173
- Digestion and Absorption of Lipids — 174
- Lipid Metabolism — 175
- Energetics — 176

13. Metabolism of Proteins — 188

- Digestion of Proteins by Enzymes — 188
- General Pathway of Protein Metabolism — 189
- Urea Synthesis — 192
- Metabolism of Glutamic Acid — 195

14. Immunochemistry — 202

- Immunity — 202
- Immune Response — 202
- Antibody-mediated Immune (Humoral) Response — 203
- Cell-mediated Immune Response — 203

Mechanisms of Antibody Production	203
Major Histocompatibility Complex	204
Free Radicals	205
Antioxidants	206
Structural and Contractile Proteins	207

15. Hormones: Outline Chemistry and Functions — 210

Classification of Hormones	211
Factors Regulating Hormone Action	212
Steroid Hormones	213
Sex Hormones	213
Peptide Hormones	215
Amine Hormones	216
Adrenal Medulla	220
Pancreatic Islet Cells	221
Adrenal Cortex	221
Gastrointestinal Hormones	221
Hypothalamic and Pituitary Hormones	222

16. Blood Chemistry — 226

Constituents of Blood	226
Functions of Blood	228
Plasma Proteins	229
Separation of Plasma Proteins	231
Regulation (Homeostasis) of pH of Blood	232

17. Urinalysis — 240

Collection of Urine	240
Composition of Urine	241
Procedure	242
Constituents of Normal Urine	242
Analysis of Normal Urine	246
Analysis of Pathological Urine	247

18. Renal Function Tests — 252

Functions of a Kidney	252
Renal Function Tests	252

19. Abnormalities of Bilirubin Metabolism: Jaundice — 258

Jaundice	258

20. Liver Function Tests — 263

Liver Function Tests	263

Part 2: Nutrition

21. Food, Nutrition and Health — 269
- History — 269
- Concepts — 269
- Nutrients — 270
- Nutrition and Health — 271
- Nutritional Problems in India — 272
- India's High Child Mortality Rate—National Shame — 273
- Factors Influencing Food Habits and Selection of Foodstuffs — 276
- Exchange Lists — 277
- Income — 278
- Functions of Food — 278
- Classification of Food — 281
- Food Guide Pyramid: A Guide to Daily Food Choice — 282
- Respiratory Quotient — 284
- Factors Affecting Energy Expenditure — 284
- Basal Metabolic Rate — 285
- Thermogenic Effect [Specific Dynamic Action (SDA)] of Food — 287
- Physical Activity — 287
- Body Mass Index/Quetelet's Index — 289

22. Carbohydrates: Sugar, Starch and Fiber — 290
- Carbohydrates — 290

23. Nutritional Aspects of Fats — 294
- Fats — 294
- Functions of Lipids — 295
- Essential Fatty Acids — 297
- Fats and Heart Ailment — 297

24. Proteins — 299
- Protein Quality — 299
- Recommended Dietary Allowance — 301
- Dietary Sources of Proteins — 302
- Functions of Proteins — 303
- Protein Deficiency — 304
- Protein-Calorie Malnutrition in Children — 305
- Effect of Excess — 306
- Nutrition — 306

25. Mineral Metabolism — 307

Macrominerals — 307
Calcium — 307
Phosphorus — 310
Sodium — 311
Potassium — 313
Chloride — 314
Sulfur — 315
Magnesium — 316
Microminerals — 316
Copper — 316
Zinc — 317
Selenium — 318
Iodine — 318
Iron — 319
Manganese — 322
Chromium — 322
Cobalt — 323
Fluorine — 323
Molybdenum — 324

26. Water Metabolism — 328

Water — 328
Electrolytes — 329
Disorders of Water and Electrolyte Balances — 330

27. Cookery Rules and Preservation of Nutrients — 332

Purpose of Cooking — 332
Aims and Objectives of Cooking Food — 332
Methods of Cooking — 333
Cooking Media — 334
Changes in Cooking — 337

28. Food Preservation: Principles and Methods — 338

Food Preservation — 338

29. Foodborne Diseases — 342

Types of Foodborne Diseases — 342

30. Food Laws and Food Standards — 345

Prevention of Food Adulteration Act, 1954 — 345
Fruit Products Order — 346
Meat Products Order — 346

Enforcement	346	
Misbranding	347	

31. Hospital Diets — 351

Types of Hospital Diets	351
Preparation of Simple Beverages and Different Types of Food	352
Light Diets	355

32. Budgeting for Balanced Diet — 357

Plans for Food Budget	357
Selection, Storage and Preparation of Food	357
Food Groups and Guidelines for Food Selection	358
Functional Classification of Foods	362
Planning of a Balanced Diet	362

33. Assessment of Nutritional Status — 365

Nutritional Assessment	365
National and International Agencies Working Towards Food/Nutrition	368

34. Role of a Nurse in Nutritional Programs — 372

Community Nutrition Programs in India	372
Objectives of Nutrition Education	374
Means for Nutrition Education	374
Methods for Nutrition Education of the Community	374
Role of Nurses in Nutritional Assessment and Nutrition Education	375

35. Nutrition in Pregnancy — 377

Energy	377
Proteins	377
Vitamins	378
Minerals	378
Iron	378
Fats	379
Nutritional Requirements during Lactation	379

36. Nutrition in Infancy — 382

Energy	382
Proteins	382
Minerals	382

Vitamins	383
Fat	383
Carbohydrates	383
Fluid	383
Breastfeeding	384
Weaning	385
Artificial Feeding	387
Preterm Babies	387
Supplementary Foods for Infants and Toddlers	388

37. Menu for Preschool, School-age Children and Adolescents — 391

Diet for a Preschool Child	391
Diet for School Children	391
Adolescent	392

38. Geriatric Nutrition — 398

Physiological Changes in Aging	398
Nutritional Requirements	399

39. Naturopathic Medicine — 407

Concepts and Principles	407
Development and its Status	408
Methods of Nature Cure	410

40. Diet Therapy — 413

Principles of Diet Therapy	413
Factors to Consider in Planning Therapeutic Diets	413
Modification of Nutrients in Therapeutic Diets	414
Types of Diet Used in Hospitals	414
Special Feeding Methods (Management of Special Diets)	415
Pre- and Postoperative Diet	417
Fever	419
Typhoid	420
Influenza	421
Tuberculosis	421
Diet in Relation to Conditions of Gastrointestinal Tract	423
Diet in Relation to Disease of the Liver and Gallbladder	427
Therapeutic Diet in Conditions of Endocrine Glands and Metabolic Disorders	431

Various Metabolic Disorders	436
Joint Diseases	437
Dietary Counseling	437
Therapeutic Diet in Conditions of the Urinary System	438
Diet Therapy in Conditions of the Circulatory System	442

Appendices 445

Appendix I: Normal Values of Important Tests	447
Appendix II: University Examination Question Papers	448

Index 485

Course Description— INC Syllabus

INC BIOCHEMISTRY SYLLABUS (REVISED: 2004)

Placement: First year
Time: Theory—30 hours

The course is designed to assist the students acquire knowledge of the normal biochemical composition and functioning of human body and understand the alterations in biochemistry in the diseases for the practice of nursing.

Unit	Time (hours)	Learning objectives	Contents	Teaching and learning activities	Assessment methods
I	3	• Describe the structure, composition and functions of a cell • Differentiate between prokaryotic cell and eukaryotic cell • Identify the techniques of microscopy	**Introduction** • Definition and significance of nursing • Review of structure, composition and functions of a cell • Prokaryotic and eukaryotic cell organization • Microscopy	• Lectures and discussions using charts and slides • Demonstrate the use of a microscope	• Short-answer questions • Objective type
II	6	• Describe the structure and functions of the cell membrane	**Structure and functions of a cell membrane** • Fluid mosaic model, tight junction, cytoskeleton • Transport mechanism: Diffusion, osmosis, filtration, active channel, sodium pump • Acid-base balance—maintenance and diagnostic tests – pH buffers	• Lectures and discussions	• Short-answer questions • Objective type
III	6	• Explain the metabolism of carbohydrates	**Composition and metabolism of carbohydrates** • Types, structure, composition and uses – Monosaccharides, disaccharides, polysaccharides and oligosaccharides	• Lectures and discussions • Demonstration of blood glucose monitoring	• Short-answer questions • Objective type

Contd...

Contd...

INC Biochemistry Syllabus

Unit	Time (hours)	Learning objectives	Contents	Teaching and learning activities	Assessment methods
			• Metabolism – Pathways of glucose: – Glycolysis – Gluconeogenesis: Cori cycle, tricarboxylic acid (TCA) cycle – Glycogenolysis – Pentose phosphate pathways (hexose monophosphate) – Regulation of blood glucose level Investigations and their interpretations		
IV	4	• Explain the metabolism of lipids	**Composition and metabolism of lipids** • Types, structure, composition and uses of fatty acids – Nomenclature, roles and prostaglandins • Metabolism of fatty acid – Breakdown – Synthesis • Metabolism of triacylglycerols • Cholesterol metabolism	• Lectures and discussions using charts • Demonstration of laboratory tests	• Short-answer questions • Objective type

Contd...

Unit	Time (hours)	Learning objectives	Contents	Teaching and learning activities	Assessment methods
			– Biosynthesis and its regulation - Bile salts and bilirubin - Vitamin D - Steroid hormones • Lipoproteins and their functions – VLDLs, IDLs, LDLs and HDLs – Transport of lipids – Atherosclerosis Investigations and their interpretations		
V	6	• Explain the metabolism of amino acids and proteins	**Composition and metabolism of amino acids and proteins** • Types, structure, composition and uses of amino acids and proteins • Metabolism of amino acids and proteins – Protein synthesis, targeting and glycosylation – Chromatography – Electrophoresis – Sequencing • Metabolism of nitrogen – Fixation and assimilation – Urea cycle – Hemes and chlorophylls	• Lectures and discussions using charts • Demonstration of laboratory tests	• Short-answer questions • Objective type

Contd...

Unit	Time (hours)	Learning objectives	Contents	Teaching and learning activities	Assessment methods

			Enzymes and coenzymes
			  – Classification
			  – Properties
			  – Kinetics and inhibition
			  – Control
			Investigations and their interpretations		

VI	2	• Describe the types, composition and utilization of vitamins and minerals	• **Composition of vitamins and minerals**
			• Vitamins and minerals
			  – Structure
			  – Classification
			  – Properties
			  – Absorption
			  – Storage and transportation
			  – Normal concentration
			Investigations and their interpretations
				• Lectures and discussions using charts
				• Demonstration of laboratory tests
					• Short-answer questions
					• Objective type

VII	3	• Describe immunochemistry	• Free radicals and antioxidants • Specialized protein: Collagen, elastin, keratin, myosin, lens protein. • Electrophoretic and quantitative determination of immunoglobulins—ELISA, etc. Investigations and their interpretations.	• Lectures and discussions using charts • Demonstration of laboratory tests	• Short-answer questions • Objective type

INC NUTRITION SYLLABUS (REVISED: 2004)

Placement: First year
Time: Theory—60 hours

The course is designed to assist the students acquire knowledge of nutrition for the maintenance of optimum health at different stages of life and its application for the practice of nursing.

INC Nutrition Syllabus

Unit	Time (hours) Theory	Time (hours) Practical	Learning objectives	Contents	Teaching and learning activities	Evaluation

I	4		• Describe the relationship between nutrition and health	**Introduction**
				• Nutrition:
				  – History
				  – Concepts
				  – Role of nutrition in maintaining health
				• Nutritional problems in India
				• National Nutrition Policy
				• Factors affecting food and nutrition: socioeconomic, cultural, traditional, production, system of distribution, life style and food habits, etc.
				• Role of food and its medicinal value
				• Classification of foods
				• Food standards
				• Elements of nutrition: macro and micro
				• Calorie, BMR
					• Lectures and discussions
					• Explaining using charts
					• Panel discussion
						• Short-answer questions
						• Objective type

II	2		• Describe the classification, functions, sources and recommended	**Carbohydrates** • Classification • Caloric value	• Lectures and discussions • Explaining using charts	• Short-answer questions • Objective type

Contd...

Contd...

Unit	Time (hours)		Learning objectives	Contents	Teaching and learning activities	Evaluation
	Theory	Practical				
			daily allowances (RDA) of carbohydrates	• Recommended daily allowances • Dietary sources • Functions • Digestion, absorption and storage, metabolism of carbohydrates • Malnutrition: Deficiencies and over-consumption		
III	2		• Describe the classification, functions, sources and recommended daily allowances (RDA) of fats	**Fats** • Classification • Caloric value • Recommended daily allowances • Dietary sources • Functions • Digestion, absorption and storage, metabolism • Malnutrition: Deficiencies and over-consumption	• Lectures and discussions • Explaining using charts	• Short-answer questions • Objective type
IV	2		• Describe the classification, functions, sources and recommended daily allowances (RDA) of proteins	**Proteins** • Classification • Caloric value • Recommended daily allowances • Dietary sources	• Lectures and discussions • Explaining using charts	• Short-answer questions • Objective type

Contd...

Contd...

INC Nutrition Syllabus

Unit	Time (hours) Theory	Time (hours) Practical	Learning objectives	Contents	Teaching and learning activities	Evaluation
				• Functions • Digestion, absorption, metabolism and storage • Malnutrition: Deficiencies and over-consumption		
V	3		• Describe the daily calorie requirement for different categories of people	**Energy** • Unit of energy—kcal • Energy requirements of different categories of people • Measurements of energy • Body mass index (BMI) and basic metabolism • Basal metabolic rate (BMR) – Determination and factors affecting it	• Lectures and discussions • Explaining using charts • Exercise • Demonstration	• Short-answer questions • Objective type
VI	4		• Describe the classification, functions, sources and recommended daily allowances (RDA) of vitamins	**Vitamins** • Classification • Recommended daily allowances • Dietary sources • Functions • Absorption, synthesis, metabolism storage and excretion	• Lectures and discussions • Explaining using charts	• Short-answer questions • Objective type

Contd...

Contd...

Unit	Time (hours)		Learning objectives	Contents	Teaching and learning activities	Evaluation
	Theory	Practical				
VII	3		• Describe the classification, functions, sources and recommended daily allowances (RDA) of minerals	• Deficiencies • Hypervitaminosis **Minerals** • Classification • Recommended daily allowances • Dietary sources • Functions • Absorption, synthesis, metabolism, storage and excretion • Deficiencies • Overconsumption and toxicity	• Lectures and discussions • Explaining using charts	• Short answers questions • Objective type
VIII	4		• Describe the sources, functions and requirements of water and electrolytes	**Water and electrolytes** • **Water:** Daily requirement, regulation of water metabolism and distribution of body water • **Electrolytes:** Types, sources and composition of body fluids	• Lectures and discussion • Explaining using charts	• Short-answer questions • Objective type

Contd...

Contd...

Unit	Time (hours) Theory	Time (hours) Practical	Learning objectives	Contents	Teaching and learning activities	Evaluation
				• Maintenance of fluid and electrolyte balance • Overhydration, dehydration and water intoxication • Electrolyte imbalances		
IX	5	15	• Describe the cookery rules and preservation of nutrients • Prepare and serve simple beverages and different types of foods	**Cookery rules and preservation of nutrients** • Principles and methods of cooking and serving – Preservation of nutrients • Safe food handling—toxicity • Storage of food • Food preservation, food additives and its principles • Prevention of Food Adulteration Act (PFA) • Food standards • Preparation of simple beverages and different types of food	• Lectures and discussions • Demonstration • Practice sessions	• Short-answer questions • Objective type • Assessment of practice sessions
X	7	5	• Describe and plan the balanced diet for different categories of people	**Balanced diet** • Elements • Food groups	• Lectures and discussions • Explaining using charts	• Short-answer questions • Objective type

Contd...

Contd...

Unit	Time (hours) Theory	Time (hours) Practical	Learning objectives	Contents	Teaching and learning activities	Evaluation
				• Recommended daily allowances • Nutritive value of foods • Calculation of balanced diet for different categories of people • Planning menu • Budgeting of food • Introduction to therapeutic diets: Naturopathy diet	• Practice session • Meal planning	• Exercise on menu planning

XI	4		• Describe the various national programs related to nutrition
			• Describe the role of a nurse in the assessment of nutritional status and nutrition education
				Role of a nurse in nutritional programs
				• National programs related to nutrition
				  – Vitamin A Deficiency Program
				  – National Iodine Deficiency Disorders (NIDD) Program
				  – Mid-day Meal Program
				  – Integrated Child Development Scheme (ICDS)
					• Lectures and discussions
					• Explaining with slides/film shows
					• Demonstration of the assessment of nutritional status
						• Short-answer questions
						• Objective type

Contd...

Contd...

Unit	Time (hours) Theory	Time (hours) Practical	Learning Objectives	Contents	Teaching and learning activities	Evaluation
				• National and international agencies working towards food/nutrition – NIPCCD, CARE, FAO, NIN, Central Food Technology and Research Institute (CFTRI), etc. • Assessment of nutritional status • Nutrition education and the role of a nurse		

Part 1
Biochemistry

1. Biochemical Perspective to Medicine
2. Chemistry of Carbohydrate
3. Chemistry of Lipids
4. Amino Acids
5. Chemistry of Proteins
6. Vitamins
7. Nucleic Acids and Nucleotides
8. Enzymology
9. Digestion and Absorption
10. Basic Concepts of Metabolism
11. Metabolism of Carbohydrates
12. Metabolism of Lipids
13. Metabolism of Proteins
14. Immunochemistry
15. Hormones: Outline Chemistry and Functions
16. Blood Chemistry
17. Urinalysis
18. Renal Function Tests
19. Abnormalities of Bilirubin Metabolism: Jaundice
20. Liver Function Tests

Part 1

Biochemistry

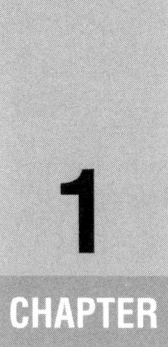

Biochemical Perspective to Medicine

The term 'Biochemistry' was introduced by Carl Neuberg in 1903. Biochemistry is the chemical language of life, basic to the understanding of biological and medical sciences. It gives us information regarding the functioning of the cells at the molecular level and also helps in finding remedies for a variety of ailments that afflict human and animals.

SCOPE OF BIOCHEMISTRY

Biochemistry is the science concerned with the chemical basis of life. It is the chemistry of the living matter in its different phases of activity, from the smallest microorganisms such as viruses to the most complex and highly evolved ones as human beings.

It is involved in finding out answers to two fundamental phenomena of nature namely:
1. How do we grow?
2. Where do we get our energy from?

The relationship of the living to their environment, such as:
1. The processes by which an exchange of chemicals takes place between the living organism and its environment through digestion, absorption and excretion.
2. The processes by which the absorbed materials are utilized for the synthetic reactions leading to growth and replenishment of tissues, and multiplication of cell and the species.
3. The metabolic breakdown of the materials to supply energy for all the above processes.
4. The mechanisms, which regulate all these processes with precision.
5. The mechanisms by means of hormonal and neuroregulatory stimuli occur. All these are the subject matter of biochemistry.

Medical biochemistry which is the sub-branch studied by doctors and nurses are covered by the following aspects of chemistry:
1. Tissues and foods.
2. Digestion and absorption.
3. Respiration.
4. Blood.
5. Cell membrane and physical chemistry.
6. Tissue metabolism.
7. Glands of internal secretion.
8. Chemistry of excretion.
9. Biochemistry disorders in disease.

Importance of Biochemistry To Nursing

Biochemistry is the language of life. The study of biochemistry by nurse is essential to understand the basic functions of the human body. This study will give information regarding the functioning of the cells at the molecular level. It helps to know how the food is digested, absorbed and used for body building and to understand how the body gets energy for day-to-day functions. She/he will be able to appreciate the close interrelation between various metabolic processes taking place in the body. It help to get a clear insight into immunity and genes from a study of biochemistry.

Modern nursing care depends on the laboratory analysis of body fluids especially the blood. A systematic study of biochemistry will give knowledge about the close relationship between disease manifestation and changes in the composition of blood and other tissues. Hence, the demarcation of abnormal from the normal values of body fluids is the primary aim of the study of biochemistry by the nurse.

Applications of the basic principles of biochemistry are essential to the nursing profession. The correct diagnosis, nursing care plans, treatment, prevention and control of infectious diseases depend on a sound knowledge of medical biochemistry. Biochemistry is perhaps the most rapidly developing branch of medicine. No wonder, the major share of Nobel Prizes in medicine has gone to research workers engaged in biochemistry.

STRUCTURE, COMPOSITION AND FUNCTIONS OF A CELL

All living organisms are composed of cells, which are minute compartments within which various processes of life occur. Microscopic organisms such as bacteria, some algae and protozoa are composed of single cells. Human body starts from a single cell, but contains about 10^{13} cells at maturity. Our body contains about 200 distinct type of cells. They are muscle cells, bone and cartilage cells, nerve cells, skin cells, visual cells in the eye and many others. Although each cell may show distinct characteristics for the particular functions performed, cells do show some fundamental characteristics. An ultrastructure of a cell is shown in Figure 1.1.

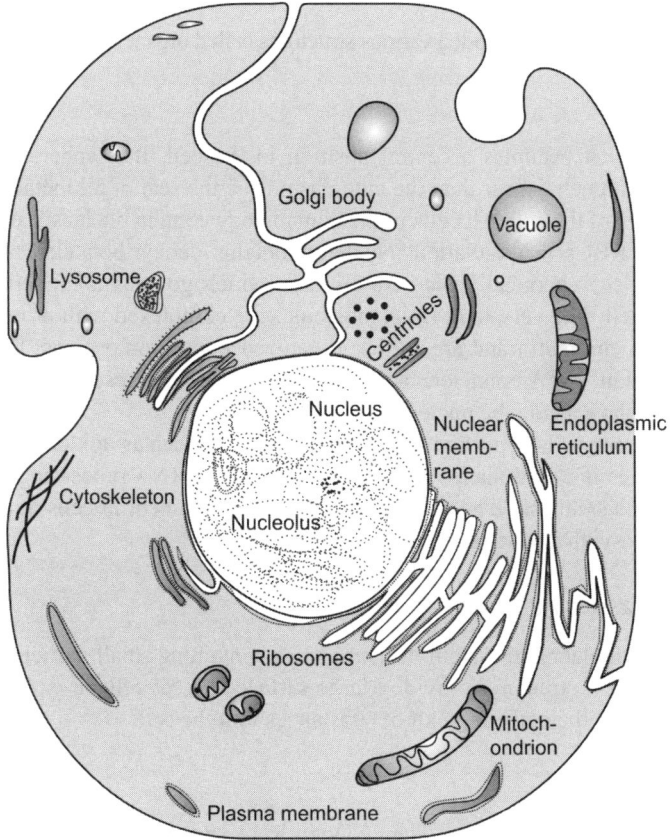

Fig. 1.1: Ultrastructure of the cell

The living matter in the cells is the protoplasm, the physical basis of life. The cell consists of an outer limiting membrane, the plasma membrane. The membranes are madeup of lipids (mainly of phospholipids), proteins and small amounts of carbohydrates in the form of glycoprotein and glycolipids. Inside the plasma membrane, there are two easily distinguishable regions, i.e. an outer watery granulated cytoplasm and an inner denser almost spherical region, the nucleus. The plasma membrane is important as it helps control the materials that go into and come out of the cell. The simple sugars, amino acids, potassium ions and water can pass through the membrane rapidly but sodium ions and other substances cannot.

Cytoplasm: Organelles

In cytoplasm are suspended various structures called organelles. These are:

Nucleus

Generally it occupies a central position in the cell. It is spherical or oval and much denser than the cytoplasm. It is the seat of all metabolic activities of the cell. All cells in the human body contain nucleus, except mature RBCs in circulation. Nucleus contains deoxyribonucleic acid (DNA), the chemical basis of the genes, which governs all functions of the cell. The very long DNA molecules are complexed with proteins to form chromatin and are further organized into chromosomes. DNA replication and ribonucleic acid (RNA) synthesis (transcription) are taking place inside the nucleus.

In some cells, a portion of the nucleus may be seen as lighter shaded area. This is called nucleolus. This is the area for RNA processing and ribosome synthesis. The nucleus will be very prominent in cells during actively synthesizing proteins.

Endoplasmic Reticulum

This is an elaborate system of membranes containing small particles of RNA. These structures provide a large surface area for cellular enzymes and control the entry and exit of substances into the cell.

Ribosomes

They are spherical bodies. They contain RNA and are especially active in the synthesis of proteins.

Mitochondria

Within the cytoplasm there are a number of rod like (3-4 μm in length) non-cellular structures called mitochondria. Their function is production of energy in cellular respiration.

Structure of the mitochondrion (Fig. 1.2): The components of the electron transport chain are located in the inner membrane. Although, the outer membrane contains special pores making it freely permeable to most ions and small molecules, the inner mitochondrial membrane is a specialized structure that is impermeable to most ions including H^+, Na^+ and K^+, small molecules such as adenosine diphosphate (ADP), adenosine triphosphate (ATP), pyruvate and other metabolites important to mitochondrial function. Specialized carriers or transport systems are required to move ions or molecules across this membrane. The inner mitochondrial membrane is unusually rich in protein, half of which is directly involved in electron transport and oxidative phosphorylation. Also it is highly convoluted. The convolutions are called cristae and serve to increase greatly the surface area of the membrane.

ATP synthetase complexes: These complexes of proteins are referred to as inner membrane particles and are attached to the inner surface of the inner mitochondrial membrane. They appear as spheres that protrude into mitochondrial matrix.

Mitochondrion is called the 'powerhouse of the cell' as it extracts energy from the oxidation of foodstuffs and traps as chemical energy with the formation of high energy chemical bonds of ATP. The final oxidation steps of carbohydrates and lipids (TCA cycle) also takes place there. Urea and heme synthesis partly take place in the mitochondria.

Cytoplasm: Cytosol

Cytosol is the liquid matrix of the cell, mostly water (cytosol + organelles except nucleus = cytoplasm) that contains salts, dissolved molecules enzymes, etc. Anaerobic glycolysis (energy metabolism) takes place in the cytosol.

Enzymes

Enzymes are special class of proteins that facilitate all the chemical reactions in the cell by providing energy, disposing waste, building proteins and creating new cells. Enzymes are molecular catalysts that initiate chemical reactions without being used up or inactivated in the process. There are thousands of different enzymes in each cell, each one specially designed to carry out the many individual processes on which life depends.

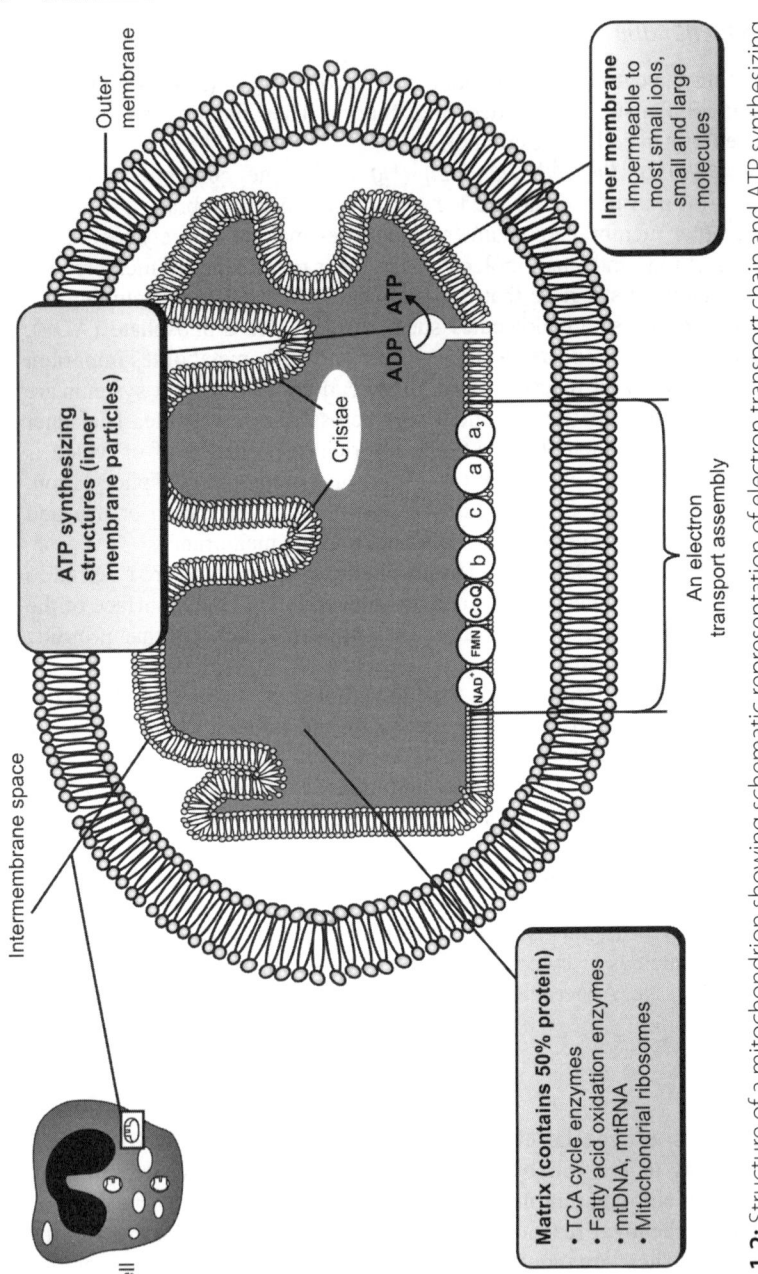

Fig. 1.2: Structure of a mitochondrion showing schematic representation of electron transport chain and ATP synthesizing structures on inner membrane (mtDNA, mitochondrial DNA; mtRNA, mitochondrial RNA).

PROKARYOTES AND EUKARYOTES

There are two basic types of cells:
1. Prokaryotes.
2. Eukaryotes.

Prokaryotes

Prokaryotic cells are small and simple but fast. The differences between prokaryotic and eukaryotic cells are listed in Table 1.1. They are more primitive, small and without organelles, e.g. bacteria, blue-green algae.

Eukaryotes

Eukaryotic cells are large and versatile but slow. They are more advanced, larger and contain organelles, e.g. all higher species: animals, plants and fungi. Human cells are of eukaryotic type.

MICROSCOPY

Light Microscopy

The resolving power of the light microscope is about half the wave length of the light being used. The light microscope used in microbiology and

TABLE 1.1: Differentiation between prokaryotic and eukaryotic cells

Prokaryotic cell	Eukaryotic cell
1. Prokaryotic cells are unicellular, e.g. bacteria	1. May be unicellular as well as multicellular, e.g. hepatocyte, erythrocyte
2. Smaller in size, ranging from 1–10 mm in diameter	2. They are approximately 10,000 times large and more complex in structure
3. They have only a single membrane, which is usually surrounded by a cell wall	3. They have cell membranes and several other membranes containing intracellular mitochondria, Golgi apparatus, etc.
4. They are similar in structure within a species	4. They vary from one tissue to another with respect to their structure as well as function, e.g. liver parenchymal cells, nerve cells, RBCs, etc.
5. There is a single chromosome and a molecule of double helical DNA, which is known as nuclear zone	5. It contains several chromosomes, which get divided into daughter chromosomes during mitosis

biochemistry generally employs a 90 power objective lens with a 10 power eye piece thus magnifying the specimen 900 times. Particles 0.2 µm in diameter are therefore magnified to about 0.2 mm and so become clearly visible. Further magnification would give no greater resolution in detail and would reduce the visible area.

Electron Microscopy

The high resolving power of the electron microscope has enabled observation of the detailed structures of prokaryotic and eukaryotic cells. The superior resolution of an election microscope is due to the fact that electrons have a much shorter wavelength than the photons of white light. The image is visualized by allowing it to impinge on a fluorescent screen and recorded on a photographic film. Viruses, with diameters of 0.01–0.2 µm can be easily visualized.

Dark Field Microscopy

Dark field microscopy is frequently performed on the same microscope on which bright field microscopy is performed. Illumination is obtained using a special condenser that blocks direct light rays and deflects light off a mirror on side of the condenser at an oblique angle. This creates a 'dark field' that contrasts against the highlighted edge of the specimens. This technique is particularly useful for observing organisms such as *Treponema pallidum*, a spirochete which is less than 0.2 µm in diameter and therefore cannot be observed with direct light.

Phase Contrast Microscopy

The phase contrast microscope takes advantage of the fact that light waves passing through transparent objects such as cells, emerge in different phases depending on the properties of the materials through which they pass. A special optical system converts differences in phase into difference in intensity so that some structures appear darker than others. Internal structures are thus differentiated in living cells.

AUTORADIOGRAPHY

If cells that have incorporated radioactive atoms are fixed on a slide, covered with a photographic emulsion and stored in the dark for a suitable period of time, traces appear on the developed film emanating from the sites of radioactive disintegration. If the cells are labeled with a weak emitter such as tritium, the tracks are sufficiently short to reveal the position of the radioactive label in the cell. The procedure called autoradiography has been particularly useful in following the replication of DNA.

FLUID MOSAIC MODEL OF CELL MEMBRANE

A theory of membrane structure called the 'fluid mosaic model' was postulated in 1972 by Singer and Nicolson, which is now widely accepted. The main postulates of this theory are:

1. A mosaic is a structure of many different small parts. Similarly, the plasma membrane is composed of different kinds of macro-molecules like phospholipids, integral proteins, peripheral proteins, glycoproteins, glycolipids and cholesterol.
2. According to this model, the matrix or continuous part of membrane structure is a polar lipid bilayer.
3. The bilayer is fluid because of the hydrophobic tails of its polar lipids consist of an appropriate mixture of saturated and unsaturated fatty acids that is fluid at the normal temperature of the cell.
4. This lipid bilayer has a dual role; it is both a solvent for integral membrane proteins and a permeability barrier.
5. Proteins are interspersed in the lipid bilayer of the plasma membrane, producing a mosaic effect.
6. The fluid mosaic model proposes that the integral proteins of membrane have hydrophobic non-polar amino acid side chain, e.g. valine and leucine, which would cause such proteins to dissolve in the central hydrophobic portion of the bilayer and thus, they are embedded within the lipid layer.
7. Peripheral membrane proteins have essential hydrophilic polar amino acid side chains, such as glutamate and serine, which are bound by electrostatic attraction to the hydrophilic electrically charged polar heads of the bilayer lipids.
8. The peripheral proteins float on the surface of 'sea' of predominantly phospholipid molecules, whereas the integral proteins are like icebergs, almost completely submerged in the hydrocarbon core.
9. There are no covalent bonds between lipid molecules of the bilayer or between the protein components and the lipids.

10. Fluid mosaic model allows the membrane proteins to move around laterally in two dimensions unless restricted by special interactions and that they are free to diffuse from place to place within the flame of the bilayer, whereas they cannot tumble from one side of the lipid bilayer to the other. Thus, there is a mosaic pattern of membrane proteins in the fluid lipid bilayer.

The Singer-Nicolson model can explain many of the physical, chemical and biological properties of membrane. Therefore, it has been widely accepted as the most probable molecular arrangement of lipids and proteins of membranes.

TRANSPORT MECHANISMS ACROSS THE CELL MEMBRANE

Movement of substances across the cell membrane is dependent on their lipid solubility. Lipid bilayer of the cell membrane allows lipid soluble solutions to pass through it.

Lipid insoluble substances are selectively transported by protein molecules present in the cell membrane called transport proteins.

Transport Proteins

Transport proteins are of two types:
1. Channel proteins.
2. Carrier proteins.

Channel Proteins

Channel proteins have watery spaces through the molecule and therefore, allow free movement of certain ions and molecules.

Carrier Proteins

Carrier proteins bind to substances that are to be transported and undergo conformational change. This causes movement of substances from one side of the membrane to the other side.

Both carrier and channel proteins are highly selective in allowing passage of ions or molecules across the membrane.

Transport Mechanisms

Transport mechanisms are of two broad types:
1. Passive transport.
2. Active transport.

Passive transport is by diffusion.

Diffusion

Diffusion is the continuous movement of molecules among one another in lipid or gaseous state. It is of two types:
1. Simple diffusion.
2. Facilitated diffusion.

Simple diffusion: This is the movement of molecules or ions through the cell membrane without the involvement of carrier proteins. Diffusion occurs from the region of higher concentration to a region of lower concentration.

Diffusion depends on:
a. Concentration of substance.
b. Velocity of kinetic motion.
c. Number of openings in the membrane.

Simple diffusion occurs through:
a. Lipid layer.
b. Protein channels.

Diffusion through lipid layer: Substances like O_2, N_2, CO_2 and alcohol dissolve directly in the lipid layer and diffuse through the cell membrane. Rate of diffusion is directly proportionate to their lipid solubility.

Diffusion through protein channels: Substances like water can easily pass through protein channels. These channels are highly selective for transport of ions or molecules. This selective permeability depends on diameter, shape and electrical charges of the channel.

Facilitated diffusion: This is also called carrier-mediated diffusion. The substance is transported with the help of a specific carrier protein, e.g. glucose and amino acids.

The characteristic features of facilitated diffusion are:
a. Carrier mechanisms can become saturated.
b. Can operate in both directions.
c. Rate of transport is more than simple diffusion.

Osmosis

Osmosis is a simple type of diffusion. It is the movement of water across a semipermeable membrane from a region of lower solute concentration to a region of higher solute concentration. Pressure required to prevent osmosis is called osmotic pressure. Osmotic pressure depends on the number of particles in the solution and not on the type or size of the particles.

QUESTION

1. Why is mitochondrion called the powerhouse of the cell?

MULTIPLE CHOICE QUESTIONS

2. The process by which solute can often pass through membrane against concentration gradient is known as:
   A. Endocytosis and exocytosis   B. Passive diffusion
   C. Active transport   D. Facilitated diffusion

3. The process by which solute can often pass through membrane against concentration gradient is known as:
   A. Emulsification   B. Passive diffusion
   C. Active transport   D. Facilitated diffusion

4. Osmosis is the flow of following through a semipermeable membrane:
   A. Solute   B. Solvent
   C. Solution   D. All the above

5. An example for colloid is:
   A. Triglycerides   B. Vitamins
   C. Nucleic acids   D. Proteins

6. Biochemistry is the study of:
   A. Immunity
   B. Action of drugs in the body
   C. Chemistry of life
   D. Structural aspects of the body

7. An eukaryotic cell differs from prokaryotic cell by the presence of:
   A. Cytoplasm   B. Nuclear membrane
   C. Nucleus   D. Mitochondria

8. All the following are cell organelles *except:*
   A. Lysosomes
   B. Golgi apparatus
   C. Ribosomes
   D. Peroxisomes
9. The technique used to separate cell organelles is:
   A. Filtration
   B. Paper electrophoresis
   C. Differential centrifugation
   D. Chromatography
10. The major complex organic biomolecules of cells are:
    A. Proteins
    B. DNA and RNA
    C. Polysaccharides
    D. All the above
11. Which of the following is the function of mitochondria?
    A. Protein synthesis
    B. Intracellular sorting of proteins
    C. Oxidative phosphorylation
    D. Glycolysis
12. The following cell organelle is involved in protein biosynthesis:
    A. Mitochondrion
    B. Nucleus
    C. Lysosome
    D. Ribosome

ANSWERS

2. (A)   3. (C)   4. (B)   5. (D)   6. (C)
7. (B)   8. (C)   9. (C)   10. (D) 11. (D)
12. (D)

CHAPTER 2

Chemistry of Carbohydrates

Carbohydrates include a large group of compounds commonly known as starch or sugars, which are widely distributed in plants and animals. Chemically, they are polyhydric alcohols having potentially active aldehyde and ketone groups. Because the ratio of hydrogen to oxygen in these compounds is often 2:1, having the empirical formula $C_n(H_2O)_n$, they are given the name carbohydrates or hydrates of carbon. In general, they are white solids, freely soluble in water with the exception of certain polysaccharides. Carbohydrates of lower molecular weights have a sweet taste.

There are practical reasons for the universal use of carbohydrates in diets. The yield of cereals, the primary source of carbohydrates, is high per unit area. Therefore they are widely available and are economic source of energy. They are easily packed and have a long shelf life when stored dry. They are mild flavored and combine well with other foods. Carbohydrate foods are easy to prepare.

BIOLOGICAL IMPORTANCE

1. Carbohydrates are the main sources of energy in the body. When carbohydrates are oxidized in the body, they liberate CO_2, water and energy. They are the least expensive source of energy to the body for muscular work. Each gram of carbohydrate provides 4 kcal of energy when oxidized. They supply the major portion of energy required by living cells. Brain cells and red blood cells (RBCs) wholly depend on glucose as energy source.
2. The body will use carbohydrates preferably as a source of energy when it is supplied in diet, thus sparing proteins for tissue building purposes.

3. The main source of energy for central nervous system (CNS) is glucose. Prolonged hypoglycemia results in irreversible damage to brain tissue.
4. All carbohydrates are digested to form glucose before they can be absorbed into bloodsteam and get transported to different tissues of the body.
5. Glucose is the sugar of the blood and is excreted in urine in glycosuria.
6. Glucose is stored as glycogen in liver and muscles.
7. Some carbohydrates are necessary in the diet so that oxidation of fats can proceed normally.
8. Lactose has several functions in the gastrointestinal tract (GIT). It promotes the growth of desirable bacteria, some of which are necessary for the synthesis of vitamin B complex.
9. Though dietary fiber yields no nutrients to the body, it adds to the stimulation of peristaltic movement of GI tract and provides ruffage to avoid constipation.
10. Carbohydrates add flavor and variety to diet.

Sources of Carbohydrates

Carbohydrates, often called starch and sugars are widely distributed in plants and animals. In plants, they are produced by photosynthesis of water from the soil and CO_2 from air. The prefix 'photo' indicates the importance of sunlight in the process. Plants are thus the primary source of food in the world.

In animal cells, carbohydrate serves as an important source of energy. Animal tissues contain glycogen and body fluids contain glucose both of which are carbohydrates. Some carbohydrates have highly specific functions such as ribose in nucleic acids, galactose in some lipids and lactose of milk.

There are three main sources of carbohydrates.
1. *Starch:* These are present in cereals, roots and tubers, e.g. rice, wheat, ragi, pulses, tapioca, yam, colocasia and potatoes.
2. *Sugars:* Disaccharides, e.g. sucrose, lactose, maltose.
3. *Cellulose:* This is the tough fibrous lining found in vegetables, fruits and cereals. It is hard to digest and has no nutrition value. However, cellulose acts as ruffage and prevents constipation.

Glucose also known as dextrose is present in fruits and honey. It is the 'sugar' of the blood. Hydrolysis of cane sugar (sucrose), maltose, lactose and starch yield glucose.

Fructose also known as levulose, is present in fruit juices and honey. It is obtained by hydrolysis of cane sugar.

Galactose is not found free in nature, its only source being hydrolysis of lactose, milk sugar. It also occurs in cerebrosides (glycolipids) present in brain and nerve tissue. Hence, it is nutritionally important.

Sucrose occurs in sugar cane, beetroot, carrot and pineapple. It is manufactured on large scale from sugar cane and beetroot.

Maltose is obtained from starch, germinating cereals and malt. Lactose is present in the milk of all mammals.

Balanced Diet

Carbohydrates rich in natural fiber should constitute 60% of energy requirements (calorie value). Proteins should give 15%–20% of daily energy needs and fats 20%–30% of the energy needs. Carbohydrates are the cheapest source of energy. Glucose derived from the digestion of carbohydrates is the main source of energy in the body. Hence, diet should contain adequate amounts of carbohydrates to meet a greater part of the energy needs.

Malnutrition for Deficiencies and Overconsumption

If the carbohydrate intake in diet is insufficient, it leads to malnutrition and other metabolic disorders. Tissue protein and fat will be used up for energy purposes. Excess carbohydrates leads to obesity.

TABLE 2.1: Monosaccharides

Simple sugars	Formula	Aldo sugars	Keto sugars
Trioses	$C_3H_6O_3$	Glycerose	Dihydroxyacetone
Tetroses	$C_4H_8O_4$	Erythrose	Erythrulose
Pentoses	$C_5H_{10}O_5$	Ribose	Ribulose
Hexoses	$C_6H_{12}O_6$	Glucose	Fructose

CHARACTERISTICS OF CARBOHYDRATES

Asymmetry

In the formula for glucose, it will be noted that a different group is attached to each of the 4 bonds of carbon atoms 2–5. A carbon atom to which 4 different atoms or groups of atoms are attached is called asymmetric carbon atom.

Isomerism

The presence of asymmetric carbon atoms in a compound makes possible the isomerism of that compound. Compounds, which are identical in composition and differ only in spatial configuration are called stereoisomers. Two such isomers of glucose, one of which is the mirror image of the other are shown below:

$$\begin{array}{cc}
\overset{O}{\underset{1}{\text{C}}}-H & H-\overset{O}{\underset{1}{\text{C}}} \\
HO-\underset{2}{\text{C}}-H & H-\underset{2}{\text{C}}-OH \\
H-\underset{3}{\text{C}}-OH & HO-\underset{3}{\text{C}}-H \\
HO-\underset{4}{\text{C}}-H & H-\underset{4}{\text{C}}-OH \\
HO-\underset{5}{\text{C}}-H & H-\underset{5}{\text{C}}-OH \\
\underset{6}{\text{CH}_2\text{OH}} & \text{HOH}_2\underset{6}{\text{C}} \\
\text{L-glucose} & \text{D-glucose}
\end{array}$$

The form in which the hydroxyl group next to the primary hydroxyl is projected to the right of the carbon chain is the D-form, and the form in which it is projected to the left is the L-form.

Optical Isomerism

The presence of asymmetric carbon atoms also gives optical activity in the compound. When a beam of polarized light is passed through a solution exhibiting optical activity, it will be rotated to the right or left in accordance to the type of the compounds, i.e. optical isomer present. A compound, which causes rotation of polarized light to the right is said to be dextrorotatory designated by plus (+) sign. Rotation of beam of light to the left is levorotatory designated by minus (−) sign.

Mutarotation

Mutarotation is defined as a change in specific rotation of optically active solution without any change in other properties.

D-glucose in aqueous solution exists as an equilibrium mixture of five isomers.

When glucose is dissolved in water, the optical rotation of the solution gradually changes and attains an equilibrium value. This change in the optical rotation is called mutarotation (invert sugar).

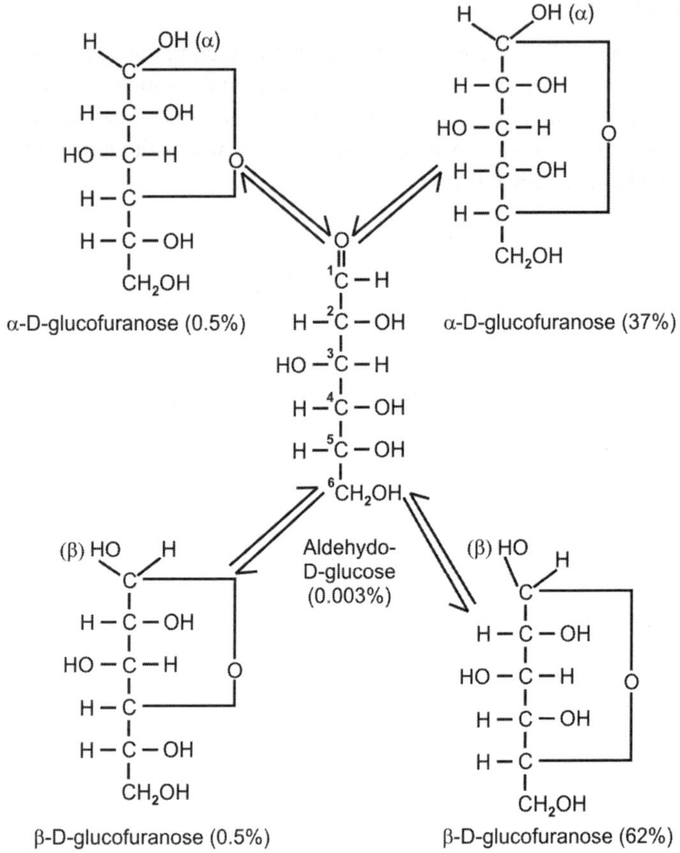

α-D-glucofuranose (0.5%)

α-D-glucofuranose (37%)

Aldehydo-D-glucose (0.003%)

β-D-glucofuranose (0.5%)

β-D-glucofuranose (62%)

Cyclic Forms of Sugars

The close proximity of an aldehyde (or ketone) group and an alcohol group in the carbohydrate facilitates their reaction to give cyclic hemiacetals (or hemiketals). This can occur with the alcohol group of either carbon 4 or carbon 5.

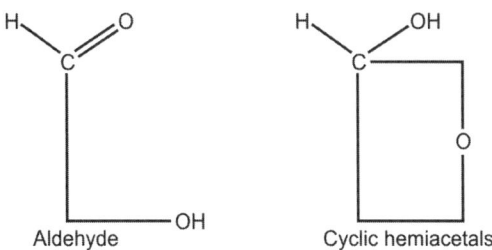

| Aldehyde | Cyclic hemiacetals |

In the first case, a ring consisting of 4 carbon atoms and one oxygen atom is created. This is called furanose ring. In the second case, the ring contains 5 carbon atoms in addition to oxygen. This is called pyranose ring.

Furan   Pyran

Because of the asymmetry present in the terminal carbon, 2 forms of each ring structure can exist.

A pyranose form of D-ribose
(α-D-ribopyranose)

A furanose form of D-fructose
(β-D-fructofuranose)

Haworth Projections

Sir Walter Haworth in 1925 established that glucose is existing in biological systems not as a rectangle, but as a pyranose ring and was awarded the Nobel Prize in 1937. To accurately represent the ring structure, the Haworth projections are used.

In Haworth projection, any group to the right of the carbon chain is written down and those to the left are written up. When there are more carbon atoms in the sugar than are involved in the ring formation, the rule is that if the ring is to the right, the extra carbon or carbon will be up.

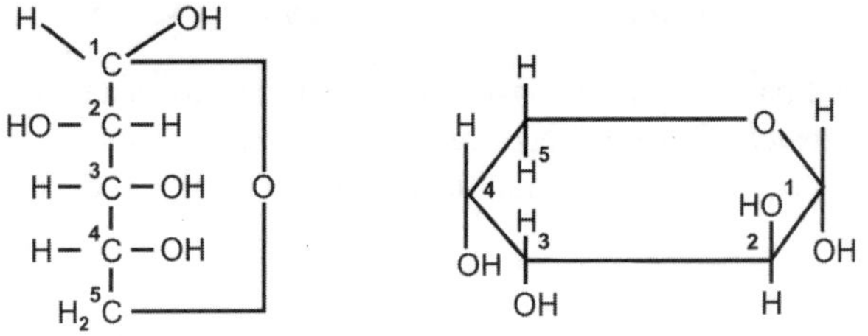

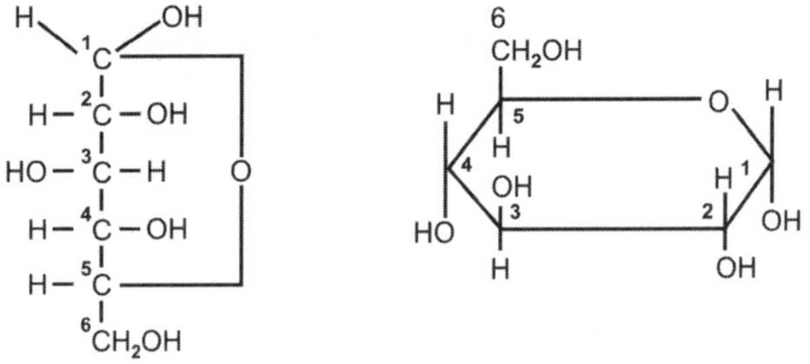

α-D-glucopyranose

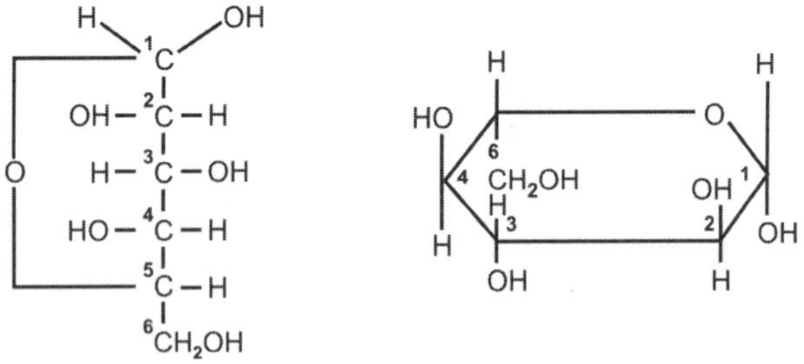

β-L-glucopyranose

REACTIONS OF CARBOHYDRATES

The carbohydrates, being polyhydroxy aldehydes and ketones, generally are capable of undergoing all of the normal reactions of aldehydes and ketones, e.g. oxidation, reduction, dehydration, esterification, ether formation and addition to the carbonyl double bond.

Test for Carbohydrates (Molisch's Test)

To 2 mL of the unknown solution, add 2 drops of fresh 1% α-naphthol reagent and mix. Pour 2 mL of concentrated H_2SO_4 so as to form a layer below the mixture. A red violet ring indicates carbohydrate.

Reducing and Non-reducing Sugars

Any free aldehyde or α-hydroxy ketone is capable of being oxidized, thus causing the reduction of some other substances. Any of the sugars in the free aldehyde or ketone form, or in any other form in equilibrium with the free aldehyde or ketone (hemiacetal forms) can be oxidized.

Carbohydrates capable of undergoing oxidation without having to be hydrolyzed first, is a reducing sugar. Sugars like sucrose and trehalose are non-reducing disaccharide.

A variety of reagents can be used to carry out the oxidation of carbohydrates and be themselves reduced. The most common is the cupric ion (Cu^{++}), which is the active ingredient in Fehling's, Benedict's and Barfoed's reagents for the detection of reducing sugars. The reaction is as follows:

$$CuSO_4 \longrightarrow Cu^{++} + SO_4^{--}$$
Cupric

Reducing sugar + $2Cu^{++}$ ⟶ Oxidized sugar + $2Cu^+$
                  Blue   Cuprous

$2Cu^+ + 2OH^- \longrightarrow 2CuOH \longrightarrow Cu_2O\downarrow + H_2O$
Cuprous   Yellow   Cuprous
                                       Oxide (red)

For example, $C_6H_{12}O_6 + 2CuO \longrightarrow C_6H_{12}O_7 + Cu_2O\downarrow$

The color of the solution or precipitate gives an approximate amount of reducing sugars present in the solution. This can be estimated by the following tests.

Benedict's Test (CuSO$_4$, Sodium Citrate and Sodium Carbonate)

To 5 mL of the reagent in a test tube, add 8 drops of the urine sample. Place in a boiling water bath for 5 minutes. Observe the colors and report:

Blue color : Nil
Green color : Up to 0.5% (+)
Yellow color : Up to 1.0% (++)
Orange color : Up to 1.5% (+++)
Red color : Up to 2.0% (++++)
Brick red precipitate : More than 2%

Barfoed's Test

Mix 5 mL of Barfoed's reagent (copper acetate in glacial acetic acid) with 0.5 mL of urine sample in a test tube.

Benedict's qualitative reagent contains cupric sulfate, sodium carbonate and sodium citrate, whereas Fehling's solution contains cupric sulfate, sodium carbonate and sodium potassium tartrate.

Sodium citrate in Benedict's reagent and sodium potassium tartrate (Rochelle salt) in Fehling's solution prevent the precipitation of cupric hydroxide or cupric carbonate by forming a deep blue solution, slightly dissociated complexes with the cupric ions. The complexes dissociate sufficiently to provide a continuous supply of readily available cupric ions for oxidation.

Osazone Formation

Heat 100°C phenylhydrazine reagent with 2 mL of a solution of sugar in a test tube for 30 minutes and examine the crystals with a microscope.

Reducing sugars can be distinguished from one another by phenylhydrazine test when characteristic osazones are formed. These osazones have characteristic crystal structures, melting points, precipitation time and show different crystalline form under a microscope.

Glucose, fructose and mannose give the same needle shaped, yellow osazone and they cannot be differentiated from one another by this test. But maltose gives sunflowered osazone while, lactose gives cotton ball-shaped osazone.

Oxidation

Oxidation of aldoses forms acids as end products. Oxidation of the aldehyde group forms aldonic acids. However, if the aldehyde group remains intact and primary alcohol group at the opposite end of the molecule is oxidized, uronic acids are formed. Heat in a boiling water bath for 5 minutes. Appearance of a red precipitation within 5 minutes indicates the presence of monosaccharides.

```
                        CHO
                        |
                    H — C — OH
                        |
   Bromine water   OH — C — H    Nitric acid
                        |
                    H — C — OH
                        |
(O)|                H — C — OH             |(O)
                        |
                      CH₂OH
                       ↓ (O)
    COOH              CHO             COOH
    |                  |                |
H — C — OH         H — C — OH      H — C — OH
    |                  |                |
HO — C — H         HO — C — H      HO — C — H
    |                  |                |
H — C — OH         H — C — OH      H — C — OH
    |                  |                |
H — C — OH         H — C — OH      H — C — OH
    |                  |                |
  CH₂OH              COOH             COOH
Gluconic acid    Glucuronic acid   Glucaric acid
                                  (saccharic acid)
```

Reduction

The monosaccharides may be reduced to corresponding alcohols by reducing agents like sodium amalgam.

```
CHO    2[H]    CH₂OH     H₂C — OH              H₂ — C — OH
|     ——→      |          |         2[H]            |
R              R          C = O    ——→         H — C = O
                          |                         |
                          R                         R
```

Glucose yields sorbitol, galactose yields dulcitol, and fructose yields mannitol and sorbitol.

CLASSIFICATION

Carbohydrates are classified into four major groups as below.

Monosaccharides

Monosaccharides, called simple sugars, are those which cannot be hydrolyzed into a simpler form. The general formula is $C_nH_{2n}O_n$. The simple sugars may be subdivided into trioses, tetroses, pentoses and hexoses depending upon the number of C atoms (Tables 2.1 and 2.2). They are aldo sugars or keto sugars depending upon the aldehyde or ketone group present (Table 2.3).

$$R-\underset{\underset{OH}{|}}{\overset{\overset{H}{|}}{C}}-\overset{\overset{O}{\|}}{C}-H \qquad R-\underset{\underset{OH}{|}}{\overset{\overset{H}{|}}{C}}-\overset{\overset{O}{\|}}{C}-R'$$

Aldehyde group   Ketone group

TABLE 2.2: Examples of pentoses

Sugars	Sources	Importance	Reactions
D-ribose	Nucleic acids	Structural elements of nucleic acids and coenzymes, e.g. ATP, NAD, NADP, flavoproteins	Reduces Benedict's, Fehling's, Barfoed's and Haynes' solutions. Forms distinctive osazones with phenylhydrazine.
D-ribulose	Formed in metabolic processes	Intermediates in direct oxidative pathways of glucose breakdown	Those of keto sugars.

Disaccharides

The disaccharides are carbohydrates that can be hydrolyzed into two units of monosaccharides. Sucrose is a non-reducing sugar while lactose and maltose are reducing carbohydrates. The general formula is $C_{12}H_{22}O_{11}$ (Table 2.4).

Maltose (2 Glucose Units)

Maltose consists of two molecules of D-glucose joined by α-1,4-glycosidic linkage. Maltose or malt sugar does not occur in free state, but is formed as an important transitory intermediate product of the digestion of starch into glycogen and glucose.

Chemistry of Carbohydrates

TABLE 2.3: Hexoses of physiologic importance

Sugars	Sources	Importance	Reactions
D-glucose dextrose	Ripe grapes and most sweet fruits and honey. Sugar of the blood. Occurs in urine of the diabetics. Hydrolysis of starch, cane sugar, maltose and lactose.	The sugar of the body, the sugar carried by the blood and the principal one used by tissues. Glucose is usually the sugar of the urine when glycosuria occurs.	As a reducing sugar, reduces Benedict's, Haynes' and Barfoed's solutions. Gives osazone with phenylhydrazine fermented by yeast.
D-fructose levulose fruit sugar	Fruit juices, honey, hydrolysis of cane sugar. Most soluble and sweetest sugar. Double sweeter than glucose.	Can be changed into glucose in the liver and so used in the body.	Reducing sugar, reduces Benedict's, Haynes' and Barfoed's solutions. Forms osazone identical with that of glucose, fermented by yeast.
D-galactose	Hydrolysis of lactose.	Can be changed to glucose in the liver and metabolized. Synthesized in the mammary gland to make lactose of mother's milk. A constituent of glycolipids.	Reducing sugar, reduces Benedict's, Haynes' and Barfoed's solutions. Forms osazone distinct from glucose and fructose, and fermented by yeast.
D-mannose	Hydrolysis of plant mannosans and gums.	Convertible to glucose in the body. A constituent of prosthetic polysaccharide of albumins and globulins.	Reducing sugar, reduces Benedict's Haynes', Barfoed's reagents. Forms same osazone as glucose.

TABLE 2.4: Disaccharides

Sugars	Occurrences	Reactions
Maltose	Hydrolysis of starch, germinating cereals and malt.	Reducing sugar, forms osazone with phenylhydrazine, fermentable. Hydrolyzed to D-glucose.
Lactose	Milk, may occur in urine during pregnancy. Formed in the body from glucose.	Reducing sugar, forms osazone with phenylhydrazine. Not fermentable by yeast. Hydrolyzed to glucose and galactose.
Sucrose	Cane and beet sugar. Carrot and pineapple.	Non-reducing sugar, does not form osazone. Fermentable, hydrolyzed to fructose and glucose.

Nutrition and Biochemistry for Nurses

```
   H-C-OH              H-C                           CHO
   |                   |                             |
   H-C-OH              H-C-OH                        H-C-OH
   |      O            |           Hydrolysis        |
  HO-C-H          O   HO-C-H     O  ─────────►      HO-C-H
   |                   |              [HOH]          |
   H-C                 H-C-OH                        H-C-OH
   |                   |                             |
   H-C                 H-C                           H-C-OH
   |                   |                             |
   H-C-OH              H-C-OH                        H-C-OH
   |                   |                             |
   H                   H                             H
 Maltose                                        2 Glucose units
```

Lactose (Glucose plus Galactose)

```
     OH              H
      \              |
   H-C              C                  CHO         CHO
   |                |                   |           |
   H-C-OH           H-C-OH              H-C-OH     H-C-OH
   |      O         |         Hydrolysis |          |
  HO-C-H       O   HO-C-H    O ────────►HO-C-H    HO-C-H
   |                |          [HOH]     |          |
   H-C             HO-C-H                H-C-OH +HO-C-H
   |                |                    |          |
   H-C              H-C                  H-C-OH    H-C-OH
   |                |                    |          |
   CH₂OH            CH₂OH                CH₂OH      CH₂OH
  Lactose                               Glucose   Galactose
```

Lactose occurs in mammalian milk. Cow's and buffalo's milk contain 4%, while human milk contains 7% lactose. It is a reducing sugar. It is formed by galactose and glucose linked by β-1,4-glycosidic linkage. As one of two aldehyde groups is free, it shows reducing properties and forms cotton ball-shaped osazone crystals.

Sucrose (Glucose plus Fructose)

Sucrose is widely distributed in plants. It is the sugar of sugar cane, sugar beets and sugar maples, the concentration is sufficient for commercial production. Sucrose is not a reducing sugar as both the –CHO and the C=O⁻ groups are involved in linkage and are not free.

$$\text{Sucrose} \xrightarrow[\text{[HOH]}]{\text{Hydrolysis}} \text{Glucose} + \text{Fructose}$$

Oligosaccharides

They yield 2–8 monosaccharide molecules on hydrolysis. Examples are raffinose, stachyose and scorodose, blood group antigens.

Polysaccharides

They yield more than 8 molecules of monosaccharides on hydrolysis. The general formula is $(C_6H_{10}O_5)_n$ and examples are starch, dextrin, glycogen.

They are further subdivided into:

a. Homopolysaccharides: They are polymers of the same monosaccharide units, e.g. starch, glycogen, cellulose, dextrin, dextran and inulin. Some homopolysaccharides serve as a sharge form of monopolysaccharides used as fuel, e.g. starch and glycogen, while some serve as structural elements in plants, e.g. cellulose.

b. Heteropolysaccharides: Polymer of different monosaccharide units or their derivatives, e.g. mucopolysaccharides (glycosaminoglycans), e.g. heparin, keratin sulfate, chondroitin sulfate, hyaluronic acid, blood group polysaccharides.

Starch

Occurs widely in the vegetable kingdom. It is a white tasteless powder insoluble in cold water.

Starch is the major storage form of carbohydrates in plants. It usually occurs in the form of compact insoluble grains inside the plant cells. The starch grains are composed of two different polysaccharides having different properties, namely amylose (19%–25%) and amylopectin (75%–83%).

Hydrolysis of starch: Starch, which is composed of several glucose units is hydrolysed to form first maltose and finally glucose molecules. Hydrolysis of starch can be brought about by both enzymes and acids.

Enzymes, which hydrolyze starch are amylases. They are present in saliva as ptyalin and in pancreatic juice as pancreatic amylase. Amylase acts on starch, hydrolysing them into fragments of dextrins, and ultimately to maltose molecules. They act at the α-1,4 glycosidic linkages. The products of hydrolysis is given in Figure 2.1.

Starch
↓
Soluble starch
↓
Amylodextrin + maltose$^+$
↓
Erythrodextrin + maltose^{++}
↓
Achrodextrin + maltose^{+++}
↓
Maltose + maltose^{++++}

Fig. 2.1: Hydrolysis of starch

Starch when completely hydrolyzed by diluted HCl solution in KI yields glucose. Starch is used for the manufacture of glucose, dextran, custard powder and sago.

Test of starch: Starch will form a blue-colored complex with iodine. This color disappears on heating, but reappears on cooling. This is a physical change and not a chemical change.

Amylose: A polysaccharide in which glucose units are joined in α-1,4-glycosidic linkages to form long slender chains.

The molecular weight of amylose is 60,000 corresponding to a chain of 300–400 glucose units. Amylose is soluble in water and is less viscous than starch.

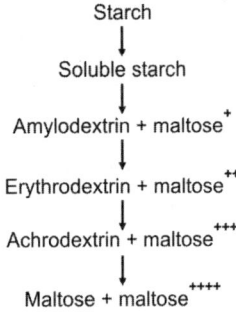

Amylopectin: This polysaccharide possesses the same basic chain as amylose, but they are larger molecules. They have molecular weights as high as 200,000 or more, corresponding to 1,000–1,300 glucose units.

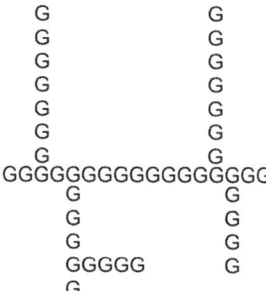

They are highly branched and soluble in warm water.

Glycogen (Animal Starch)

Glycogen is the major carbohydrate reserve in animals. In most mammals, deposits of glycogen are maintained especially in the liver and in the skeletal muscles. Liver may store 200 g and muscles 350 g of glycogen.

The structure of the glycogen is essentially the same as amylopectins, except that there is much more extensive branching. This gives an increased solubility. Glycogen is quite readily put into suspension even in cold water.

Cellulose

Cellulose forms the chief constituent of the structure of cell wall of plants. It is similar in structure to amylose, except that all of the glucose are held together by β-1,4-glycosidic linkages.

It is highly insoluble and resistant to hydrolysis. There is no enzyme in the human beings to break the β-1,4-glycosidic linkage. It therefore passes through the human digestive tract without being attacked by the enzymes. Cellulose is consumed but not digested. Cellulose forms the bulk of fecal matter. When cellulose is not sufficient in the diet, constipation results.

In industry, cellulose is used for manufacture of rayon and explosives.

Dextran

Dextran is a polysaccharide, closely related to starch and glycogen. It has a molecular weight of approximately 50,000. It is a polymer of D-glucopyranose units. It is synthesized from sucrose by certain bacteria. It is used as a blood substitute in extensive loss of blood. It is a blood volume extender. It can maintain the osmotic pressure of the blood, but has an adverse effect on blood clotting process.

Inulin

Inulin is a polysaccharide, each molecule of which is composed of about 80 D-fructose units. It occurs as a reserve carbohydrate in the tubers and roots of chicory, dahlia, dandelions, and in the bulb of onions and garlic. It is a white crystalline powder, sweet to taste. It is readily soluble in hot water and does not give any color with iodine. It has no reducing property.

Inulin is not hydrolyzed by enzymes of the gastrointestinal tract and does not undergo any metabolic change in the body. When injected intravenously, it is excreted quantitatively by glomerular filtration within a short time. It does not undergo any reabsorption in the tubules. This property of inulin clearance is made use of in the determination of the rate of glomerular filtration or inulin clearance in an individual (urine).

Mucopolysaccharides

Proteoglycans or carbohydrates containing uronic acid and amino sugars are present in connective tissues. They are viscous and act as lubricants and shock absorbers.

Mucopolysaccharides represent a variety of polysaccharides present largely in the ground substance of connective tissue along with mucoproteins. They are acidic substances containing amino sugars or their derivatives. They are divided into the following subgroups.

1. Neutral mucopolysaccharides, such as immunologically important blood group substances, which contain only an N-acetylhexosamine and a hexose.
2. The second group has a hexuronic acid (e.g. D-glucuronic acid) along with an N-acetylhexosamine. The group includes hyaluronic acids, which are found as components of connective tissues. They are straight chain polymers with D-glucuronic acid and N-acetylglucosamine alternatively in the chains.
3. The third group is a complex one in which a polysaccharide may contain hexoses, amino sugars (free and acetylated) hexuronic acids and sugar sulfates. Examples are chondroitin sulfate of cartilage (N-acetylgalactosamine, glucuronic acid and sulfate esters of these sugars) and heparin, the natural anticoagulant of blood (glucosamine

N-sulfate, glucuronic acid and their sulfate esters).

Glycosidic linkages involving uronic acids or amino sugars are highly resistant to hydrolysis. Hence, polysaccharides containing these units are extremely stable and are present where chemical resistance and physical strength are needed, e.g. in skin, connective tissues, insect exoskeletons, umbilical cord, etc.

QUESTIONS

1. What are carbohydrates? What are their functions in living organisms?
2. Classify carbohydrates with examples. What is an asymmetric carbon atom?
3. What are the differences between mono, di and polysaccharides?
4. What are the differences between cellulose and starch?
   Ans: In starch, the glucose units are linked by α (1-4) linkages. In cellulose the glucose units are linked by β-1,4 glycosidic linkages.
5. Write short notes on:
   A. Mucopolysaccharides.
   B. Mutarotation and its causes.
   C. Benedict's test.
6. What is the difference between starch and glycogen?

   Starch
   1. Plant origin.
   2. It is a branched molecule. Branching occurs after every 20–24 glucose units.
   3. Blue color with iodine solution.

   Glycogen
   1. Animal origin.
   2. More branched than starch molecules. Branching occurs after every 8–10 glucose units.
   3. Red color with iodine solution.

MULTIPLE CHOICE QUESTIONS

7. Carbohydrates are the compounds of:
   A. C, H, N and O
   B. C, H and O
   C. C, N and H
   D. N, H and O
8. Which of the following is a monosaccharide?
   A. Glucose
   B. Lactose
   C. Sucrose
   D. Maltose
9. Monomer of cellulose is:
   A. Lactose
   B. Maltose
   C. Fructose
   D. Glucose

10. **Invert sugar is a mixture of:**
    A. Sucrose and glucose
    B. Glucose and fructose
    C. Maltose and glucose
    D. Lactose and maltose
11. **A carbohydrate can be defined as:**
    A. Polyhydroxy alcohol
    B. Hydrates of carbon
    C. Aldehydes or ketone bodies
    D. All of the above
12. **Which one of the sugars is a ketose?**
    A. Xylose
    B. Fructose
    C. Arabinose
    D. Erythrose
13. **Glucose is the constituent of:**
    A. Insulin
    B. DNA
    C. Collagen
    D. Starch
14. **Sorbitol is:**
    A. Sterol
    B. An amino alcohol
    C. A glycerol derivative
    D. A sugar alcohol
15. **Inverted sugar is:**
    A. Sucrose
    B. Fructose
    C. Glucose
    D. A mixture of glucose and fructose
16. **All the following are reducing sugars *except*:**
    A. Fructose
    B. Sucrose
    C. Maltose
    D. Lactose
17. **All the following are mucopolysaccharides *except*:**
    A. Chondroitin sulfates
    B. Hyaluronic acid
    C. Amylodextrin
    D. Heparin
18. **Which of the following statement is correct?**
    A. Cellulose is a heteropolysaccharide
    B. Sucrose can form osazone
    C. Oligosaccharides contains 5–10 monosaccharide units
    D. Glycogen is the storage form of glucose in human beings
19. **Dextrins are polysaccharides formed as intermediate compounds during the hydrolysis of:**
    A. Cellulose
    B. Starch
    C. Dextran
    D. Glycogen
20. **Glucose and fructose form the same osazone because both are:**
    A. Monosaccharides
    B. Soluble in water
    C. Differing in carbon 1 and 2, carbon 1 and 2 are involved
    D. Differing in carbon 5 and 6, carbon 1 and 2 are involved

Chemistry of Carbohydrates

21. **Shape of maltosazone is:**
    A. Sunflower shaped
    B. Needle/broom shaped
    C. Cotton ball shaped
    D. Powder puff shaped

22. **One of the following carbohydrates is not digested in the human gastrointestinal (GI) tract:**
    A. Starch
    B. Cellulose
    C. Lactose
    D. Sucrose

23. **Following polysaccharide is naturally occurring anticoagulant:**
    A. Hyaluronic acid
    B. Chondroitin sulfate
    C. Heparin
    D. Keratin sulfate

24. **Blood group substances consist of N-acetyl-glucosamine, galactosamine, fucose, sialic acid and:**
    A. Glucose
    B. Fructose
    C. Galactose
    D. Sucrose

25. **Following are homopolysaccharides *except:***
    A. Cellulose
    B. Starch
    C. Glycogen
    D. Heparin

ANSWERS

7. (B)	8. (A)	9. (D)	10. (B)	11. (D)
12. (B)	13. (D)	14. (D)	15. (D)	16. (B)
17. (C)	18. (D)	19. (B)	20. (C)	21. (A)
22. (B)	23. (C)	24. (C)	25. (D)	

3 Chemistry of Lipids

Lipids are defined as a group of naturally occurring substances consisting of higher fatty acids, their naturally occurring compounds and substances found normally in association with them. They are insoluble in water, but soluble in organic solvents like ether, chloroform, benzene and acetone.

They include fatty acids, triacylglycerols, ketone bodies, cholesterol, phospholipids and sphingolipids.

The terms 'fats' and 'oils' are commonly used to denote crude lipid mixtures, which are obtained from natural sources. Fats are solids and oils are liquids at room temperature (15°C).

OCCURRENCE

Fats are widely distributed in plants and animals. In plants, they are present in nuts, seeds and oils. The nervous system of animals is rich in lipids like cholesterol, phospholipids and glycolipids. Blood contains lipoproteins. The fat depots such as subcutaneous tissues, mesenteric tissues, fatty tissues around the kidney and yellow bone marrow contain large amounts of fat. Food sources rich in fat are milk, egg, meat, liver, fish oils, nuts, seeds and oils.

BIOLOGICAL SIGNIFICANCE OF FATS

1. Lipids form one of the three main types of foodstuffs and act as fuel in the body. It yields more heat and energy than proteins and carbohydrates. Their caloric value is 9 kcal/g.
2. Deposits of fat underneath the skin exert insulating effect to the body. They protect the body from excessive heat or cold. Fat people can withstand heat or cold better than thin people.

3. The mesenteric fat around organ like kidney provides padding and protect the internal organs.
4. Building materials: Breakdown products of fats can be utilized for building biologically active material like cholesterol, which in turn can be utilized for synthesis of certain hormones.
5. Lipids supply the essential fatty acids, which cannot be synthesized in the body.
6. The nervous system is particularly rich in lipids.
7. Vitamins A, D, E and K are fat soluble, hence lipid is needed for absorbing these vitamins.
8. Lipoproteins and phospholipids are important constituents of many natural membranes like cell walls and mitochondrion.

An adult ingests almost 60–150 g of lipids per day of which more than 90% is triacylglycerol (TAG). Balance is cholesterol, cholesteryl esters, phospholipids and free fatty acids (FFA).

CLASSIFICATION OF LIPIDS

Simple Lipids

Simple lipids are esters of fatty acids with various alcohols. Neutral fats are triesters of fatty acids with glycerol.

The alcohol in fats is glycerol and the alcohol in waxes is anything other than glycerol.

Compound Lipids

Compound lipids contain some other chemical groups in addition to alcohol and fatty acids. There are four subdivisions under this group:
1. *Phospholipids:* They contain fatty acids, glycerol, phosphoric acid and a nitrogenous compound. For example, lecithin, cephalin, sphingomyelin.
2. *Glycolipids:* They are lipids containing carbohydrate and nitrogen, but no phosphoric acid and glycerol (also called cerebrosides).
3. *Sulfolipids:* Lipids containing sulfate groups.
4. *Lipoprotein:* They are attached to proteins. They are present in plasma and tissues.

Derived Lipids

These are substances derived from groups mentioned above by hydrolysis. They are fatty acids, alcohols other than glycerol, glycerides and bases. Bases include: choline, sphingosine, glycerides and serine.

Substances Associated with Lipids

1. Carotenoids.
2. Tocopherols.
3. Vitamins A, D, E and K.
4. Steroids (cholesterol).

CHEMICAL COMPOSITION OF FATS

Animals and vegetable fats are complex mixtures of glycerides, i.e. they are esters of glycerol and fatty acids. Neutral fats in the form of triglyceride are composed of 3 molecules of fatty acids, esterified to glycerol. A triglyceride is formed by the condensation of one molecule of glycerol with 3 molecules of fatty acids:

$$\begin{array}{c} CH_2-[OH+H]-O-\overset{O}{\overset{\|}{C}}-R_1 \\ | \\ CH-[OH+H]-O-\overset{O}{\overset{\|}{C}}-R_2 \\ | \\ CH_2-[OH+H]-O-\overset{O}{\overset{\|}{C}}-R_3 \end{array} \longrightarrow \begin{array}{c} CH_2-O-\overset{O}{\overset{\|}{C}}-R_1 \\ | \\ CH-O-\overset{O}{\overset{\|}{C}}-R_2 +3H_2O \\ | \\ CH_2-O-\overset{O}{\overset{\|}{C}}-R_3 \end{array}$$

Glycerol Fatty acid Triglyceride (neutral fat)

Common fatty acids present in natural fats are:
Palmitic acid $CH_3(CH_2)_{14}COOH$
Stearic acid $CH_3(CH_2)_{16}COOH$
Oleic acid $CH_3(CH_2)_7 CH=CH (CH_2)_7 COOH$

ESSENTIAL FATTY ACIDS (POLYUNSATURATED FATTY ACIDS)

1. Linoleic acid
   Present in corn, peanut, cotton seed and soyabean oil.
   $CH_3-(CH_2)_4-CH=CH_2-CH=CH(CH_2)_7-COOH$

2. Linolenic acid
   Present in linseed oil.
   $CH_3-CH_2-CH=CH-CH_2-CH=CH-CH_2CH=CH(CH_2)_7-COOH$

Polyunsaturated fatty acids like linoleic acid (C-18, 2 double bonds), linolenic acid (C-18, 3 double bonds) and arachidonic acid (C-20, 4 double bonds) are not synthesized by the body and hence should be taken in diet. Linseed, cotton seeds, peanut and corn oils are good sources. Essential fatty acids reduce blood cholesterol levels. About 3% of energy requirements of the body come from polyunsaturated fatty acids. Fatty acids with more than one unsaturated bond cannot be synthesized by the body. However, mammalian tissues can convert linoleic acid to linolenic and arachidonic acids. Hence, linoleic is the only fatty acid, which is absolutely indispensable.

PROPERTIES OF FATS

Physical Properties

1. They are greasy to touch and leave an oily impression on paper.
2. They are insoluble in water, but soluble in organic solvents.
3. They have less specific gravity than water. Specific gravity of solid fat (0.86) is less than liquid fat (0.95).
4. Pure glycerides are tasteless, odorless, colorless and neutral in reaction. But after exposure to air for some time, they become acidic and develop a yellow color due to partial hydrolysis and oxidation of unsaturated fatty acids in them.
5. The flavor of butter is due to the presence of bacterial flora, which is carefully controlled to impart special flavor to butter. The color of butter, human fat and egg yolk are due to the presence of carotene and xanthophil contained in them.
6. The hardness or consistency depends upon the relative amounts of saturated and unsaturated fatty acids present. Fats containing saturated fatty acids are solids at room temperature. Fats containing unsaturated fatty acids are liquids at room temperature and these are oils.
7. Fats have definite melting points. The melting point of a fat is always higher than the temperature at which it solidifies.
8. When a liquid fat is placed on water, it spreads uniformly over the surface of water and if the quantity is sufficiently small, it will form a layer of one molecule thickness. The effect is to lower the surface tension and help the transport of fat.
9. Though fats are insoluble in water, they can be broken down into minute droplets and dispersed in water. This is emulsification.

Chemical Properties

Acrolein Formation

When glycerol is heated in the presence of a dehydrating agent such as potassium bisulfate, acrolein is produced.

$$\begin{array}{c} CH_2OH \\ | \\ CH-OH \\ | \\ CH_2OH \\ \text{Glycerol} \end{array} \xrightarrow[-2H_2O]{KHSO_4, \Delta} \begin{array}{c} CHO \\ | \\ CH \\ || \\ CH_2 \\ \text{Acrolein} \end{array}$$

Acrolein has a characteristic unpleasant odor and is easily identified on the basis of this smell. This reaction occurs whether glycerol is in free or esterified form as in the triglycerides.

Hydrogenation

Unsaturated fats can be hydrogenated by the addition of hydrogen across the double bonds of the fatty acids in the presence of nickel as catalyst, to give saturated fats. This process is called 'hardening' of oils whereby vegetable oils are hydrogenated to produce commercial cooking fats (dalda).

Saponification

Hydrolysis of a fat by alkali is called saponification. The products of hydrolysis are glycerol and alkali salts of fatty acids called soaps. Soaps are cleansing agents. Since the common fats contain palmitic, stearic and oleic acids predominantly, soaps used for washing consist largely of sodium salts of these acids. While the fatty acids are insoluble in water (scraps), their sodium and potassium salts are soluble in water. Potassium salts are bathing soaps.

$$\begin{array}{c} CH_2OCOR \\ | \\ CH-OCOR \\ | \\ CH_2OCOR \\ \text{Fat} \end{array} + 3NaOH \xrightarrow{\text{Hydrolysis}} \begin{array}{c} CH_2OH \\ | \\ CH-OH \\ | \\ CH_2-OH \\ \text{Glycerol} \end{array} + 3RCOONa \quad \text{Soap}$$

Rancidity

Rancidity is a chemical change resulting in unpleasant odor and taste on storage when fats are exposed to light, heat, air and moisture. Rancidity may be due to hydrolytic or oxidation change taking place at the double bonds of the unsaturated fatty acids resulting in short-chain aldehydes or ketones, which have unpleasant odor.

Rancidity is more rapid at high temperature. Substances like ascorbic acid (vitamin C) and vitamin E prevent rancidity and are called antioxidants. Antioxidants are added to food fats to improve their storage qualities. Many natural fats and oils contain antioxidants like vitamin E, which prevent rancidity. Therefore vegetable fats can be preserved for longer time than animal fats.

CHARACTERISTICS OF FATS

Saponification Number

Saponification number is defined as the number of milligrams of potassium hydroxide required to saponify 1 g of fat. It is an indication of the molecular weight of the fat and is inversely proportional to it. Saponification number of a fat decreases with increase in molecular weight. Human fat has a saponification number of 194–196, butter 210–230 and coconut oil 253–262.

Iodine Number

Iodine number of a fat is defined as the number of grams of iodine taken up by 100 g of fat. It is an index of unsaturation and is directly proportional to the content of unsaturated fatty acids. Higher the iodine number, the higher is the degree of unsaturation. Different types of fats and their iodine numbers are given in Table 3.1.

TABLE 3.1: Different fats and their iodine numbers

Fat/Oil	Iodine number
Human fat	65–69
Butter	26–28
Coconut oil	6–10
Sunflower oil	124–136
Groundnut oil	84–100
Palm oil	44–58

STRUCTURAL LIPIDS OR MEMBRANE LIPIDS

a. Phospholipids.
b. Glycolipids.
c. Sterols (cholesterols).

Phospholipids (Phosphoglycerides and Sphingomyelins)

Any lipid containing phosphorus is called phospholipid. Phospholipids are good emulsifying agents. They are found in cell membranes and in subcellular structures where lipids and water soluble materials interact.

```
GLYCEROL ──Fatty acid              CH₂–O–C(=O)–R
         ──Fatty acid              CH –O–C(=O)–R₁
         ── P – N                  CH₂–O–P(=O)(OH)–N compound
Phospholipid
or phosphoglycerides
```

The most common phospholipid is the glycerol phospholipids. They contain glycerol phosphate, two fatty acids and a nitrogen compound that may be choline, ethanol amine or serine. Lecithins and cephalins are examples of phospholipids. Phospholipid content of blood is given in Table 3.2.

Phosphatidyl Cholines (Lecithins)

This is the most common form of phospholipids and has choline as the nitrogen compound.

TABLE 3.2: Fatty contents in blood (100 mg)	
Triglycerides	80–240 mg
Phospholipids	150–250 mg
Cholesterol	130–260 mg
Free (non-esterified) fatty acids	8–30 mg

$$\begin{array}{l}CH_2O-\overset{O}{\underset{\|}{C}}-OR_1\\ |\\ CHO-\overset{O}{\underset{\|}{C}}-OR_2\\ |\\ CH_2O-\overset{O}{\underset{\|}{P}}-O-CH_2CH_2\overset{+}{N}(CH_3)_3\\ \quad\quad\;\; |\\ \quad\quad\;\; OH\end{array}$$
Choline phosphoglyceride

Free choline is a compound with an alcohol group. Its linkage to the phosphate portion of a lecithin like that of the glycerol to the phosphate, is that of a phosphate ester.

$$HO-CH_2-CH_2-N^+(CH_3)_2$$
Choline

Lecithins are required for the normal transport and utilization of other lipids especially in the liver. Anything, which interferes with the synthesis of choline also will block the synthesis of lecithins and thus interrupt the normal transportation of lipids to and from liver. This usually results in the accumulation of lipid material in the liver giving rise to a condition called fatty liver.

Cephalins

$$\begin{array}{l}CH_2O-\overset{O}{\underset{\|}{C}}-OR_1\\ |\\ CHO-\overset{O}{\underset{\|}{C}}-OR_2\\ |\\ CH_2O-\overset{O}{\underset{\|}{P}}-O-CH_2-CH_2-NH_2\\ \quad\quad\;\; |\\ \quad\quad\;\; OH\end{array}$$
Cephalin
(ethanolamine phosphoglyceride)

Cephalin differs from lecithins with respect to base attached to phosphoric acid. If the base is ethanolamine, then it is called phosphatidyl ethanolamine or ethanolamine cephalin. If the base is amino acid serine, then it is called phosphatidylserine or serine cephalin.

Cephalin on hydrolysis yields glycerol, fatty acids, phosphoric acid, ethanolamine or serine. They are found in nerve tissues. Cephalins are important in clotting of blood and as sources of phosphoric acid for the formations of new tissues.

Plasmalogens

These compounds structurally resemble lecithin and cephalins, with the result that the normal ester is replaced by the ether linkage on the C_1 atom. On treatment with acid, they give rise to a phosphoryl choline or phosphoryl ethanolamine. These compounds constitute as much as 10% of the phospholipids of the brain and the muscles.

$$\begin{array}{l} CH_2-O-CH=CH-R_1 \\ | \\ CH-O-\overset{\overset{O}{\|}}{C}-OR_2 \\ | \\ CH_2-O-\overset{\overset{O}{\|}}{\underset{\underset{O^-}{|}}{P}}-O-Base \end{array}$$

Plasmalogen

Sphingomyelins

They are found in large quantities in brain and nerve tissue. No glycerol is present. On hydrolysis yield a fatty acid, phosphoric acid, choline and a complex aminoalcohol, sphingosine (in place of glycerol).

$$H_3C-(CH_2)_{12}-CH=CH-\underset{\underset{OH}{|}}{CH}-\underset{\underset{NH_2}{|}}{CH}-CH_2-OH$$

Sphingosine

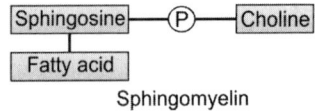

Sphingomyelin

Cerebrosides (Glycolipids)

Glycolipids are carbohydrate-glyceride derivatives containing sugar, sphingosine and a fatty acid. These compounds do not contain phosphoric acid. If the sugar component is galactose, the lipid is termed as galactolipid. The term cerebroside is used because it is found in large quantities in brain tissues particularly in white matter.

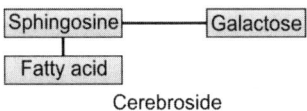
Cerebroside

Steroids

Steroids are non-saponifiable lipids, biological compounds with diverse physiological activities. All steroids are compounds having a cyclopentanoperhydrophenanthrene ring system. The structures of a number of different types of steroids having greatly varying biological activities are shown below:

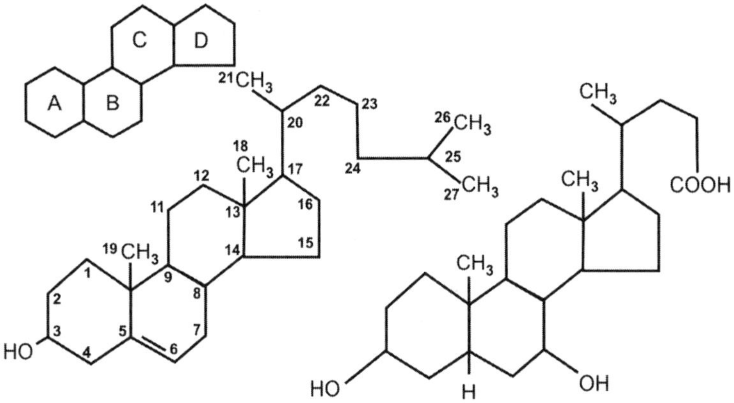

Cholesterol   Cholic acid

When a steroid has only a hydroxyl group (–OH) as its functional group, it is called sterol, e.g. cholesterol.

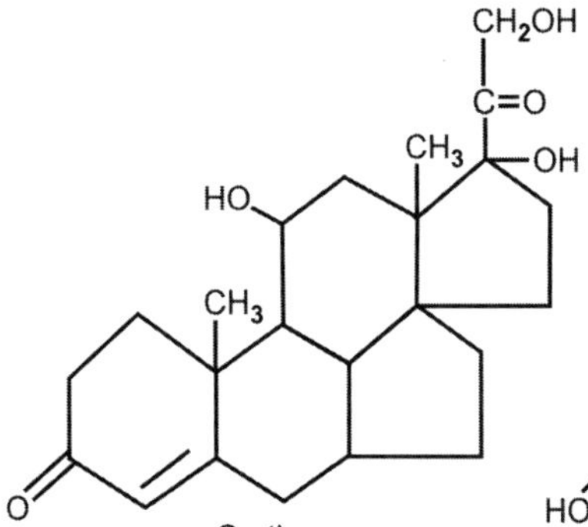

Cortisone 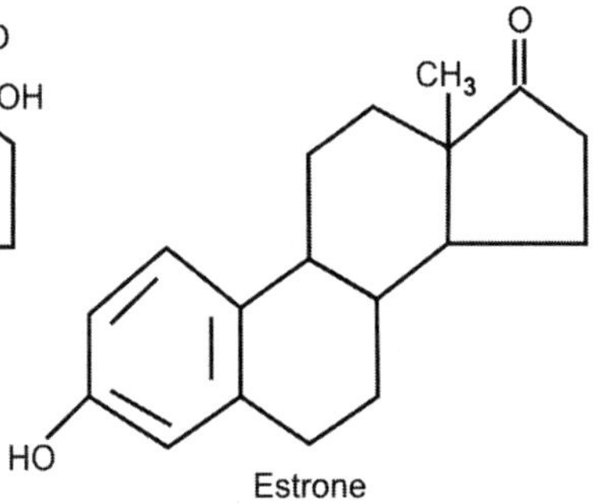   Estrone

Cholesterol is a light yellow crystalline solid. It is soluble in chloroform and other fat solvents. The –OH group in the 3rd position can be esterified with fatty acids to form cholesterol esters. Polyunsaturated acids (essential fatty acids) tend to lower the plasma cholesterol level. This is how cholesterol level in the body is regulated. The level of cholesterol in body fluids is of primary importance due to its role in the development of atherosclerosis. Cholesterol is the most abundant lipid in the human body. It is synthesized mainly in the liver, adrenal cortex, intestines, testes and skin. Acetyl-CoA is the precursor of all the C atoms in cholesterol. In addition, cholesterol plays an important role as a component of biomembranes and has a modulating effect on the fluid state of membranes.

Cholesterol in body fluids can be estimated by color reactions, e.g. Liebermann-Burchard reaction. A solution of cholesterol in chloroform gives a blue or green color, when acetic anhydride and concentrated sulphuric acid are added. This reaction is the basis of a colorimetric estimation of blood cholesterol (Liebermann-Burchard reaction).

FUNCTIONS OF CHOLESTEROL

1. Cholesterol is an important tissue component. It has a modulating effect on the fluid state of the membrane and its integrity and permeability.
2. Because of its low conductivity, cholesterol plays an important role in insulating nerves and brain structure.
3. For the transport of fatty acids in the body through the formation of esters of fatty acids. It is a part of lipoproteins.
4. Cholesterol neutralizes the hemolytic action of a number of agents, such as snake venoms and bacterial toxins.
5. Cholesterol gives rise to provitamin 'D'.
6. It is a precursor of cholic acid in the body and also bile salts.
7. It gives rise to sex hormones.

Cholesterol level in blood is increased in:
- Diabetes mellitus
- Atherosclerosis
- Hyperthyroidism
- Obstructive jaundice
- Nephrotic syndrome

- Myxedema
- Xanthomatosis

LIPOPROTEINS

Lipoproteins are conjugated proteins involved in transport and delivery of lipids to tissues. Lipids such as cholesterol and triglycerides are not soluble in water and are thus need to be complexed to water soluble carrier proteins for transporting them in the blood between different organs.

Plasma lipoproteins consist of a neutral lipid core of triglyceride and cholesterol ester that is surrounded and stabilized by free cholesterol protein and phospholipid. The relative proportion of non-polar lipid, protein and polar lipid determine the density, size and charge of the resulting lipoproteins. The density of lipoproteins has been used to classify them as shown in Table 3.3.

The total plasma lipid is 700–1,000 mg/dL. Roughly 1/3 is triglycerides, another 1/3 is cholesterol and rest 1/3 is phospholipids. These are complexed with proteins to form lipoproteins.

The plasma cholesterol is distributed in different protein fractions. In normal persons, cholesterol level varies from 150 to 220 mg/dL with 70% being esterified cholesterol and 30% free. In the average normal adult male, the plasma cholesterol should be preferably below 200 mg/dL. The females have a lower level because of the high estrogen level, which also affords protection against atherosclerosis.

Normally, almost 60% of total cholesterol is LDL, 22% HDL, 13% VLDL and 5% chylomicrons.

TABLE 3.3: Types of Lipoprotein

Type	Density g/mL	Protein	Triglycerides	Cholesterol Free	Cholesterol Ester	Phospho-lipids (PL)
Chylomicrons	Less than 0.95	1	85–95	1–2	1–2	3–6
Very low-density lipoproteins (VLDL)	0.95–1.006	10	50–60	4–8	10	15–20
Low-density lipoproteins (LDL)	1.006–1.063	22	10	10	38	20
High-density lipoproteins (HDL)	1.063–1.21	45–60	3	5	15–20	25–30

Functions of Lipoproteins

Chylomicrons are the lipoprotein particles lowest in density and largest in size. It contain the most of lipid and smallest percentage of protein. They transport mainly TAG and smaller amounts of PL, cholesterol ester and fat soluble vitamins from intestines to liver and adipose tissues. The lipids carried by chloromicrons principally are dietary lipids. They are formed in the intestinal mucosa. VLDL are composed mainly of TAG and are more enriched in cholesterol esters than are chylomicrons. VLDLs are synthesized in the liver and released into blood. They transport triacylglycerides synthesized in the liver and cholesterol esters from liver to peripheral tissues including adipose tissue for storage (Table 3.4).

Fatty liver occurs in conditions in which there is an imbalance between hepatic triacylglyceride synthesis and the secretion of VLDL by the liver. Diseases such as diabetes mellitus and chronic ethanol ingestion can cause fatty liver.

As VLDL passes through the circulation, their structure is altered to LDL.

LDL provides cholesterol for cellular needs. LDL promotes coronary heart disease by first penetrating the coronary artery wall and then depositing cholesterol to form atherosclerosis plaque.

Elevated LDL levels have been associated with increased risk of developing coronary artery disease, whereas elevated HDL levels reduce the risk. Women have higher HDL levels than men (55 vs 45 mg/dL) and this may account for women's lower rate of heart disease. Aerobic exercise increases HDL levels (Marathon runners average 65 mg/dL).

TABLE 3.4: Site of synthesis and function of lipoproteins

Types	Site of synthesis	Functions
Chylomicrons	Intestine	Transport of dietary lipids from intestine to peripheral tissue
VLDL	Liver	Transport of endogenous triacylglycerol from liver to peripheral tissue
LDL	Plasma	Transport free form of cholesterol from liver to peripheral tissue
HDL	Liver and intestine	Transport free cholesterol from peripheral tissue to the liver where it can be catabolized (reverse cholesterol transport)

ESTIMATION OF PLASMA LIPIDS

For clinical purposes, the lipid portions in plasma estimated are total cholesterol, HDL cholesterol and triglycerides.

Total cholesterol is estimated colorimetrically.

1. Serum is used for Liebermann-Burchard reaction. Cholesterol in presence of concentrated H_2SO_4, acetic acid and acetic anhydride is oxidized to cholesterol polyenes to give blue-green color.
2. More modern is the enzymatic cholesterol oxidase method. Cholesterol is oxidized. The H_2O_2 produced in this reaction is split by peroxidase to produce nascent oxygen, which is used to oxidize a colorless chromogen to a colored product.

HDL and LDL

HDL cholesterol is estimated after precipitating LDL and VLDL. The LDL cholesterol can be calculated from total cholesterol, HDL cholesterol and serum triglycerides.

LDL cholesterol = Total cholesterol - (HDL cholesterol + TAG/5)

1/5 of the triglyceride value is believed to represent VLDL in fasting plasma. The sample serum should be taken after 14–16 hours of fasting.

QUESTIONS

1. What are lipids? Classify them by giving suitable examples.
2. Describe the chemistry and functions of phospholipids.
3. Describe the chemistry and functions of cholesterol.
4. What are plasma lipoproteins? What are their functions?
5. Write short notes on:
   A. Essential fatty acids.
   B. Rancidity.
   C. Saponification number.
   D. Lipoproteins.
   E. Phospholipids.
6. What is the relationship between polyunsaturated fatty acids and cholesterol?

MULTIPLE CHOICE QUESTIONS

7. **Lipids are:**
   A. Structural components of cell membrane
   B. Components having high energy value
   C. Soluble in non-polar solvents
   D. All of the above

8. **An example of a simple lipid is:**
   A. Triglyceride (triacylglycerol)   B. Cephalin
   C. Fatty acids   D. Glycerol

9. **Glycerol is a:**
   A. Compound lipid   B. Simple lipid
   C. Derived lipid   D. Aliphatic alcohol

10. **All the following are polyunsaturated fatty acid *except*:**
    A. Linolenic acid   B. Palmitic acid
    C. Arachidonic acid   D. Linoleic acid

11. **Which compound facilitates emulsification of fats?**
    A. Bile salts   B. Bile pigments
    C. Bile acids   D. Steroids

12. **Hydrolysis of fat by an alkali is known as:**
    A. Esterification   B. Saponification
    C. Emulsification   D. Peroxidation

13. **Iodine number indicates:**
    A. Total number of fatty acids in fat
    B. Level of rancidity of fat
    C. Measure of the degree of unsaturation in fat
    D. Number of volatile fatty acids in fat

14. **The main lipid present in cell membrane bilayer is:**
    A. Cholesterol   B. Triglyceride
    C. Phospholipid   D. Fatty acid

15. **Major storage form of lipid is:**
    A. Esterified cholesterol   B. Glycerophospholipids
    C. Triglycerides   D. Sphingolipids

16. **The highest phospholipid content is found in:**
    A. Chylomicron   B. VLDL
    C. LDL   D. HDL

17. Which of the following transport endogenous triacylglycerol and cholesterol from liver to tissues?
    A. VLDL, HDL
    B. VLDL, LDL
    C. VLDL, LDL, IDL
    D. VLDL, IDL
18. Which of the following transport endogenous cholesterol from tissues to liver?
    A. LDL
    B. IDL
    C. HDL
    D. VLDL

ANSWERS

7. (D)	8. (A)	9. (C)	10. (B)	11. (A)
12. (B)	13. (C)	14. (C)	15. (C)	16. (D)
17. (C)	18. (C)			

CHAPTER 4

Amino Acids

The principal source of amino acids is hydrolysis of proteins. Proteins are high molecular weight substances found in all living tissues. Upon acid, base or enzyme-catalyzed hydrolysis, they are broken up into thousands of amino acid molecules. Most proteins produce approximately 20 different α-amino acids.

Alpha-amino acids have both an amino and a carboxylic acid group attached to the same α-carbon.

$$R-\underset{\underset{COOH}{|}}{\overset{\overset{H}{|}}{C^{\alpha}}}-NH_2$$

UTILIZATION OR METABOLISM OF PROTEINS

Amino acids from digested proteins are absorbed rapidly into blood and passed on to different tissues to meet their needs. Some non-essential amino acids are synthesized in the liver and released into circulation. The major anabolic pathway for amino acids is the synthesis of all needed body proteins. The N_2 portion of amino acids is used for the synthesis of non-protein nitrogen containing (NPN) compounds. If the intake of carbohydrates and fats are inadequate, the amino acids will be catabolized to produce glucose or usable energy [Adenosine triphosphate (ATP)].

Semi-essential Amino Acids

Arginine and histidine are synthesized partially by the body, but not at the rate to meet the requirement in growing children, pregnant or lactating women.

Non-essential Amino Acids

Non-essential amino acids can be synthesized by the body and may not be required in the diet. These amino acids are derived from the carbon skeletons of lipids and carbohydrates during their metabolism or from the transamination of essential amino acids, e.g. alanine, aspartic acid, serine, proline.

Essential Amino Acids

There are 8 amino acids not synthesized by the body and therefore must be taken in the diet.
1. Leucine.
2. Isoleucine.
3. Threonine.
4. Tryptophan.
5. Phenylalanine.
6. Valine.
7. Methionine.
8. Lysine.

Mnemonic
Pvt. Tim hall

Pvt. Tim Hall	H-histidine
563 427 18	A-arginine

Adequate amounts of essential amino acids are required to maintain the proper nitrogen balance in the body.

Deficiency of one or more essential amino acids in the diet reduces protein synthesis leading to failure in growth of the child, negative nitrogen balance in adults and fall in plasma proteins and hemoglobin levels.

The body can make only 11 of the amino acids. The human body requires 20 amino acids for synthesis of proteins. There are 9 amino acids called essential amino acids that are supplied through food, e.g. beef, lamb, pork, poultry, fish, egg, milk and milk products. If proteins of the food supply enough essential amino acids, they are called complete proteins. If proteins of the food do not supply enough essential amino acid they are called incomplete proteins, e.g. grain, fruits and vegetables.

Essential amino acids cannot be synthesized by the body and they must be taken in diet. They are:
1. **Methionine:** It is one of the sulfur-containing amino acids. Methionine forms cysteine, but cysteine cannot be converted into methionine.
2. **Threonine:** It is important in the formation of some non-essential amino acids.
3. **Tryptophan:** 60 parts of tryptophan are equal to one part of niacin (B-complex vitamin). This is called niacin equivalent. Milk is an excellent source of tryptophan.

4. Valine: It is branched chain amino acid and it is good for renal and liver tissues.
5. Isoleucine: Parenteral nutrition preparations are derived from methionine, leucine and isoleucine. These amino acids are recommended to manage bowel problems.
6. Leucine: It is one of the branched chain amino acids and it is good for the welfare of renal tissues.
7. Phenylalanine: Tyrosine, a non-essential amino acid is formed from phenylalanine.
8. Lysine: It is a limiting amino acid in rice. It is converted into carnitine, but there is some limitation in the form of carnitine in infants.

ABSORPTION OF PROTEINS (AMINO ACIDS)

Amino acids are absorbed by blood from small intestine by active transport and diffusion. Rate of absorption depends on:
1. Total load of amino acids released from digestion.
2. The proportion of various amino acids.
3. Availability of carrier.
4. Uptake of amino acids by tissues.
5. Essential amino acids.
6. Branched chain amino acids.
7. Amino acids in the blood.

Active Transport and Specific Carrier

Amino acids are absorbed by active transport, but some diffusion of amino acids also takes place. Some amino acids are absorbed rapidly than others. Methionine, leucine, isoleucine and valine have the highest rate of absorption than threonine. So protein must contain an excess of rapidly absorbed amino acids.

CLASSIFICATION AND STRUCTURE OF AMINO ACIDS

Amino acids can be classified into three groups depending upon their reaction in solution, i.e:
1. Neutral.
2. Acidic.
3. Basic.

Basic is the largest group and can be further subdivided into aliphatic, aromatic, heterocyclic and sulfur-containing amino acids.

FUNCTIONS OF AMINO ACIDS

1. Building blocks of proteins.
2. Specific amino acids give rise to specialized products.
   For example:
   a. Tyrosine forms thyroid hormones T_3, T_4 and a pigment called melanin.
   b. Tryptophan can synthesize a vitamin called niacin.
   c. Glycine, arginine and methionine synthesize creatinine.
   d. Glycine and cysteine help in the synthesis of bile salts.
   e. Cysteine and methionine are sources of sulfur.

OCCURRENCE OF AMINO ACIDS

All the amino acids in Table 4.1 are present in proteins. Cereals are rich in acidic amino acids, aspartic acid and glutamic acid. Collagen is rich in basic amino acids and also proline and hydroxy proline.

PROPERTIES OF AMINO ACIDS

Physical Properties

Colorless crystalline substances, more soluble in water than in organic solvents like ether (this is due to Zwitterion form). High melting points, usually more than 200°C and high dielectric constants.

Chemical Properties

Properties Due to Carboxylic Group (-COOH)

1. Formation of esters with alcohols.
2. Reduction to amine alcohol in presence of lithium aluminum hydride.
3. Formation of amines by decarboxylation.
4. Formation of amides.

TABLE 4.1: L-α-amino acids found in protein

Groups	Trivial names	Abbreviations	Chemical names	Structural formula
I.	Neutral amino acids			
	With aliphatic side chains			
	Glycine	Gly	Aminoacetic acid	H–CH–COOH | NH$_2$
	Alanine	Ala	α-aminopropionic acid	CH$_3$–CH–COOH | NH$_2$

	Valine	Val	α-aminoisovaleric acid	H$_3$C
				    \>CH–CH–COOH
				H$_3$C |
				           NH$_2$

	Leucine	Leu	α-aminoisocaproic acid	H$_3$C
				    \>CH–CH$_2$–CH–COOH
				H$_3$C |
				                   NH$_2$

	Isoleucine	Ile	α-amino-β-methylvaleric acid	CH$_3$–CH$_2$
				          \>CH–CH–COOH
				    H$_3$C |
				                NH$_2$

Contd...

Contd...

Groups	Trivial names	Abbreviations	Chemical names	Structural formula
II.	With side chains containing hydroxyl groups (-OH)			
	Serine	Ser	α-amino-β-hydroxypropionic acid	$CH_2-CH-COOH$ $\quad\vert\quad\quad\vert$ $\;OH\;\;NH_2$
	Threonine	Thr	α-amino-β-hydroxybutyric acid	$CH_3-CH-CH-COOH$ $\quad\quad\;\;\vert\quad\quad\vert$ $\quad\quad OH\;\;NH_2$
III.	With side chains containing sulfur atoms			
	Cysteine (cystine is formed by the linkage of two cysteine side chains through a disulfide bond)	Cys	α-amino-β-mercaptopropionic acid	$CH_2-CH-COOH$ $\quad\vert\quad\quad\vert$ $\;SH\;\;NH_2$
	Methionine	Met	α-amino-γ-methylthio-n-butyric acid	$\overset{\gamma}{CH_2}-\overset{\beta}{CH_2}-\overset{\alpha}{CH}-COOH$ $\;\vert\quad\quad\quad\quad\;\;\vert$ $S-CH_3\;\;\;\;NH_2$
IV.	Containing aromatic rings			
	Histidine	His	α-amino-β-imidazole propionic acid	HN⟩—$CH_2-CH-COOH$ $\quad\quad\quad\quad\quad\;\;\vert$ $\quad\quad\quad\quad\;\;NH_2$
	Phenyl alanine	Phe	α-amino-β-phenylpropionic acid	⟨◯⟩—$CH_2-CH-COOH$ $\quad\quad\quad\quad\quad\;\;\vert$ $\quad\quad\quad\quad\;\;NH_2$

Contd...

Contd...

Groups	Trivial names	Abbreviations	Chemical names	Structural formula
	Tyrosine	Tyr	α-amino-β-(hydroxyphenyl) propionic acid	$OH{-}\bigcirc{-}CH_2{-}CH{-}COOH$ with $-NH_2$
	Tryptophan	Trp	α-amino-β-3-indolepropionic acid	indole$-CH_2{-}CH{-}COOH$ with $-NH_2$
V.	Proline	Pro	Pyrrolidine-2-carboxylic acid	pyrrolidine ring with $-COOH$
	4-hydroxy proline	Hyp	4-hydroxypyrrolidine-2-carboxylic acid	$HO-$ pyrrolidine (positions 1,2,3,4) with $-COOH$
VI.	Acidic amino acids with side chains containing acidic groups or their amides			
	Aspartic acid	Asp	α-aminosuccinic acid	$HOOC{-}CH_2{-}\overset{\alpha}{C}H{-}COOH$ with $-NH_2$
	Asparagine	Asn	α-amide of α-aminosuccinic acid	$H_2N{-}\overset{\gamma}{C}{-}\overset{\beta}{C}H_2{-}\overset{\alpha}{C}H{-}COOH$ with $=O$ and $-NH_2$

Contd...

Amino Acids

Contd...

Groups	Trivial names	Abbreviations	Chemical names	Structural formula
	Glutamic acid	Glu	α-aminoglutaric acid	$\overset{\alpha}{HOOC-CH_2-CH_2-CH-COOH}$ $\quad\quad\quad\quad\quad\quad\quad\quad\quad\quad\;\; \mid$ $\quad\quad\quad\quad\quad\quad\quad\quad\quad\quad NH_2$
	Glutamin	Gln	δ-amide of α-aminoglutaric acid	$\overset{\delta}{H_2N-C}-\overset{\gamma}{CH_2}-\overset{\beta}{CH_2}-\overset{\alpha}{CH}-COOH$ $\quad\;\; \parallel \quad\quad\quad\quad\quad\quad\quad\quad\;\; \mid$ $\quad\;\; O \quad\quad\quad\quad\quad\quad\quad\quad\; NH_2$
VII.	Basic amino acids with chains containing basic group Arginine	Arg	α-amino-δ-guanidinovaleric acid	$H-N-CH_2-CH_2-CH_2-CH-COOH$ $\;\;\mid \quad\quad\quad\quad\quad\quad\quad\quad\quad\quad\quad\;\; \mid$ $\;C=O \quad\quad\quad\quad\quad\quad\quad\quad\quad\; NH_2$ $\;\;\mid$ $\;NH_2$
	Lysine	Lys	α-ε-diaminocaproic acid	$CH_2-CH_2-CH_2-CH_2-CH-COOH$ $\;\mid \quad\quad\quad\quad\quad\quad\quad\quad\quad\quad\quad\; \mid$ $NH_2 \quad\quad\quad\quad\quad\quad\quad\quad\quad\quad NH_2$
	Hydroxylysine histidine (refer group IV)	Hyl	α-ε-diamino-δ-hydroxy-n-caproic acid	$CH_2-CH-CH_2-CH_2-CH-COOH$ $\;\mid \quad\;\;\; \mid \quad\quad\quad\quad\quad\quad\quad\quad\;\; \mid$ $NH_2 \;\; OH \quad\quad\quad\quad\quad\quad\quad\; NH_2$

Contd...

Properties Due to Amino Group (-NH$_2$)
1. Salt formation with acids like HCl.
2. Liberation of N$_2$ when reacting with nitrous acid (HNO$_2$).
3. Reaction with formaldehyde.

Sørensen, a Danish biochemist who originated the use of the pH scale as a measure of acidity of solutions, found that addition of large excess of formaldehyde ties up amino groups, permitting the attainment of sharp end points when titrating amino acids with alkali. Such a titration is called formol titration and is used for the estimation of free carboxyl group in amino acids and mixture of amino acids.

The isoelectric pH of an amino acid is that pH at which it has no net charge and hence does not move in an electric field.

Zwitterion formation: The acidic and basic group within the same molecule of an amino acid react with each other.

$$R-CH(NH_2)-COOH \rightleftharpoons R-CH(NH_3^+)-COO^-$$

Such a doubly charged ion is known as an inert salt, or a zwitterion or a dipolar ion. Amino acids exist over 50% in the dipolar or zwitterion form. This gives them a salt-like character, as revealed by their large solubility in water and insolubility in ether, benzene, etc. and by their relatively high melting points.

Ninhydrin reaction: Ninhydrin, a powerful oxidizing agent, causes oxidative decarboxylation of α-amino acids, producing CO_2, NH_3 and an aldehyde with one less carbon atom than parent amino acids. The reduced ninhydrin then reacts with the liberated amino acids forming a blue complex (blue-purple color).

The intensity of the blue-purple color produced under standard conditions is the basis of a quantitative estimation of α-amino acids. Amines other than α-amino acids also react with ninhydrin, forming blue-purple color, but without evolving CO_2. The evolution of CO_2 is thus indicative of an α-amino acid. Proline and 4-hydroxyproline produce a yellow color with ninhydrin.

Amino Acids

```
R—CH—COOH
    |
    NH₂           + 2 [Ninhydrin]  →Heat→
Amino acid
```

$$\text{Amino acid} + 2 \text{ Ninhydrin} \xrightarrow{\text{Heat}} \text{Blue-purple color} + R\text{-CHO} + CO_2\uparrow$$

Amino acid + 2 molecules of ninhydrin $\xrightarrow{\text{Heat}}$ Aldehyde with 1 carbon atom less + CO_2 + blue-purple complex

Isomerism

Stereoisomerism: All amino acids except glycine (no asymmetric C atom) exist as D and L-isomers. In D-amino acids–NH_2 group is on the right.

```
    COOH              COOH
    |                 |
H₂N—C—H           H—C—NH₂
    |                 |
    R                 R
L-amino acid      D-amino acid
```

Optical isomerism: All amino acids except glycine have asymmetric C atom. Consequently, all except glycine exhibit 'optical' activities and rotate the plane of polarized light and exist as dextrorotatory (d) and levorotatory (l) isomers. Optical activity depends on pH and side chain.

 QUESTIONS

1. **Classify amino acids with examples.**
2. **Give the names of essential amino acids.**

3. Short notes on:
   A. Essential amino acids.
   B. Properties of amino acids.
   C. Amphoteric nature of amino acids.

MULTIPLE CHOICE QUESTIONS

4. Which class of amino acids contain only non-essential amino acids?
   A. Aromatic
   B. Basic
   C. Sulfur containing
   D. Acidic
5. The high intake of which amino acid can prevent pellagra in people consuming a niacin-deficient diet:
   A. Lysine
   B. Methionine
   C. Threonine
   D. Tryptophan
6. Which one of the following is an acidic amino acid?
   A. Palmitic acid
   B. Aspartic acid
   C. Pyruvic acid
   D. Lysine
7. A basic amino acid is:
   A. Phenyl alanine
   B. Serine
   C. Arginine
   D. Glutamic acid
8. Which one of the following is not a sulfur-containing amino acid?
   A. Histidine
   B. Cysteine
   C. Cystine
   D. Methionine
9. All the following are essential amino acids *except:*
   A. Phenyl alanine
   B. Tryptophan
   C. Tyrosine
   D. Isoleucine
10. The semi-essential amino acids are:
    A. Histidine and alanine
    B. Arginine and glycine
    C. Proline and methionine
    D. Arginine and histidine
11. An example for neutral amino acid:
    A. Tyrosine
    B. Proline
    C. Lysine
    D. Leucine
12. Test for L-amino acid is:
    A. Molisch's test
    B. Biuret test
    C. Ninhydrin test
    D. Murexide test

13. **Which amino acid is important in the buffering action of proteins at physiologic pH?**
    A. Tyrosine
    B. Histidine
    C. Lysine
    D. Glutamic acid

ANSWERS

| 4. (D) | 5. (D) | 6. (B) | 7. (C) | 8. (A) |
| 9. (C) | 10. (D) | 11. (D) | 12. (C) | 13. (B) |

5 Chemistry of Proteins

BIOLOGICAL IMPORTANCE

The word protein is derived from the Greek word 'proteios', which means primary. Proteins are high molecular weight (5,000–2,500,000) substances. About half the dry weight of living materials is protein. They are the source to replace nitrogen as almost 30 g of nitrogen is lost everyday by an adult chiefly as urinary urea.

COMPOSITION OF PROTEINS

In addition to C, H and O, which are present in carbohydrates and lipids, proteins contain N. They are macromolecules. They are all polymers, i.e, they are chain-like molecules produced by the linking together of a number of small units, chiefly almost 20 α-amino acids belonging to L form.

$$R-CH(NH_2)-C(=O)-OH$$
α-amino acid

These units are joined through the peptide bonds (CO–NH$^-$). The peptide linkage is formed between two amino acids by the release of one water molecule. The amino group of the first amino acid and the carbonyl group of the next amino acid are involved in the formation of peptide bonds.

Peptide Bonds

When two amino acids are joined together by the peptide bond the resulting compound is called dipeptide.

Proteins contain more than 100 amino acid residues, polypeptides (100 or less than 100).

$$H_2N-\underset{R_1}{\underset{|}{\overset{H}{\overset{|}{C}}}}-CO\text{-}OH + H\text{-}HN-\underset{R_2}{\underset{|}{\overset{H}{\overset{|}{C}}}}-COOH \longrightarrow H_2N-\underset{R_1}{\underset{|}{\overset{H}{\overset{|}{C}}}}-CO-\underset{}{\overset{H}{\overset{|}{N}}}-\underset{R_1}{\underset{|}{\overset{H}{\overset{|}{C}}}}-COOH + H_2O$$

Dipeptide

A tripeptide consists of 3 amino acids linked by 2 peptide bonds.

A tripeptide composed of glycine, alanine and serine.

A polypeptide consists of a large number of amino acids joined together by peptide bonds. Each polypeptide can have any number of any one or different types of amino acids, which can be present in any sequence. The individual amino acid of a peptide is called the amino acid residue. Each polypeptide has one free carboxylic acid group (-COOH) at one end, which is called the C-terminal and a free amino group at the other end called N-terminal.

BIOMEDICAL IMPORTANCE OF PROTEINS

1. Proteins are the main dietary constituents for supply of nitrogen and sulfur.
2. Biochemical catalysts known as enzymes are proteins.
3. Proteins called immunoglobulins are the frontline of defence against bacterial and viral infections.
4. Structural proteins furnish mechanical support for the movement of muscles.
5. Several hormones are proteins.
6. Some proteins present in cell membrane, cytoplasm and nucleus of the cell act as receptors. They bind specific substances such as vitamins, hormones, etc. and mediate their circular action.
7. The transport proteins carry out the function of transporting specific substances either across the membrane or in body fluids.

8. Storage proteins bind with specific substances and store them, e.g. iron is stored as ferritin.
9. Some proteins are constituents of respiratory pigments present in the electron transport chain or respiratory chain, e.g. cytochromes, myoglobin and hemoglobin.
10. Proteins by means of exerting osmotic pressure help in maintenance of electrolyte and water balance in the body.

STRUCTURE OF PROTEINS

Proteins exhibit four levels of organization.
1. Primary structure: Refers to amino acid sequence.
2. Secondary structure: Refers to folding of polypeptide chain into specific coiled structure, which is repetitive.
3. Tertiary structure: Refers to arrangement and interrelationship of twisted chain into a three-dimensional structure
4. Quaternary structure: Refers to the association of different monomeric subunits into a composite polymeric protein.

Primary Structure

The primary structure is the sequence in which the amino acids are arranged in a protein. The amino acid sequence of a protein determines the function of the protein. Even a change of just one amino acid in sequence drastically alters properties of the entire protein molecule. For example, the hemoglobin molecule has 574 amino acid residues. Changing one specific amino acid in the sequence results in a defective hemoglobin found in patients suffering from sickle cell anemia.

–Val–His–Leu–Thr–Pro–Glu–Glu–Lys
Normal hemoglobin
–Val–His–Leu–Thr–Pro–Val–Glu–Lys
Sickle cell hemoglobin

Insulin has 51 amino acids present in two polypeptide chains. These chains are cross linked at two places by disulfide bonds. One chain contains 21 amino acid units and the other has 30 amino acids. The molecular weight of insulin is 5,733.

Secondary Structure

Secondary structure determines (Fig. 5.1) the coiling of the polypeptide chain into a helical structure because of folding or twisting of polypeptide chains into a coiled or spiral forms due to hydrogen bonding. The hydrogen bonding arises due to the bonding between the carbonyl oxygen and amide nitrogen. Since peptide bonds occur at regular intervals, the hydrogen bonding of the secondary structure also occurs regularly. The right-handed helix, i.e. the alpha-helix is the most preferred configuration. The diameter of the helix is 10Å.

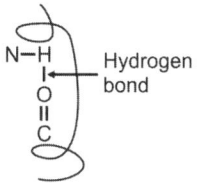

Fig. 5.1: Secondary structure

Tertiary Structure

Tertiary structure refers to the coiling of several helical portion of single helix into three-dimensional structure (Fig. 5.2). Interaction among amino acids relatively widely separated in primary position yield tertiary structure. The tertiary structure of proteins is stabilized by:

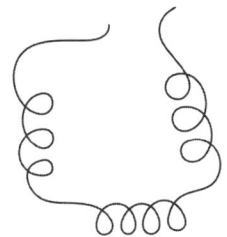

Fig. 5.2: Tertiary structure

1. Hydrogen bonding.
2. Disulfide bonding.
3. Ionic interaction.
4. Hydrophobic interaction.
5. van der Waals forces.

The tertiary structure acquired by native protein is always thermodynamically most stable.

Quaternary Structure

Quaternary structure is the molecular structure arising from the interaction of individual peptide chains to form a specific aggregate. Numerous globular proteins and enzymes possess quaternary structure. They are composed of a number of subunit peptide chains linked together by any or all of the forces that can act between amino acid side-chains.

Hemoglobin, the oxygen transporting protein of blood is an example of quaternary structure. This protein consists of four peptide chains of two types. Each of these subunits is itself complexly folded. The two pairs of folded peptides interact with each other to give a quite stable, compact bundle, which is the active protein, hemoglobin.

Quaternary structure is essential for the activity of protein enzymes.

DENATURATION OF PROTEINS

Native state is the conformation of protein in the most stable form as it exists in the cells or tissues of the living organism. If a protein is exposed to different set of environmental conditions, its conformation may change, with attendant alterations in its physical properties and most significantly, in the ability of the proteins to perform its biological role. Such a change in a protein is termed as denaturation. A number of relatively weak secondary bonds are broken and new bonds are formed during denaturation.

The boiling of an egg is an example of denaturation. Raw egg white is a globular protein, a soluble form and on boiling gets converted into a fibrous form, which coagulates and hardens.

The formation of cheese is another example. When the pH of milk is brought down to 4–5 or below, casein (milk protein) precipitates and cheese, an insoluble form of milk protein is formed.

During denaturation, the protein molecule uncoils from an ordered and specific configuration into a more random configuration and thus precipitates from the solution.

Denatured protein molecules often tend to form large aggregates and precipitates from solution—a process described as 'coagulation'.

CLASSIFICATION OF PROTEINS

Based on Solubility

Fibrous Proteins

The fibrous proteins are insoluble in water and include the following:
Collagens: Present in bone, teeth, tendons, skin and soft connective tissue. When such tissue is boiled with water, the portion of its collagen that dissolves is called gelatin.
Elastins: It is found in ligaments, the walls of blood vessels and the necks of the grazing animals. Elastin is rich in hydrophilic side chains. Cross links between elastin strands are important for its recovery after stretching.
Keratins: Present in hair, wool, animal hooves, nails and porcupine quills.
Myosins: The proteins in contractile muscles.
Fibrin: The protein of a blood clot. During clotting, it forms fibrin from its precursor, fibrinogen by series of complex reactions.

Globular Proteins

Globular proteins are soluble in water or in water with 5% NaCl and include the following:

Albumins: Present in egg white and in blood. Albumins serve many functions. Some are buffers, some carry water insoluble molecules of lipids or fatty acids. Some carry metal ions.

Globulins: It includes the γ-globulin that are part of body's defense mechanism against disease. The globulins need the presence of dissolved salt (5% NaCl) to be soluble in water.

Based on Nutritional Level

From nutritional points of view, proteins are classified as:
1. Complete proteins, e.g. fish, egg albumin, casein (milk).
2. Partially incomplete proteins.
3. Incomplete proteins, e.g. grain, fruits and vegetables.

Based on Composition

Proteins are classified into three groups as per their composition:
1. Simple proteins.
2. Conjugated proteins.
3. Derived proteins.

Simple Proteins

On hydrolysis, yield only amino acids and their derivatives.

Conjugated Proteins

On hydrolysis, give amino acids and a non-conjugated proteins.

Derived Proteins

Produced by the action of chemical, enzymatic and physical forces on the other two classes of proteins. They include proteoses, peptones, polypeptides, tripeptides and dipeptides.

Based on Conjugated Proteins

As per the nature of the prosthetic group, conjugated proteins are subdivided as:

Glycoproteins: Proteins with sugar units, e.g. gamma globulin.
Hemoproteins: Proteins with heme units such as hemoglobin, myoglobin and certain cytochromes (enzymes that help cell use oxygen).
Lipoproteins: Proteins that carry lipid molecules including cholesterol.
Metalloproteins: Proteins that incorporates a metal ion like many enzymes.
Nucleoproteins: Proteins bound to nucleic acids such as ribosomes and certain viruses.
Phosphoproteins: Proteins with a phosphate ester to a side chain—OH group, such as in serine, e.g. casein.

Based on Biological Function

Proteins on the basis of their function, are grouped as follows:
Enzymes: The body catalysts.
Contractile muscle: With stationary filaments—myosin and moving filaments—actin.
Hormones: Such as growth hormone, insulin and others.
Neurotransmitters: Enkephalins and endorphins.
Storage proteins: Those that store nutrients that organism will need such as seed proteins in grains, casein in milk or albumin in egg white and ferritin, the iron storage protein in human spleen.
Transport proteins: Those that carry things from one place to another. Hemoglobin and the serum albumins. Ceruloplasmin is copper-carrying protein.

PROPERTIES OF PROTEINS

Ninhydrin Reactions

Ammonia, many amines, peptides and any protein will give a blue-purple color, when boiled with ninhydrin, a benzene type compound.

Colloidal Nature

Proteins form colloidal dispersions in water. Being colloidal, proteins will pass through a filter paper, but not through a membrane. Serum proteins cannot pass through cell membranes. Thus, there should be no protein material present in the urine. Proteinuria indicates damage to the membranes in the kidneys—possibly nephritis.

Denaturation

Denaturation of a protein refers to the unfolding and rearrangement of the secondary and tertiary structure of protein without breaking the peptide bonds (primary structure). Protein that is denatured loses its biological activity.

Reagents and conditions that cause denaturation are:
1. Heat.
2. Salts of heavy metals (addition of positive ions).
3. Salting out.
4. Alcohol.
5. Alkaloidal reagents.
6. Oxidizing and reducing agents.
7. pH.
8. Radiation.

Heat

Gentle heating causes reversible denaturation of proteins whereas vigorous heating denatures proteins irreversibly by disrupting several types of bonds.

Egg white, a substance containing high percentage of protein, coagulates on heating. Heat coagulates and destroys proteins present in bacteria. Hence, sterilization by heat in microbiology. The presence of protein in urine can be detected by heating a sample of urine, which will cause the coagulation of any protein material that is present (usually albumin).

Precipitation Reactions

For many estimations, it is necessary to get protein-free filtrate from blood and other biological fluids. Precipitation of protein is called deproteinization. Precipitation reactions are also employed in the isolation of proteins and precipitation of protein derivatives. Proteins may be precipitated and separated from solution by the following methods:

Addition of Neutral Salt Solution

Proteins are precipitated from solution by the addition of concentrated salt solutions like ammonium sulfate and sodium sulfate. This process is also called salting out. Lesser concentration of salt is required for protein molecules of larger size and higher concentration is required for protein molecules of smaller size.

Fractionation by Solvents

Precipitation by salting out introduces the difficult problem of the added salt, particularly when pure fraction of plasma proteins are required for clinical purposes. This problem is overcome by alcohol fractionation at low temperature and drying the protein precipitated in vacuum. Addition of alcohol to an aqueous solution of protein lowers its dielectric constant, thus reducing the solubility of the proteins resulting in its precipitation.

Addition of Positive Ions

The commonly used positive ions for precipitation of proteins are those of heavy metals such as Zn^{2+}, Hg^{2+}, Fe^{2+}, Cu^{2+} and Pb^{2+}. These ions precipitate proteins in alkaline solution, where the proteins are negatively charged and combine with the positively charged heavy metals to form insoluble metallic proteinate. Antidote for $AgNO_3$ and $HgCl_2$ taken internally is egg white.

Addition of Negative Ions

Proteins are positively charged in acid medium and combine with negatively charged complex alkaloidal reagents like picric acid, sulfosalicylic acid, tannic acid and phosphotungstic acid and get precipitated.

Dialysis

Protein molecules being large in size may be dialyzed. This involves removal of smaller sized crystalloidal constituents from plasma other than proteins by selective diffusion through a semipermeable membrane. Dialysis is the process of separating crystalloids from colloids by diffusion through a semipermeable membrane by osmotic force.

COLOR REACTIONS (TESTS) OF PROTEINS

Color tests for the presence of proteins depend on the presence of certain amino acids in that protein. These tests, which are generally common to amino acids, peptides and proteins—are useful for detection and sometimes for their quantitative estimation.

Xanthoproteic Test

The word 'xanthoproteic' means yellow proteins. The test consists of adding concentrated HNO_3 to a protein. The protein will then turn yellow and get precipitated. Anyone who has spilled nitric acid on hand will recall the yellow color produced by the reaction of HNO_3 with the protein of the skin. The test is answered only by proteins consisting of amino acids with a benzene ring, such as tyrosine, phenylalanine or tryptophan.

Ninhydrin Test

When proteins are boiled with ninhydrin (a benzene type compound), a blue-purple color and CO_2 are produced. The test indicates the presence of α-amino acids or peptide groups.

Biuret Test

When urea is heated, it forms biuret. The compound biuret contains two peptide linkage.

$$\begin{array}{c}NH_2\\|\\C=O\\|\\NH_2\\+\\NH_2\\|\\C=O\\|\\NH_2\\\text{Urea}\end{array} \xrightarrow{\Delta} \begin{array}{c}NH_2\\|\\C=O\\|\\NH + NH_3\\|\\C=O\\|\\NH_2\\\text{Biuret}\end{array}$$

If biuret or any similar structure having two peptide bonds linked by not more than one carbon atom, is made alkaline with NaOH solution and $CuSO_4$ solutions added, a violet color is produced. Any peptide having three amino acid units or more will give biuret test positive. The dipeptides and free amino acids do not give the biuret test. Biuret test is due to coordination of cupric ions with unshared electron pairs of peptide nitrogen and the oxygen of water to form a colored coordination complex.

$$CH_2 \overset{|}{\underset{R}{\vphantom{|}}} \overset{O}{\underset{\|}{C}} -NH-\underset{R}{CH}-\overset{O}{\underset{\|}{C}} \overset{|}{\vphantom{|}} NH-\underset{R}{CH}-\overset{O}{\underset{\|}{C}}-OH$$

The required unit for biuret test is shown between broken lines in the above chemical structure.

The biuret reaction is used widely both as a qualitative test for proteins and as a quantitative measure of protein concentrations.

QUESTIONS

1. Describe the classification of proteins with suitable examples.
2. What are proteins? Give their biological importance.
3. Describe the structure of proteins. Discuss how proteins are precipitated.
4. Short notes:
   A. Two color reactions of proteins.
   B. Denaturation of proteins.

MULTIPLE CHOICE QUESTIONS

5. **Number of amino acids in insulin is:**
   A. 21
   B. 31
   C. 41
   D. 51

6. **Two polypeptide chains in insulin are cross linked as:**
   A. One sulfide link
   B. One disulfide link
   C. Two disulfide links
   D. Three disulfide links

7. **Protein can have the following structure:**
   A. Fibrous
   B. Sheet
   C. Globular
   D. All the above

8. **Structure of protein is stabilized by:**
   A. Hydrogen bonding
   B. Ionic bonding
   C. Covalent bonding
   D. All the above

9. **Number of amino acids present in protein are:**
   A. 10
   B. 20
   C. 100
   D. 200

10. **The amino acids found in biological protein are of:**
    A. D-configuration and dextrorotatory
    B. L-configuration and levorotatory
    C. D-configuration and levo or dextrorotatory
    D. L-configuration and dextro or levorotatory

11. **Which amino acid does not occur in proteins of biological system:**
    A. Ornithine
    B. Arginine
    C. Cystine
    D. Histidine

12. **Albumin and globulins are:**
    A. Simple proteins
    B. Conjugated protein
    C. Primary derived proteins
    D. Secondary derived proteins

13. **All the following are conjugated proteins *except*:**
    A. Metallo proteins
    B. Hemoproteins
    C. Histones
    D. Lipoproteins

14. **Which one of the following is a fibrous protein?**
    A. Collagen
    B. Myoglobin
    C. Hemoglobin
    D. None of the above

15. **Plasma proteins can be separated into different fractions by:**
    A. Chromatography
    B. Electrophoresis
    C. Dialysis
    D. Centrifugation

16. **Denaturation of protein involves:**
    A. Changes in primary structure
    B. Loss of biological activity
    C. Irreversible changes
    D. None of the above
17. **In a quaternary structure, subunits are linked by:**
    A. Peptide bonds
    B. Disulfide bonds
    C. Covalent bonds
    D. Non-covalent bonds
18. **A coagulated protein is:**
    A. Insoluble
    B. Biologically non-functional
    C. Unfolded
    D. All the above
19. **During denaturation of proteins, all the following are disrupted** *except:*
    A. Primary structure
    B. Secondary structure
    C. Tertiary structure
    D. Quaternary structure
20. **The largest protein amongst the following is:**
    A. Fibrinogen
    B. Globulin
    C. Albumin
    D. Hemoglobin
21. **A disulfide bond can be formed between:**
    A. Two methionine residue
    B. Two cystine residue
    C. A methionine and cystine residue
    D. All the above
22. **Aromatic amino acids in protein can be detected by:**
    A. Sakaguchi reaction
    B. Millon-Nasse reaction
    C. Hopkins-Cole reaction
    D. Xanthoproteic reaction
23. **The least soluble protein among the following is:**
    A. Albumin
    B. Globulin
    C. Casein
    D. Collagen

ANSWERS

5. (D)	6. (C)	7. (D)	8. (A)	9. (B)
10. (D)	11. (A)	12. (A)	13. (C)	14. (A)
15. (B)	16. (B)	17. (D)	18. (C)	19. (A)
20. (A)	21. (B)	22. (D)	23. (D)	

CHAPTER 6

Vitamins

DEFINITION

Vitamins are defined as organic compounds, occurring in natural food either as such or as utilizable precursors, which are required in minute quantities for normal growth, maintenance and reproduction.

Vitamins differ from hormones in that they are supplied with the diet whereas hormones are produced by glands in the body. Most vitamins and hormones, however, are involved in affecting enzyme activity directly or indirectly. Several vitamins are coenzymes or prosthetic groups of enzymes in both plants and animals.

Vitamins differ from other organic foodstuffs in following aspects:
1. Vitamins do not enter tissue cultures unlike proteins.
2. Unlike carbohydrates, proteins and lipids, vitamins do not undergo degradation for providing energy.

CLASSIFICATION

Vitamins belong to several chemical groups. They are classified according to their solubility. Vitamins A, D, E and K are fat soluble. Vitamins B and C are water soluble. In humans there are 13 vitamins four fat soluble (A, D, E, K) and nine water soluble (eight B complex vitamins and one vitamin C).

Differences Between Fat-soluble and Water-soluble Vitamins

1. Water-soluble vitamins function as precursors for coenzymes whereas fat-soluble vitamins do not form coenzymes.

2. Water-soluble vitamins are non-toxic since excess amounts of these vitamins are excreted in the urine. Fat-soluble vitamins are not excreted in urine, being not water soluble and are toxic in excessive quantities.
3. Water-soluble vitamins are not stored extensively except vitamin B_{12}. Hence, they have to be taken frequently as compared to fat-soluble vitamins, which are stored.

VITAMINS NOT ACTING AS COENZYMES OR FAT-SOLUBLE VITAMINS

Vitamin A

Vitamin A is a complex primary alcohol with empirical formula $C_{20}H_{29}$OH and exists in two forms: vitamin A_1 or retinol and vitamin A_2 or dehydroretinol.

Sources

Vitamin A occurs only in animal tissues—in cod liver oil, butter, eggs, cheese. Its precursor β-carotene occurs in green vegetables and yellow-colored vegetables like carrots, tomatoes, apricots, sweet potatoes and corn; also yellow fruits papaya, mango and pumpkin. It is stable to heat, acid and alkali, but is destroyed by oxidation (when butter turns rancid). Ordinary cooking does not destroy vitamin A.

Conversion of Beta-carotene to Retinal (Vitamin A Aldehyde)

Beta-carotene, the yellow pigment present in vegetables is the precursor, which can be converted into vitamin A in human liver. One molecule of β-carotene can give rise to two molecules of vitamin A.

Requirements

Recommended dietary allowance (RDA) is the average daily dietary intake that meets the nutrient requirement of more than 97% of the healthy population.

Daily requirements of vitamin A for adults is 750 µg. The requirements for infants and young children is 300 µg. Women during pregnancy and lactation need 1,200 µg/day.

Functions

1. Vitamin A is indispensable for normal vision. It contributes to the production of retinal pigment rhodopsin, needed for vision in dim light.
2. In the maintenance of proper health of epithelial tissues.
3. For the stability and integrity of cellular and subcellular membranes, which line intestinal, respiratory and urinary tracts as well as skin and eyes.

[Chemical structures showing β-carotene being converted by 2 [O] to 2 moles of retinal (vitamin A aldehyde), then by Retinal reductase with NADH + H⁺ → NAD to Retinol (vitamin A) / CH_2OH]

4. Necessary for the synthesis of mucopolysaccharides.
5. In the nucleic acid metabolism.
6. Involved in the electron transport chain and oxidative phosphorylation.
7. It increases the release of calcium and phosphate in the bones and is necessary for normal growth and development especially skeletal growth.
8. It is anti-infective. There is increased susceptibility to infection and lowered immune response in vitamin A deficiency.

9. It may protect against some epithelial cancers and bronchial cancers.

An early sign of vitamin A deficiency in man is inability to see objects in dim light, especially after exposure to bright light. This condition is known as night blindness or nyctalopia.

Vitamin A and Vision

Wald's visual cycle

The overall mechanism through which vitamin A takes active part in visual system is known as Wald's visual cycle. Rhodopsin was discovered by George Wald for which he was given the Nobel Prize in 1967.

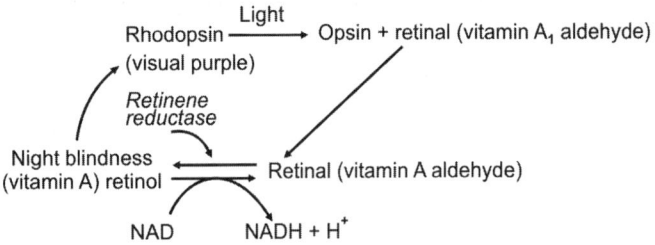

Retina contains two types of receptor cells:

Cones: These are specialized for color and detailed vision in bright light.
Rods: These are specialized for visual activity in dim light (night vision).

Light waves striking these receptors produce chemical changes, which in turn give rise to nerve impulses. Vitamin A plays a significant role in the photochemical phase of this process.

The retinal pigment rhodopsin or visual purple, which has long been recognized in the rod cells of the retina, is a conjugated protein with a molecular weight of approximately 40,000. When light strikes the retina, rhodopsin is split into its protein component opsin and the associated non-protein carotenoid, retinal (vitamin A_1 aldehyde). Retinal is slowly converted by reduction to the alcohol, retinol. The regeneration of retinal from retinol is done by the oxidation of the terminal alcohol group by the enzyme retinene reductase involving NAD as a coenzyme. The retinal can then combine with opsin to regenerate rhodopsin in the cycle. If there is a lack of vitamin A, rhodopsin is regenerated very slowly causing night blindness.

Deficiency Diseases of Vitamin A

1. Keratinization: Lack of vitamin A causes shrinking and hardening of epithelial tissues of the membranes in the eye, digestive tract,

respiratory tract and urinary tract. Such a hardening is called keratinization.

When keratinization occurs in the lining of the respiratory tract, the patient is more likely to suffer from cold, pneumonia and other respiratory infections because of the drying of the membranes.

2. Xerophthalmia: When keratinization occurs in the eyes, the tear ducts become keratinized and are no longer be able to secrete tears to wash the eyes. When this occurs, bacteria are able to attack the corneal tissue of the eyes, producing an infection called xerophthalmia and Bitot's spot, in this disease the cornea becomes cloudy and does not allow light to pass through, so sight is lost permanently.
3. Failure of growth in children.
4. Nerve lesions.
5. Faulty bone modeling.
6. Increased pressure of CSF.
7. Abnormalities of reproduction including degeneration of testes, abortion, producing malformed offspring, etc.
8. Certain forms of skin cancers.

Vitamin A Toxin

Hypervitaminosis A: An excess accumulation of vitamin A in the liver can lead to toxicity, which manifests in bone pain, hepatosplenomegaly, nausea and diarrhea, night blindness, increases susceptibility to infections, dry and scaly skin, loss of smell and appetite, fatigue, defective teeth and gums, retarded growth.

Vitamin D

Vitamin D is called solar vitamin, because its synthesis involves the ultraviolet irradiation of sterols, such as 7-dehydrocholesterol in human skin. People not exposed to sunlight, e.g. people hospitalized for long time, people living in polar region or ladies in purdah suffer from vitamin D deficiency.

Sources

Eggs, butter, liver, fatty fish and fish oils such as cod liver oil and vitamin D fortified milk are good natural sources. Humans exposed to bright sunlight year round do not require dietary vitamin D. Daily requirement for adult is 5 μg. Pregnant and lactating mothers and children may need up to 10 μg/day.

Physiological Action

The principal action of vitamin D is to increase the absorption of calcium and phosphorus from small intestine. It also increases the release of calcium and phosphate in the bones and is necessary for normal growth and development. Vitamin D is required for the proper activity of the parathyroid hormone and so it is used therapeutically in the treatment of hypoparathyroidism.

A lack of vitamin D may cause hypocalcemia and hypophosphatemia.

Deficiency

Vitamin D deficiency in children, known as rickets is most common in areas lacking sunshine. Rickets deforms the growing bones of children. Rickets is characterized improper mineralizing during development of bones that result in soft bones. If it begin before the child learns to walk, the spine may become abnormally curved. If it begins or continues after child starts to walk, the legs may become bowed by the weight of the body. Phosphorus and vitamin D deficiency in adults, is called osteomalacia—adult form of rickets. A lack of calcium and vitamin D can cause osteoporosis in adults. This disease, like osteomalacia, is characterized by decalcification and softening of bones, but to a much greater extent.

Hypervitaminosis D

Excess of vitamin D causes loss of appetite, vomiting, growth failure, weight loss, drowsiness, polyurea, increased calcium deposit in soft tissues blood vessels and kidneys.

Vitamin E

Vitamin E consists of a group of tocopherols, the α-tocopherols being most active.

Source

Vitamin E occurs so widely in vegetable oils that it is almost impossible not to obtain enough of it. It also occurs in grains and leafy vegetables. Daily requirement is 6 mg. The richest sources are soyabean oil and corn oil (50–150 mg/100 g). Palm and sunflower oil has 20–70 mg/100 g. Coconut and olive oils are relatively low in vitamin E (1–10 mg/100 g).

Function

Vitamin E protects the polyunsaturated fats and vitamin A from oxidation. As an antioxidant, it also protects the erythrocytes.

Deficiency

In the absence of vitamin E, activities of certain enzymes are reduced and red blood cells hemolyze more readily. Anemia and edema are reported in infants with vitamin E deficiency. It can also contribute to an increased susceptibility to sudden heart attacks, especially in males under stress.

Hypervitaminosis E

Excess leads to interference with utilization of vitamins A and K, prolonged prothrombin time, intestinal irritability, headache, dizziness and fatigue.

α-tocopherol

Vitamin K (Coagulation Vitamin)

Vitamin K is a group of naphthoquinones with long, branched hydrocarbon side chains. Vitamin K is an antihemorrhagic vitamin.

Sources

Vitamin K is present in fish liver oils, green leafy vegetables and deficiencies are rare.

Function

Vitamin K works as a cofactor in the blood clotting mechanism.

Deficiency

Deficiency leads to generalized bleeding, prolonged clotting time in adults and hemorrhagic diseases of the newborn.

Hypervitaminosis K

Excess leads to hyperbilirubinemia in infants and newborn.

WATER-SOLUBLE VITAMINS

Vitamin C or Ascorbic Acid

Vitamin C or ascorbic acid (a special case of sugar acid) is a white crystalline substance highly soluble in water. It aids in utilization of iron and production of collagen. It acts as a cementing material between endothelial cells of the blood vessels and maintain their integrity.

Sources

Fresh fruits and vegetables, including oranges, lime, lemons, green chillies, grapefruits, gooseberries, guava, berries, melons, tomatoes, raw cabbages and leafy green vegetables. It is destroyed by extended cooking. Even when vitamin C is kept in regrigerator in well-capped bottles, it slowly deteriorates.

Function

Vitamin C is an antioxidant like vitamin E. It prevents scurvy. It is involved in the metabolism of amino acids, synthesis of some adrenal hormones, and resistance to infection and healing of wounds. Sufficient dosages, i.e. up to several grams per day is believed to prevent common cold. The vitamin is non-toxic at these high levels. Maximum daily requirement is 60 mg.

Deficiency

The deficiency disease is scurvy (bleeding gums). Children of 6–12 months fed on bottled milk and not fruit/vegetables and widowers who prepare their food may show deficiency of vitamin C (bachelor scurvy).

Hypervitaminosis C

Excess intake may lead to kidney stones, polyneuritis mental confusion, muscular weakness, calf tenderness, loss of deep jerk, cardiac enlargement, etc.

Excess may also lead to rapid pulse, headache, weakness, irritability and insomnia. When taken in large doses, vitamin C can cause diarrhea in health adults.

Relatively large doses of vitamin C may cause indigestion when taken on an empty stomach.

B Complex Group of Vitamins

B complex group of vitamins are chemically not related. They are grouped together because all the vitamins of B complex group function in the cells as coenzymes.

Thiamine (Vitamin B_1)

Thiamine consists of a substituted pyrimidine ring joined by a methylene bridge to substituted thiazole ring.

Sources: Good sources are lean meats, legumes and whole grains. It is stable when dry, but destroyed by alkaline conditions or prolonged cooking. Thiamine is not stored and excess is excreted in the urine. Daily requirement is 1.5 mg for adults and children. Parboiled rice is superior to raw (polished) rice (also white bread) as this form has bran containing vitamin B_1 and looses only 30% of vitamin B_1 on washing whereas raw rice has no bran and has no vitamin B_1 and looses 80% on washing. Vitamin B_6 is also lost during polishing of grains.

Function: Thiamine is needed for the breakdown of carbohydrates. Its deficiency disease is beriberi, a disorder of the nervous system.

Deficiency: Thiamine deficiency leads to dry and wet type of beriberi.

Dry beriberi: The main feature of dry (paralytic or nervous) beriberi is peripheral neuropathy. Early in the course of the neuropathy 'burning feet syndrome' may occur. Other symptoms include abnormal (exaggerated) reflexes, diminished sensation and weakness in the legs and arms. Muscle pain and tenderness and difficulty in rising from a squatting position have been reported. Severely thiamine-deficient individuals may experience seizures.

Wet beriberi: In addition to neurological symptoms, wet (cardiac) beriberi is characterized by cardiovascular manifestations of thiamine deficiency, which include rapid heart rate, enlargement of the heart, severe swelling (edema), difficulty in breathing and ultimately congestive heart failure.

Whole wheat flour of 100 g contains 0.55 mg of thiamine, while 100 g of wheat flour contains only 0.06 mg of thiamine.

Riboflavin (Vitamin B_2) or Lactoflavin

Riboflavin is an orange yellow crystalline compound. It is relatively heat stable, but is destroyed by light. It occurs in bound forms as flavin adenine nucleotide or as flavoproteins.

Riboflavin exists as component of two coenzymes called flavin mononucleotide (FMN) and flavin adenine dinucleotide (FAD), which act as coenzymes or prosthetic groups.

Sources: Milk and certain meats like kidney, liver and heart are the sources. Daily requirement is 1.5 mg. During pregnancy and lactation additional 0.2–0.4 mg are required. People aged above 60 years may also need more.
Function: Riboflavin is required by a number of oxidative processes in metabolism.
Deficiency: Leads to the inflammation and breakdown of tissue around the mouth (glossitis), tongue and nose, a scaliness of the skin and burning itchy eyes. Wound healing is impaired.
Hypervitaminosis B_2: Excess causes ulcer, elevated blood glucose levels and increased uric acid levels in blood.

Pyridoxine (Vitamin B_6)

Vitamin B_6 refers to a group of pyridoxine, pyridoxal and pyridoxamine compounds having similar biological activity. All these change in the body to the active form, pyridoxal phosphate.
Sources: Vitamin B_6 is required in proportion to protein intake. It is present in meat, wheat, yeast, corn, vegetables and nuts. It is relatively stable to heat, light and alkali.
Function: The activities of at least 60 enzymes involved in the metabolism of various amino acids depend on pyridoxal phosphate. Adults need 2 mg/day, during pregnancy and lactation, the requirement is increased to 2.5 mg/day.
Deficiency: Vitamin B_6 deficiency is found in many pregnant women and also in alcoholics as well as after chronic administration of B_6 antagonists such as isoniazid and penicillamine. Its features include hypochromic anemia, peripheral neuropathy, irritability, convulsions and glossitis. Vitamin B_6 deficiency can lead to niacin deficiency, because B_6 is required to convert tryptophan to niacin.

Hypervitaminosis B_6: Excess leads to bloating, depression, headache, fatigue, irritability and brain damage.

Niacin (Vitamin B_3) or Nicotinic Acid

Both nicotinic acid and nicotinamide are essential for nearly all biological oxidation.

Source: It is found in liver, kidney and heart as well as in yeast, peanuts, cereals, milk, leafy vegetables and wheat germ.

Functions: Nicotinamide along with thiamine and riboflavin serves as a coenzyme in tissue oxidation. It functions in the mitochondria in the form of NAD^+ and $NADP^+$. Recommended daily intake of niacin is 16–19 mg for males and 13–15 mg for females with a slight increase in requirements for adolescents and during pregnancy and lactation. It is needed by every cell of the body every day.

Deficiency: Its deficiency disease is pellagra, a deterioration of the nervous system and the skin. Pellagra is particularly a problem where corn (maize) is the major item of the diet as in Rajasthan and Central America.

Nicotinic acid (niacin)   Nicotinamide

Maize is deficient in tryptophan. Humans convert a fraction of their dietary tryptophan to nicotinamide and hence deficiency of tryptophan causes pellagra. Pellagra can cause 3D's, i.e. dermatitis (browning of the skin), diarrhea and dementia. If untreated it may cause death.

Hypervitaminosis B_3: Excess of niacin leads to ulcer, liver dysfunction, elevated blood glucose levels, increased blood and uric acid levels, diarrhea, nausea and blushing.

Folacin or Folic Acid (Vitamin B_9)

Sources: Good sources are fresh leafy green vegetables (spinach, broccoli and lettuce), asparagus, fruits (bananas, melons), liver and kidney. Relatively unstable to heat, air and ultraviolet light, its activity is lost by cooking and storage. Daily requirement for male, 200 µg and 180 µg for female.

Functions: Vitamin B_9 is needed for the synthesis of nucleic acids and heme.

Deficiency: It causes macrocytic anemia. Excess causes diarrhea, insomnia, irritability, masking of vitamin B_{12} deficiency. Its deficiency disease is megaloblastic anemia. Several drugs, including alcohol, cause folic acid deficiency.

$$\text{H}_2\text{N} - \text{Pteridine nucleus (with OH)} - \text{CH}_2\text{NH} - \text{PABA} - \overset{\text{O}}{\underset{}{\text{C}}} - \text{NH} - \overset{\text{CO}_2\text{H}}{\underset{}{\text{CH}}}\text{CH}_2\text{CH}_2\text{COH}_2 \quad \text{Glutamic acid}$$

Pantothenic Acid (Vitamin B_5)

Sources: This vitamin is supplied by liver, kidney, egg yolk, whole grain cereals, legumes and skimmed milk and its deficiency is rare. Its requirement is 4–7 mg/day.

Functions: Pantothenic acid is used to make coenzyme A (symbol: CoASH), which the body needs to metabolize fatty acids. Pantothenic acid, a B complex vitamin combines with ATP and cysteine in the liver to generate CoASH.

$$\underset{\text{CH}_3\ \text{OH}}{\overset{\text{HO}\quad \text{CH}_3}{\text{CH}_2 - \text{C} - \text{CH} - \overset{\text{O}}{\text{C}} - \overset{\text{H}}{\text{N}} - \overset{\text{H}}{\underset{\text{H}}{\text{C}}} - \overset{\text{H}}{\underset{\text{H}}{\text{C}}} - \text{COOH}}}$$

Deficiency: It disease is paresthesia (sensation of offensive smell or bitter taste).

Hypervitaminosis B_5: Excess causes increased need of thiamine, occassionally diarrhea and water retention.

Table 6.1 details the sources and other features of all vitamins.

Biotin (Vitamin B_7)

Sources: Humans acquire biotin, a B complex vitamin, both from the diet and from intestinal bacteria. Egg yolk, liver, tomatoes and yeast are its good sources.

Functions: Biotin ($C_{10}H_{16}N_2O_3S$) is required for all pathways in which CO_2 is temporarily used as a reactant as in synthesis of fatty acids. Biotin is necessary for cell growth, production of fatty acids and for metabolism of fats and amino acids. It plays an important role in citric acid cycle. It is helpful for a steady blood sugar level. Biotin is often recommended for strengthening hair and nails and so it is

TABLE 6.1: Sources, RDA, functions and deficiency diseases of vitamins

Name	Sources	Recommended daily allowance (RDA)	Functions	Deficiency diseases
Fat-soluble vitamins				
Vitamin A	Fish liver oils, butter, milk, kidneys and muscle meat. β-carotene is present in yellow fruits and leafy green vegetables.	Adults: 750 µg Children: 300 µg Women during pregnancy and lactation:1,200 µg	Helps vision, keeps skin healthy	Xerophthalmia, nyctalopia
Vitamin D (cholecalciferol); 'Sunshine' vitamin	Eggs, butter, fatty fish, fish liver oils; humans exposed year round to bright sunlight do not require dietary vitamin D	Adult: 5 µg Children: 10 µg Lactation: 10 µg	Needed for strong teeth and bones	Rickets, osteomalacia, osteoporosis
Vitamin E (tocopherol)	Green leafy vegetables—spinach, cabbage, alfalfa, putrefied fish meal, liver, eggs and cheese	6 mg	Keeps skin and RBCs healthy antioxidant prevents oxidation of vitamin A and unsaturated	Muscular weakness creatinuria and fragile RBCs
Vitamin K (coagulation vitamin)	Green leafy vegetables—spinach, cabbage, alfalfa, putrefied fish meal, fish liver oils, liver, eggs and cheese	Adult: 50–100 µg Children: 1 µg/kg	Needed for blood clotting. Essential for the synthesis of clotting factors including prothrombin by liver.	Retarded/delayed blood clotting

Contd...

Contd...

Name	Sources	Recommended daily allowance	Functions	Deficiency diseases
Water-soluble vitamins				
B complex vitamins				
Thiamine (B_1)	Lean meats, legumes and whole grains	1–1.5 mg	Needed for healthy nerves	Beriberi, a disorder of the nervous system with dependent edema involving the trunk and extremities
Riboflavin (B_2)	Liver, dried yeast, egg, whole milk, milk powder, fish, whole cereals, legumes and green leafy vegetables	Adult: 1.5 mg Pregnancy and lactation: 1.72 mg	Yellow crystalline compound helps cells use energy in foods. FMN and FAD are coenzymes required for oxidation reaction in metabolism.	Inflammation and break down of tissue around the mouth, tongue and nose, wound healing is impaired
Niacin (B_3) formerly known as nicotinic acid	Liver, kidney, heart, yeast, peanuts and wheat germ. Amino acid tryptophan can supply much of body's need of niacin, 60 mg of tryptophan can produce 1 g niacin.	Adult: 20 mg Pregnancy: 22 mg Lactation: 25 mg	Helps cells use energy in foods. Niacinamide along with thiamin and riboflavin, serves as a coenzyme in tissue oxidation. It functions in the mitochondria in the form of NAD^+ and $NADP^+$.	Pellagra, a deterioration of the nervous system and skin rashes and glossitis

Contd...

Contd...

Name	Sources	Recommended daily allowance (RDA)	Functions	Deficiency diseases
Folic acid	Liver, kidney and fresh leafy vegetables, cauliflower	Male: 200 µg Female: 180 µg	In reactions involving transfer of methyl groups as in the synthesis of hemoglobin, nucleic acids and methionine	Megaloblastic anemia and gastrointestinal disturbances
Biotin	Liver, egg yolk, kidney, yeast and milk	200–300 µg	As a coenzyme for carboxylation reactions in the formation of fatty acids	Delay dermatitis, muscle pains, nausea and depression
Pyridoxine	Yeast, liver, egg yolk and the germs of the various grains and seeds, less in milk and leafy vegetables	Male: 2.0 mg Female: 1.6 mg Pregnancy and lactation: 2.5 mg	Pyridoxal phosphate and pyridoxamine serve as coenzymes for decarboxylation of amino acids. Takes part in the reactions occurring in gray matter of the CNS. Pyridoxine is involved in the absorption of zinc by the intestine.	Epileptic seizures
Pantothenic acid	Egg yolk, yeast, kidney, lean meats, skimmed milk, sweet potatoes and molasses	4–7 mg	One of the constituents of coenzymes A (CoA), which is involved in the metabolism of carbohydrates, fats and proteins and in the synthesis of cholesterol	Normally there is no deficiency as the RDA is easily met with an ordinary diet

Contd...

Contd...

Name	Sources	Recommended daily allowance (RDA)	Functions	Deficiency diseases
Cobalamin (vitamin B_{12}, antipernicious anemia factor)	Liver, kidney, fish, eggs, milk, oysters and clams. It contains the element cobalt (4.35%).	2.0 µg	In the transfer of methyl groups, in the maintenance of the myelin sheath, in the synthesis of nucleic acids and hemoglobin, in the metabolism of carbohydrates and lipids	Pernicious anemia, similar to folic acid deficiency
Vitamin C (ascorbic acid)	Amla, guava, gooseberry, orange, lemons, lime, papaya, tomatoes, green chillies, green leafy vegetables	50 g	Tissue healing increased, resistance to infection, antioxidant	Scurvy, poor wound healing, bleeding gums, mucous membranes loose teeth

found in many cosmetic and health products for hair and skin.
Deficiency: Developmental delay, dermatitis, muscular pain, nausea and depression.

Cobalamin (Vitamin B_{12})

Sources: The central portion of the molecules consists of four reduced and extensively substituted pyrrole rings surrounding a single cobalt atom. This deficiency is very rare as liver, kidney, lean meats, eggs and milk products are good sources of B_{12}. A strict vegetarian diet, which excludes milk and eggs has virtually no B_{12}. The liver stores relatively large amounts of this vitamin. Strict vegetarians in India may continue for decades without developing vitamin B_{12} deficiency because with a normal stomach and terminal ileum, they reabsorb most of the B_{12} they excrete into the bile. Vitamin B_{12} is synthesized exclusively by microoganisms and is stored in liver of animals. Also in meat (liver and shellfish), milk and eggs.

Functions: Vitamin B_{12} normally involved in the metabolism of every cell of the body, especially affecting the DNA synthesis and regulation, but also fatty acid synthesis and energy production. However, many effects of the functions of B_{12} can be replaced by corresponding effects of folic acid, since B_{12} is need to regenerate folate deficiency in the body.

Deficiency: Most of the B_{12} deficiency symptoms are similar to that of folate deficiency. Pernicious anemia, megaloblastosis, leukopenia and thrombocytopenia, which are due to poor synthesis of DNA, when the body does not have a proper supply of folate for the production of thiamine.

Deficiency manifestations: Pernicious anemia—persons with subnormal serum concentration of vitamin B_{12} develop symptoms like glossitis and peripheral sensory disturbances. Gross deficiency of vitamin B_{12} causes pernicious anemia, which manifests the same abnormalities of blood formation as in folic acid deficiency, namely evidences of accumulation of megaloblasts and myeloblasts. Peripheral blood picture shows macrocyptic type of anemia. Other characteristics of pernicious anemia are:

1. Atrophy of the mucous membrane of mouth and tongue with inflammation resulting in glossitis, stomatitis and pharyngitis.
2. Degenerative lesions of the posterior and lateral columns of the spinal cord, resulting in peripheral sensory disturbances, hyperactive reflexes and paralysis.

Pernicious anemia arises due to failure of the secretion of the intrinsic factor by the gastric fundus in adequate quantity to facilitate absorption of vitamin B_{12} from the intestines. Pernicious anemia may occur in patients following surgical removal of the stomach (total gastrectomy) and extensive resection of small intestines, the latter causing the problem of reduced surface area for absorption of the vitamin.

QUESTIONS

1. Name the water-soluble vitamins. Describe the chemistry and role of thiamine.
2. Describe the source, daily requirements, functions and deficiency symptoms of vitamin A.
3. What are B complex vitamins? Describe the role of any one of them.
4. Name the fat-soluble vitamins. Describe the chemistry and functions of vitamin D.
5. Write the coenzyme forms of the following vitamins with two examples.
   A. Riboflavin.
   B. Niacin.
   C. Pyridoxine.
6. Define vitamins. How are they classified? Give a note on vitamin K.
7. Describe the deficiency diseases, daily requirements and biochemical role of vitamin D.
8. Describe the sources, daily requirements and biochemical role of vitamin A.
9. Describe the sources, daily requirements, physiological action and deficiency diseases associated with vitamin C.
10. Describe the sources, function, daily requirements and deficiency diseases associated with niacin.

MULTIPLE CHOICE QUESTIONS

11. Retinol is transported in the blood as attached to:
    A. Albumin
    B. α_1-globulin
    C. α_2-globulin
    D. β-globulin
    E. γ-globulin

12. Increased carbohydrate consumption increases the dietary requirement of:
    A. Thiamine
    B. Riboflavin
    C. Pyridoxine
    D. Folic acid
    E. Niacin

13. The disease pellagra is due to the deficiency of:
    A. Vitamin B_6
    B. Nicotinic acid
    C. Pantothenic acid
    D. Folic acid
    E. Biotin
14. The deficiency of one of the following vitamins causes creatinuria:
    A. Vitamin E
    B. Vitamin K
    C. Vitamin A
    D. Vitamin B_6
    E. Vitamin B_1
15. Which of the following vitamin is associated with synthesis of coagulation factor prothrombin?
    A. Vitamin A
    B. Vitamin C
    C. Vitamin K
    D. Vitamin E
    E. Vitamin D
16. Vitamins are:
    A. Accessory food factors
    B. Required in small quantities
    C. Not used to provide energy
    D. All of the above
17. Which is the fat-soluble vitamin?
    A. Riboflavin
    B. Folic acid
    C. Vitamin K
    D. Vitamin C
18. The provitamin of vitamin A is:
    A. Cholesterol
    B. Torcopherol
    C. Retinol
    D. β-carotene
19. Which form of vitamin A participates in Wald's visual cycle (rhodopsin cycle)?
    A. Retinal
    B. Retinoic acid
    C. Retinol
    D. None of the above
20. Vitamin A is stored mainly in:
    A. Kidneys
    B. Liver
    C. Brain
    D. Spleen
21. All the following are deficiency symptom of vitamin A *except*:
    A. Keratomalacia
    B. Nyctalopia
    C. Xerophthalmia
    D. Osteomalacia
22. Hypervitaminosis A results in:
    A. Skin disorders
    B. Metastatic calcification
    C. Hepatolenticular regeneration
    D. Night blindness
23. Pyridoxal phosphate is a coenzyme for:
    A. Oxidative decarboxylation
    B. Transamination
    C. CO_2 fixation
    D. Decarboxylation

24. **Biologically active form of vitamin D is:**
    A. 7-dehydrocholesterol
    B. 25 (OH) cholecalciferol
    C. 1,25-dihydroxycholecalciferol
    D. 24,25-dihydroxycholecalciferol
25. **Provitamin D is:**
    A. 7-dehydrocholesterol
    B. 25 (OH) cholecalciferol
    C. 1,25-dihydroxycholecalciferol
    D. 24,25-dihydroxycholecalciferol
26. **Renal calculi may be due to the deficiency of:**
    A. Vitamin A
    B. Vitamin D
    C. Vitamin K
    D. Folic acid
27. **FMN and FAD can accept:**
    A. Two hydrogen atoms
    B. Two electrons
    C. One hydrogen atom
    D. One electron
28. **People consuming polished rice as their staple food are prone to:**
    A. Beriberi
    B. Pellagra
    C. Scurvy
    D. None of the above
29. **Poor souce of vitamin D is:**
    A. Liver
    B. Eggs
    C. Milk
    D. Butter
30. **Retinal is reduced to retinol by retinene reductase in presence of the coenzyme:**
    A. NAD^+
    B. NAD + NADP
    C. $NADH + H^+$
    D. $NADPH + H^+$
31. **Nicotinic acid is essential for normal function of :**
    A. Skin
    B. Intestinal tract
    C. Neurons system
    D. All of the above
32. **Increased protein intake is accompanied by an increased dietary requirement of:**
    A. Ascorbic acid
    B. Nicotinic acid
    C. Pantothenic acid
    D. Folic acid
33. **Pantothenic acid exists in tissues as:**
    A. Coenzyme A
    B. β-mercaptoethylamine
    C. Pantonic acid
    D. β-alanine
34. **One of the amino acids is constituent of vitamin folic acid is:**
    A. Aspartic acid
    B. Arginine
    C. Glutamic acid
    D. Histidine
35. **Vitamin D deficiency causes:**
    A. Decrease of Ca and P
    B. Increase of Ca and P
    C. Decrease of Ca and increase of P
    D. Increase of Ca and decrease of P

36. **People whose staple food is maize suffer from deficiency of vitamin:**
    A. Riboflavin
    B. Pyridoxin
    C. Niacin
    D. Pantothenic acid

37. **Active coenzyme form of folic acid is:**
    A. Folate
    B. Dihydrofolate
    C. Trihydrofolate
    D. Tetrahydrofolate

38. **The metal ion present in cobalamin is:**
    A. Iron
    B. Cyanide
    C. Cobalt
    D. Calcium

39. **Bran layer of cereals is rich sources of vitamin:**
    A. Riboflavin
    B. Niacin
    C. Folic acid
    D. Thiamine

40. **Intake of which vitamin is associated with the intake of unsaturated fatty acid.**
    A. Vitamin A
    B. Vitamin D
    C. Vitamin E
    D. Vitamin K

41. **Biologically active form of thiamine (vitamin B).**
    A. Thiamine monophosphate
    B. Thiamine diphosphate
    C. Thiamine triphosphate
    D. Thiamine pyrophosphate

42. **Which of the following vitamins is also called as childbearing vitamins?**
    A. Vitamin E
    B. Vitamin K
    C. Vitamin D
    D. Vitamin C

43. **Antioxidant property of vitamin E is due to:**
    A. Phenolic hydroxyl group
    B. Active reducing group
    C. Alcoholic group
    D. Sulfhydryl group

ANSWERS

11. (B)	12. (A)	13. (B)	14. (A)	15. (C)
16. (D)	17. (C)	18. (D)	19. (A)	20. (B)
21. (D)	22. (A)	23. (B)	24. (C)	25. (A)
26. (A)	27. (A)	28. (A)	29. (B)	30. (C)
31. (D)	32. (C)	33. (A)	34. (C)	35. (C)
36. (C)	37. (D)	38. (C)	39. (D)	40. (C)
41. (D)	42. (B)	43. (A)		

7

CHAPTER

Nucleic Acids and Nucleotides

NUCLEIC ACIDS

Nucleic acids like proteins and polysaccharides are another class of biological polymers or macromolecules that are present in all living cells. Also, a nucleic acid is an essential component of all viruses. The main function of DNA is the storage, transmission and use of genetic information upon which the continuation of cell structure depends.

Each chromosome is made up of long strands of DNA. A gene is a specific segment of the DNA that contains instructions for making proteins. There are about 30,000 genes in 23 pairs of chromosomes. Project 'genome' has recently located these genes on the chromosomes.

The fundamental components of nucleic acids are the pyrimidine and purine bases, the pentose sugars (ribose and 2-deoxyribose) and phosphoric acid (Fig. 7.1).

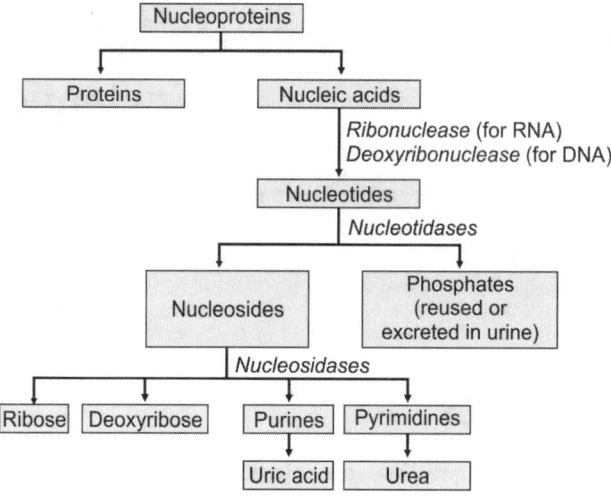

Fig. 7.1: Components of nucleoproteins

Pyrimidines of Nucleic Acids

The pyrimidine bases contain the six membered ring with two nitrogen atoms, that constitutes the compound pyrimidine. The three major pyrimidines found in humans are cytosine, uracil and thymine.

Purines of Nucleic Acids

The purine bases consist of pyrimidine ring fused to an imidazole ring.

NUCLEOSIDES (NITROGEN BASE + SUGAR)

When a heterocyclic nitrogenous base is connected through one of the nitrogen atoms to the glycosidic carbon of a sugar, the resulting compound is called nucleoside. If the sugar is a ribose, the compound is a ribonucleoside or a riboside then deoxyribose gives a deoxyriboside.

NUCLEOTIDES (NITROGEN BASE + SUGAR + PHOSPHATE)

A nucleotide is a phosphate ester of a nucleoside. The structure of the 5'-deoxyribotide of adenine is an example of a purine nucleotide.

The monomeric unit of the nucleic acids is termed as nucleotide. This monomer can undergo further hydrolysis giving three subunits: a nitrogen-containing ring compound (a nitrogen base), a pentose and molecule of phosphoric acid. On the basis of hydrolysis there are two types of nucleic acids. One of these yields D-ribose as the only sugar component and is called ribonucleic acid (RNA). The other yields D-2-deoxyribose and is called deoxyribonucleic acid (DNA).

DNA is found in the cells as a major component of the chromosomes of the nucleus. Small amounts of DNA are present in the chloroplasts of green plants and in the mitochondrial particles of cell cytoplasm. Certain viruses have DNA protein particles.

The RNA of cells are of three types, ribosomal RNA occurs in combination with proteins in the small subcellular particles called ribosomes. These particles are distributed throughout the cell, chiefly in the cytoplasm. The second type is the soluble RNA found in free form in the cytoplasm. A third type of RNA, messenger RNA occurs in small quantities, associated with ribosomes. RNA molecules in conjunction with proteins are major components of many viruses.

Structure of DNA

The three-dimensional structure of DNA molecules was elucidated by James Watson and Francis Crick in Cambridge in 1953. Their results were based on the X-ray diffraction patterns obtained from DNA by Maurice Wilkins in London. A DNA chain consists of two strands of polynucleotide chains coiled around each other in the form of a double helix. The nucleotides of each strand of DNA are connected by phosphate ester bonds. This forms the backbone of each DNA strand from which the bases extend. The bases are held in position by the hydrogen bonding between them.

The bases of one strand of a DNA molecule are held in position by the bases of the other strand to which they are bound by strong hydrogen bonds. The two strands of the DNA molecule are said to be complementary to each other in the sense that the sequence of bases in one strand automatically controls (or decides) that of the other. This specific base pairing is the most important principle of the structure of the DNA molecule. Watson, Crick and Wilkins were jointly awarded the Nobel Prize in chemistry (1962).

Secondary Structure of RNA

Free RNA generally occurs as a single polyribotide chain probably lacking fixed secondary structure. However, each chain is free to fold back upon itself many times in numerous ways.

Size of Nucleic Acids

The nucleic acids are truly macromolecules. The smallest, the soluble RNA molecules have molecular weights of about 30,000. The single RNA chain of a tobacco mosaic virus (TMV) particle has a molecular weight of over 2 million, corresponding to 6,500 nucleotide units.

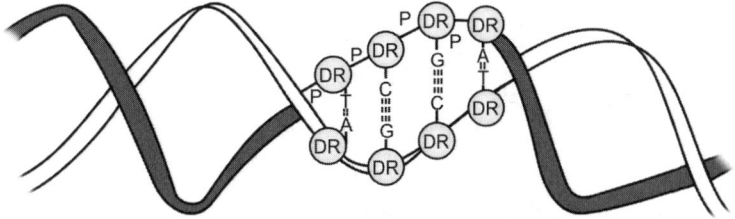

Fig. 7.2: A representation of the double helix structure of a DNA molecule. A, adenine; T, thymine; G, guanine; C, cytosine; P, phosphate; DR, deoxyribose.

The molecular weight of the DNA duplex of T_2 bacteriophage is 130 million. The DNA of the chromosome of the bacterium *Escherichia coli* is one unit with molecular weight of about 10^9.

Functions of Nucleic Acids

Nucleic acids perform two important functions namely replication (DNA) and protein synthesis (RNA). Replication of DNA takes place whenever a cell divides. The genetic information for the cell is contained in the sequence of the bases A, T, G and C in the DNA molecule. During replication both the strands of the DNA get separated and act as a template (mold) for the synthesis of a new strand. A new strand complementary to each of the parent strands is produced. Thus, two double helical molecules are formed. The specificity of base pairing ensures the exact duplication of the sequence of the bases in the newly synthesized strand of DNA. This process is called replication. RNA has only one strand and does not replicate.

NUCLEOTIDES OF BIOLOGICAL IMPORTANCE

Free Nucleotides

Besides the nucleotides, which form integral components of nucleic acids, the following nucleotides exist in free state in the tissues.

Adenosine nucleotide coenzymes:
- Adenosine monophosphate (AMP)
- Adenosine diphosphate (ADP)
- Adenosine triphosphate (ATP).

These are the body's energy compounds. They are involved in various metabolic, processes involving storage and release of energy from their phosphate bonds.

Nucleic Acids and Nucleotides

[Structure of Adenosine triphosphate (ATP)]

[Structure of Adenosine monophosphate (AMP)]

The ultimate purpose of tissue respiration is the phosphorylation of ADP to produce ATP. The overall direction of cellular metabolism is regulated by this process. ATP, ADP and AMP form a system of coenzymes that have the function of influencing the direction of flow of metabolic pathways. Both ADP and AMP act as transfer agents for the phosphate group and are involved in oxidative phosphorylation. ATP serves as a source of high energy phosphates.

Cyclic AMP: Adenosine-3',5'-cyclophosphate, is an unusual cyclic derivative of adenosine-5'-monophosphate. It is involved in the activation of phosphorylation.

Coenzyme A: It is a coenzyme of pantothenic acid, having as part of its structure a molecule of AMP. Coenzyme A is required for a number of metabolic reactions in which organic acids are involved.

$$\underset{\beta\text{-mercaptoethylamine}}{\text{HS}-CH_2-CH_2-NH-\overset{O}{\overset{\|}{C}}}-\underset{\text{Pantothenic acid}}{CH_2-CH_2-NH-\overset{O}{\overset{\|}{C}}-\overset{OH}{\underset{|}{CH}}-\overset{CH_3}{\underset{CH_3}{\overset{|}{C}}}-CH_2-O}-\underset{\text{Pyrophosphate}}{\overset{O}{\overset{\|}{\underset{OH}{\underset{|}{P}}}}-O-\overset{O}{\overset{\|}{\underset{OH}{\underset{|}{P}}}}-O-CH_2}\;\text{-Adenine-ribose-phosphate}$$

Coenzyme A

Coenzyme A is a complex molecule, which contains a free sulfhydryl (–SH) group. This group can react with a carboxyl group to form a thioester. In acetyl-coenzyme A, an acetyl group is linked to the S-atom. In the body, cholesterol is synthesized from acetyl-coenzyme A.

Oxidation-reduction Nucleotides

$NAD^+/NADP^+$ and Their Reduced Forms NADH/NADPH

They are involved in many dehydrogenase reactions in the mitochondrion, cytosol and endoplasmic reticulum of the cell. They are water soluble and are usually free to diffuse away from the enzyme, after conversion to the oxidized or reduced form to take part in another dehydrogenase reaction catalyzed by another enzyme.

Nicotinamide adenine dinucleotide (NAD^+) and nicotinamide adenine dinucleotide phosphate ($NADP^+$) are derived from vitamin niacin or nicotinamide (B_3). These coenzymes can accept two electrons and a proton (a hydride ion H^-) to get converted to reduced forms, NADH and NADPH respectively.

If the –OH of the carbonyl group of niacin (vitamin B_3) is replaced by $-NH_2$, nicotinamide is produced. When nicotinamide is attached to ribose and phosphate, and linked to AMP, NAD^+ is formed.

NAD and NADP are coenzymes to dehydrogenases. They serve as agents transferring hydrogen atoms from one substrate to another in biological oxidations, e.g. when a carbonyl group is oxidized to a carboxyl group or an alcohol group is oxidized to carbonyl (i.e. aldehyde or ketone). NAD^+ is one of the compounds, which living organisms have evolved to act as intermediates in oxidation-reduction reactions under physiological conditions.

Pyrophosphate nicotinamide adenine dinucleotide (NAD), diphosphopyridine nucleotide (DPN+), i.e. oxidized form, electrons removed

Flavin Nucleotide Coenzymes: FMN and FAD

Flavin mononucleotide (FMN) and flavin adenine dinucleotide (FAD) are two other coenzymes participating in oxidation-reduction reactions.

They are derivatives of vitamin B_2 (riboflavin). These compounds can accept two protons and two electrons, and get reduced to $FMNH_2$ and $FADH_2$.

FAD is the coenzyme involved in the dehydrogenation reaction such as:

$$-\underset{\underset{H}{|}}{\overset{\overset{H}{|}}{C}}-\underset{\underset{H}{|}}{\overset{\overset{H}{|}}{C}}- + FAD \rightleftharpoons -\overset{\overset{H}{|}}{C}=\overset{\overset{H}{|}}{C}- + FADH_2$$

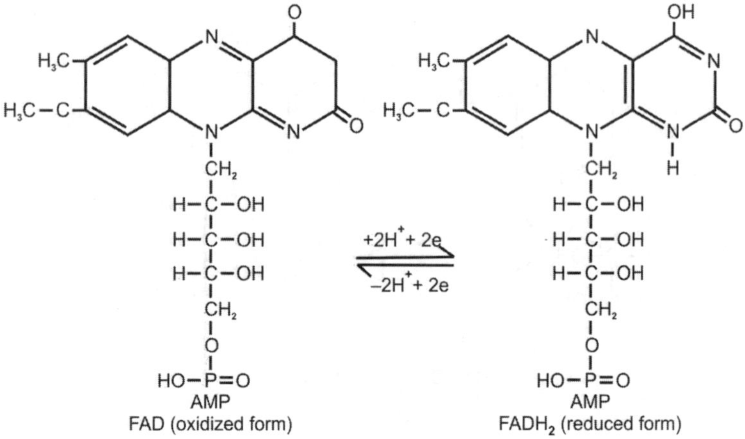

QUESTIONS

1. What are nucleic acids?
2. What are the bases present in DNA and RNA?
3. What are the sugars present in DNA and RNA?
4. What are the functions of DNA and RNA?
5. Name the purine base in DNA and also a biologically important nucleotide.
6. What vitamin is a part of ?
   A. NAD$^+$
   B. FAD
   C. CoA
7. What nitrogenous base is present in:
   A. NAD$^+$
   B. FAD
   C. CoA
8. What function does each of the following perform?
   A. NAD$^+$
   B. FAD
   C. CoA

MULTIPLE CHOICE QUESTIONS

9. **Nucleic acids are:**
   A. Small molecules
   B. Polymeric in nature
   C. Compounds of C, H and O
   D. Special types of proteins

10. The sugar present in nucleic acids is:
    A. Glucose
    B. Fructose
    C. Ribose
    D. Ribose or deoxyribose
11. Structure of DNA molecule is:
    A. Linear
    B. Branched
    C. Single helix
    D. Double helix
12. Function of DNA is:
    A. To store genetic information
    B. In replication
    C. In protein synthesis
    D. All the above
13. Nucleoprotein are:
    A. Simple proteins
    B. Conjugated protein
    C. Primary derived protein
    D. Secondary derived protein
14. Following base is present only in DNA:
    A. Adenine
    B. Guanine
    C. Cytosine
    D. Thymine
15. Nucleotides are composed of:
    A. Base + Phosphoric acid
    B. Sugar + Phosphoric acid
    C. Base + Phosphoric acid
    D. Base + Sugar + Phosphoric acid
16. The number of hydrogen bonds present between guanine and cytosine are:
    A. One
    B. Two
    C. Three
    D. Four
17. RNA is synthesized from DNA in the process of:
    A. Translation
    B. Transcription
    C. Replication
    D. Reverse transcription
18. The number of hydrogen bonds present between adenine and thymine are:
    A. One
    B. Two
    C. Three
    D. Four
19. Gene is a segment of the DNA molecule containing base pairs about:
    A. 300
    B. 400
    C. 500
    D. 600
20. In nucleotides, phosphate is attached to sugar by:
    A. Salt bond
    B. Hydrogen bond
    C. Ester bond
    D. Glycosidic bond
21. The number of nucleotides of RNA molecule are:
    A. 40–4,000
    B. 50–5,000
    C. 60–6,000
    D. 70–7,000

22. The number of nucleotides in DNA molecule are:
    A. 800–4,000
    B. 1,000–6,000
    C. 1,200–8,000
    D. 800–9,000
23. The purine nucleotides act as components of :
    A. FAD
    B. NAD⁺
    C. NADP
    D. All the above
24. The pyrimidine nucleotides act as the high energy intermediates in:
    A. UDPG
    B. ATP
    C. ADP
    D. AMP
25. Nucleic acids are:
    A. Structural molecules
    B. Information molecule
    C. Second messengers
    D. Communication molecules
26. The base present in DNA but not present in RNA is:
    A. Guanine
    B. Uracil
    C. Cytosine
    D. Thymine
27. Which of the following bases is a constituent of RNA but not DNA?
    A. Thymine
    B. Cytosine
    C. Adenine
    D. Uracil
28. Molecule of genetic information is:
    A. Protein
    B. DNA
    C. RNA
    D. Enzyme
29. Two strands of double helical DNA are linked by:
    A. Peptide bonds
    B. Phosphodiester bonds
    C. Glycosidic bonds
    D. Hydrogen bonds
30. DNA can be denatured by:
    A. Acid
    B. Alkali
    C. Heat
    D. All of the above
31. Proteins present in nucleoproteins are:
    A. Histones
    B. Albumin
    C. Histidine
    D. Globulins

ANSWERS

6. A. Vitamin B_3 (nicotinamide)
   B. Vitamin B_2 (riboflavin)
   C. Pantothenic acid
7. A. Adenine
   B. Adenine
   C. Adenine

8. A. Coenzyme to hydrogenases.
   B. Coenzyme participating in oxidation-reduction reaction.
   C. Coenzyme of pantothenic acid, having AMP as part of its molecule. Acetyl CoA is the precursor of cholesterol.

9. (B)	10. (D)	11. (D)	12. (D)	13. (B)
14. (C)	15. (D)	16. (C)	17. (B)	18. (B)
19. (D)	20. (C)	21. (C)	22. (D)	23. (D)
24. (A)	25. (B)	26. (D)	27. (D)	28. (B)
29. (D)	30. (D)	31. (A)		

CHAPTER 8

Enzymology

Enzymes are biological catalysts, which bring about chemical reactions in living cells. They are produced by the living organisms and are present in very small amounts in various cells.

Almost all the functions of the body such as digestion, breathing, synthesis and breakdown of carbohydrates, fats and proteins are catalyzed and controlled by specific enzymes. Most chemical reactions of the living cells would have occurred very slowly had it not been catalyzed by enzymes.

The substance upon which an enzyme acts is called substrate. The enzyme will convert the substrate into the product or products. The enzymes are generally named by adding the suffix 'ase' to the name of the substrate. Thus, the enzyme lactase acts on the substrate lactose, and the products glucose and galactose are formed.

All enzymes are proteins. Enzymes follow the physical and chemical reactions of proteins.

They are heat-labile, soluble in water, precipitated by protein precipitating reagents (ammonium sulfate or trichloroacetic acid) and contain 16% weight nitrogen.

GENERAL PROPERTIES OF ENZYMES

1. All enzymes are proteins.
2. They accelerate the reaction, but
   a. Do not alter the reaction equilibrium.
   b. Not consumed in overall reaction.
   c. Required only in very small quantities.
3. They have enormous power for catalysis.
4. Enzymes are highly specific for their substrates.

5. Enzymes possess active sites at which interaction with substrate takes place.
6. Enzymes lower activation energy.
7. They form substrate complex as intermediates during their action.
8. Some enzymes are regulatory in function.

CLASSIFICATION OF ENZYMES

As per the International Union of Biochemists, enzymes are divided into six major classes.

1. *Oxidoreductases:* One compound oxidized, another reduced, e.g. tyrosinase, urease, lactic dehydrogenase, catalase and peroxidase.

$$A + B \rightleftharpoons A + B$$
$$\text{Reduced oxidized} \quad \text{Reduced oxidized}$$

$$\text{Lactate} \xrightarrow[\text{NAD} \quad \text{NADH} + H^+]{\text{Lactate dehydrogenase}} \text{Pyruvate}$$

2. *Transferases:* This class of enzymes transfer group containing C, N or S from the substrate to another substrate. They are important in biological synthesis, e.g. transaminase, hexokinase, transacylase, transaldolase.

$$\text{Serine} \xrightarrow[\text{Methyltransferase}]{\text{Serine dehydrogenase}} \text{Glycine}$$

3. *Hydrolases:* They catalyze hydrolysis of esters, ether, peptide or glycosidic bond by addition of water molecules across the bond which is split, e.g. esterase, peptidase. The digestive enzymes, amylase, pepsin, trypsin and chymotrypsin are all hydrolases.

$$\text{Urea} + H_2O \xrightarrow{\text{Urease}} CO_2 + 2NH_3$$

4. *Lyases:* They catalyze the addition or removal of groups without hydrolysis, oxidation or reduction, producing double bonds at times, e.g. decarboxylase, carboxylase, carbonic anhydrase.

$$\text{Fructose-1,6-biphosphate} \xrightarrow{\text{Aldolase}} \text{Glyceraldehyde 3P + Dihydroxyacetone phosphate}$$

$$\text{Pyruvate} \xrightarrow{\text{Pyruvate dehydrogenase}} \text{Acetaldehyde} + CO_2$$

5. *Isomerases:* These can produce optical, geometric or position isomers of substrates by intermolecular rearrangement, e.g. racemase, epimerase, isomerase.

$$\text{Glucose-6-phosphate} \xrightarrow{\text{Glucosephosphate isomerase (GPI)}} \text{Fructose-6-phosphate}$$

$$\text{Methylmalonyl-CoA} \xrightarrow{\text{Mutase}} \text{Succinyl-CoA}$$

6. *Ligases:* These enzymes also called synthetases link two substrates together usually with the linking of pyrophosphate bound in ATP (ligare = to bind), e.g. glutamine synthetase.

$$A + B + ATP \longrightarrow AB + ADP + Pi$$

$$\text{Glutamate} + NH_3 + ATP \xrightarrow{\text{Glutamine synthetase}} \text{Glutamine} + ADP + Pi$$

$$\text{Pyruvate} \xrightarrow[\text{ATP} \quad \text{ADP} + Pi]{\text{Pyruvate carboxylase}} \text{Oxaloacetate}$$

ENZYME SPECIFICITY

Some enzymes are very specific and show activity with only one substrate. Some others are much less particular. Generally three types of enzymatic specificities are observed.

1. *Stereospecificity:* Some enzymes show specificities only with a specific group of a substrate, *e.g.* urease catalyzes the hydrolysis of urea.

$$H_2N-\underset{\underset{O}{\|}}{C}-N_2H + 2H_2O \xrightarrow{\text{Urease}} (NH_4)_2 CO_2$$

The catalysis does not take place when structure of urea is altered, e.g. N-methyl urea and thiourea are not hydrolyzed by urease.

$$H_2N-\underset{\underset{O}{\|}}{C}-NH-CH_3 \qquad H_2N-\underset{\underset{S}{\|}}{C}-NH_2$$
$$\text{N-Methyl urea} \qquad \qquad \text{Thiourea}$$

D-amino acid-oxidase acts only on the D-form of amino acid and not on L-form.

2. *Substrate specificity:* Some enzymes catalyze similar type of reaction, but differ in their action due to substrate specificity, e.g.

a. Pepsin hydrolyses peptide bonds involving aromatic amino acids like phenylalanine and tyrosine.
b. Trypsin hydrolyses peptide bonds involving carboxyl groups of basic amino acids like arginine or lysine.
3. *Reaction specificity:* A substrate can undergo many reactions, but in reaction specificity, one enzyme can catalyze only one of the various reactions. For example, oxalic acid can undergo different reactions, but each of these reactions is catalyzed by separate enzymes.

MECHANISM OF ENZYME ACTION

According to Michaelis and Menten, the enzyme molecule (E) first combines with a substrate molecule (S) to form an enzyme-substrate (ES) complex, which further dissociates to form product (P) and enzyme (E) back.

$$E + S \rightleftharpoons ES \longrightarrow E + products$$

Enzyme once dissociated from the complex is free to combine with another molecule of the substrate.

The site at which a substrate can meet with the enzyme molecule is extremely specific and is called active site or catalytic site. Normally the molecular size and shape of the substrate molecule is extremely small compared to the enzyme molecules. The active site is made up of several amino acid residues, that come together as a result of the foldings of secondary and tertiary structures of the enzymes. So the active site possesses a complex three dimensional form and shape, provides a predominantly non-polar cleft or crevice to accept and bind the substrate.

Factors Affecting Enzyme Activity

Substrate Concentration

At a low substrate concentration the initial velocity of an enzyme catalyzed reaction is proportional to the substrate concentration. However, as the substrate concentration is increased, the initial velocity increases less as it is no longer proportional to the substrate concentration. With a further increase in the substrate concentration and the velocity assumes a constant rate as a result of enzyme being saturated with its substrate.

It was Michaelis and Menten who suggested an explanation for these findings by postulating that at low substrate concentrations, the enzyme is not saturated with the substrate and the reaction is not

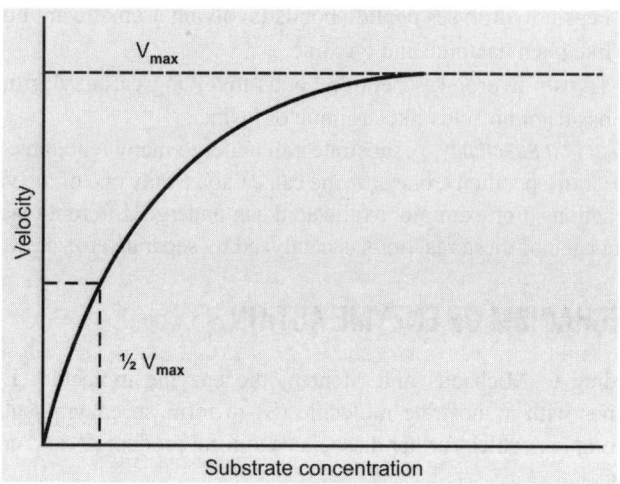

Fig. 8.1: Enzyme activity and substrate concentration

proceeding at maximum velocity, whereas, when the enzyme is saturated with substrate, maximum velocity is observed. The enzyme combines with the substrate to form an enzyme-substrate complex and the rate of decomposition of the substrate is proportional to the enzyme-substrate complex. The velocity of the reaction at this high substrate concentration is termed as maximum velocity (V_{max}). The substrate concentration at which the velocity is half of the maximum velocity is called Michaelis' constant (K_m). K_m indicates the affinity of the substrate towards the enzyme and is inversely proportional to the affinity.

$$K_m \,\alpha\, \frac{1}{\text{Affinity}}$$

Higher the affinity the smaller will be the K_m and lower the affinity, the higher will be the K_m (Fig. 8.1).

The Michaelis-Menten equation is given by the expression:

$$V_o = \frac{V_{max}\,[S]}{V_m + [S]}$$

Where V_o = Initial velocity
  V_m = Maximum velocity
  K_m = Michaelis constant
  [S] = Substrate concentration

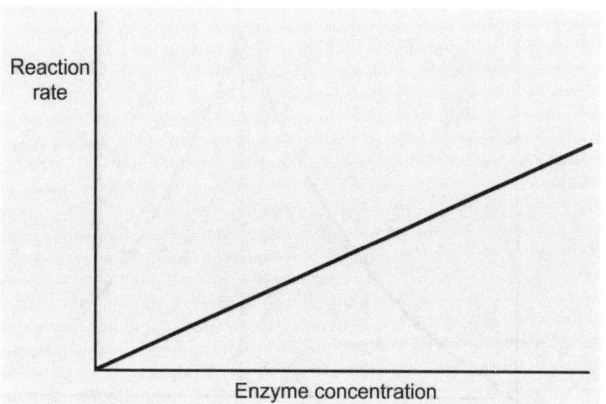

Fig. 8.2: Enzyme activity and enzyme concentration

When the initial velocity is exactly half the maximum velocity,

$$½ V_{max} = \frac{V_{max} [S]}{K_m + [S]}$$

$$K_m + [S] = 2[S]$$
$$K_m = [S]$$

Therefore, K_m is equal to substrate concentration at which the velocity is half the maximum.

Effect of Enzyme Concentration

The rate of an enzyme catalyzed reaction is directly proportional to concentration of the enzyme. The greater the concentration of enzyme, the faster will be reaction taking place (Fig. 8.2).

Effect of pH

The enzyme activity is maximum at a particular pH, which is called optimum pH. This is due to the changes in the net charge on enzymes resulting from changes in pH. Excessive changes in pH brought on by addition of strong acids or bases may completely denature and inactivate enzymes (Fig. 8.3).

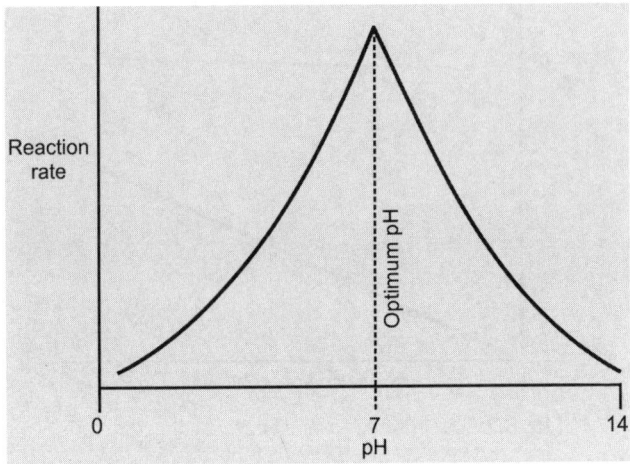

Fig. 8.3: Enzyme activity and pH

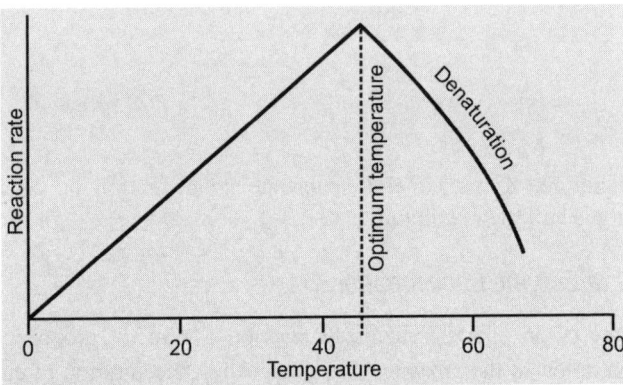

Fig. 8.4: Enzyme activity and temperature

Effect of Temperature

The velocity of enzyme reaction increases when temperature of the medium is increased; reaches a maximum and then falls. The temperature at which maximum amount of substrate is converted to the product per unit time is called optimum temperature (Fig. 8.4).

As temperature is increased, more molecules get activation energy or molecules are at increased rate of motion and so their collision probabilities along with the reaction rate is increased. Above this temperature the reaction rate decreases as enzymes being protein in nature are denatured by heat and become inactive.

Effect of Time

The time required for completion of an enzyme reaction increases with decrease in temperature from its optimum. Under the optimum conditions of pH and temperature, time required for enzyme reaction is less.

Enzyme Inhibition

Enzymes are proteins and they can be inactivated by the agents that denature them. The chemical substances, which inactivate the enzymes are called inhibitors and the process is called enzyme inhibition. Most of the substances commonly referred to as poisons are harmful in that they inhibit one or more essential enzymes.

The inhibitors may be classified in two broad groups. First, compounds or ions, which are specific in their effect, inhibiting only one enzyme or several closely related enzymes. And second, substances, which are non-specific, inhibiting many enzymes.

Specific Inhibition

The inhibitor molecule is a structural analog of the normal substrate of the enzyme, i.e. it is chemically similar to the substrate. The inhibitor is capable of combining with the active site by virtue of its similar structure. As long as the active site is bound to the inhibitor, the enzyme is not a catalyst. Since, both are competing for combination with the same active site, the term competitive inhibition (Fig. 8.5) is used.

An important example is provided by the sulfa drugs. These are structural analogs of para-aminobenzoic acid, a compound required by many bacteria for synthesizing their food (vitamin) tetrahydrofolic acid (THFA), but which is not used by higher organisms such as man. The

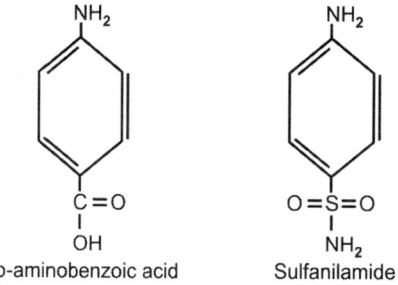

Fig. 8.5: Competitive inhibition

sulfa drugs inhibit growth of the bacteria in man by competing with the para-aminobenzoic acid for the active site of some bacterial enzyme.

Non-specific Inhibition

Every protein molecule has a number of reactive groups present on the side chains of the constituent amino acids, groups such as $-CO_2H$, $-SH$, $-NH_2$, etc. Any substance capable of combining with a common group of this type is a potential inhibitor of all. Heavy metal ions are non-specific inhibitors. They can bind to a number of protein groups in particular $-SH$ and $-CO_2H$ at the active site inhibiting the normal catalytic activity. In sufficient concentration, heavy metal ions will inhibit most enzymes and are therefore poisonous to all living things. However, some of these heavy metal ions Cu^{++}, Zn^{++}, Co^{++} are absolute requirements in low concentrations for cells as cofactors for a variety of enzymes. Thus, classification of a metal ion as poison depends on its concentration. Mostly non-specific inhibition is non-competitive in nature.

COENZYMES

Coenzymes are molecules that cooperate in the catalytic action of an enzyme. A coenzyme may be tightly bound to the protein or it make free to diffuse away from the enzyme acting essentially as an additional substrate NAD^+ in many dehydrogenase reactions. If tightly bound to an enzyme, it is called prosthetic group. The term cofactor refers rather non-specifically to various materials required for full enzyme activity, e.g. cations, Mg^{++}, Zn^{++}. Water-soluble vitamins function as coenzymes or as components of coenzyme molecules.

Many enzymes require the presence of small non-protein organic molecules for their efficient performance. Only when both enzyme and coenzyme are present, catalysis will occur. Coenzymes are low molecular weight, non-protein organic compounds that are heat resistant and function as cosubstances. Usually, it binds loosely and can be easily separated from its enzyme by dialysis, but when it binds tightly, it is considered as a prosthetic group of the enzyme. Co-factor differs from a coenzyme only because it usually is a metallic ion (Fe^{++}, Mg^{++}, Zn^{++}, Cu^{++}) rather than an organic molecule. Water-soluble vitamins (vitamin B complex and vitamin C) form coenzymes.

The term apoenzyme refers to the protein part of the enzyme. The apoenzyme with its prosthetic group (or coenzyme) constitute a complete enzyme or holoenzyme.

Conjugated protein enzyme ⇌ Protein + prosthetic group
OR
Holoenzyme ⇌ Apoenzyme + coenzyme
(Protein part) (non-protein part/prosthetic group)

Classification of Coenzyme

Coenzymes for group transfer are given in Table 8.1.

Water-soluble Vitamins as Coenzymes

Vitamins of B complex and vitamin C (ascorbic acid) act as coenzymes as shown in Table 8.2.

DIAGNOSTIC VALUE OF PLASMA ENZYMES

When a tissue is injured, some cells of that tissue are destroyed and their contents including enzymes are released into the blood stream. The increase of enzymes in blood stream will indicate the disease (Table 8.3).

Urinary Elevation

N-acetyl glucosaminidase in the urine can be used to indicate renal transplant rejection.

TABLE 8.1: Coenzymes with the groups they transfer

Coenzymes for groups other than H	Coenzymes for transfer of H
ATP and its relatives	NAD^+, $NADP^+$
Sugar phosphates	FMN, FAD
CoA	Lipoic acid
Thiamine pyrophosphate	Coenzyme Q
B_6 phosphate	
Folate coenzyme	
Biotin	
Cobamide (B_{12}) coenzyme	
Lipoic acid	

TABLE 8.2: Relationship among water-soluble vitamins, their coenzyme forms and metabolic reactions in which they participate

Vitamins	Coenzymes	Types of reactions
Thiamine (B_1)	Thiamine pyrophosphate (TPP)	Decarboxylation of α-keto acid, certain reactions of keto sugars
Riboflavin (B_2)	Flavin mononucleotide (FMN), flavin adenine dinucleotide (FAD)	Several kinds of oxidation-reduction reactions
Pyridoxine (B_6)	Pyridoxal phosphate	Several kinds of reactions involving amino acids, e.g. decarboxylation, transamination
Niacin (B_3)	Nicotinamide adenine dinucleotide (NAD+), nicotinamide adenine dinucleotide phosphate (NADP+)	Numerous oxidation-reduction reactions
Pantothenic acid	Coenzyme A	Many reactions of fatty acids, particularly those involving transfer of acetyl groups
Biotin	Enzyme bound biotin	Certain carbon dioxide fixation reactions
Folic acid	Tetrahydrofolic acid	Various reactions involving single carbon compounds
Cyanocobalamine	Several 'cobamide' coenzymes	Carbon chain isomerizations, certain methyl group transfers

TABLE 8.3: Increase of different enzymes in diseases

Enzymes	Increased in
Amylase	Acute pancreatitis
Acid phosphatase (optimum pH = 5)	Prostatic carcinoma
Alkaline phosphatase (optimum pH = 10)	Liver disease, rickets
Aspartate transaminase (AST) (previously GOT)	Myocardial infarction
Alanine transaminase (ALT) (previously GPT)	Liver disease especially with liver cell damage
Lactate dehydrogenase (LDH)	Myocardial infarction, but also increased in liver disease and some blood disease
Creatine kinase (CK)	Myocardial infarction and skeletal muscle diseases (muscular dystrophy, dermatomyositis)
γ-glutamyl transferase (γ-GT)	Diagnosis of liver disease, particularly biliary obstruction and alcoholism

QUESTIONS

1. Define an enzyme. Classify the enzymes and add a brief note on the factors influencing enzyme activity.
2. Name the enzymes catalyzing the following reactions:
   A. Glucose-6-phosphate to Glucose.
   B. Glucose-6-phosphate to Fructose-6-phosphate.
3. Short essay on transaminases.
4. Write the coenzyme forms of the following vitamins with examples:
   A. Riboflavin.
   B. Niacin.
   C. Pyridoxine.
5. Differentiate between coenzymes and isoenzymes.

MULTIPLE CHOICE QUESTIONS

6. The enzyme maltase can act on:
   A. Glucose
   B. Maltose
   C. Starch
   D. Cellulose
7. An enzyme is specific:
   A. For a substrate
   B. For reaction, which it can catalyze
   C. Both A and B are correct
8. Coenzymes:
   A. Alter the equilibrium of reactions
   B. Are consumed by reactions
   C. Usually consist of polypeptides
   D. Include Mg^{++}, Zn^{++} and Fe^{++}
9. Which of the following coenzymes is not derived from vitamins?
   A. CoA-SH
   B. Pyridoxal phosphate
   C. TPP
   D. Lipoamide
10. Which vitamin cannot serve as antioxidant?
    A. Vitamin A
    B. Vitamin C
    C. Vitamin E
    D. Vitamin K
11. Which of the following non-proteins can act as an enzyme?
    A. DNA
    B. Phospholipids
    C. Glycolipids
    D. RNA

12. The enzymes regulated by phosphorylation-dephosphorylation (e.g. covalent binding and later cleavage of the phosphate by the enzyme) include all the following *except:*
    A. Glucose-6-phosphatase
    B. Glycogen synthase
    C. Pyruvate dehydrogenase
    D. Glycogen phosphorylase

13. A non-competitive enzyme inhibitor will do all the following *except:*
    A. Decrease V_{max}
    B. Act independently of substrate
    C. Decrease K_m
    D. Not attach to a substrate binding site

14. Enzymes are:
    A. Biocatalysts
    B. Proteins except ribozymes
    C. Products of germs
    D. All of the above

15. Lactate hydrogen belongs to the class of:
    A. Ligases
    B. Lyases
    C. Oxidoreductases
    D. Isomerases

16. All the following gastrointestinal enzymes are secreted as zymogens *except:*
    A. Ribonucleases
    B. Pepsin
    C. Chymotrypsin
    D. Trypsin

17. An example of an intracellular enzyme is:
    A. Glucokinase
    B. Pancreatic amylase
    C. Hexokinase
    D. Glucose-6-phosphatase

18. All the following are coenzymes *except:*
    A. NAD^+
    B. TPP
    C. ALT (SGPT)
    D. Pyridoxal phosphate

19. The function of a coenzyme in a enzymatic reaction is to:
    A. Act as cosubstrate
    B. Activate the substrate
    C. Raise the activation energy of the coenzymatic reaction
    D. Enhance the specificity of the substrate

20. A cofactor in an enzymatic reaction is:
    A. An organic molecule
    B. A metal ion
    C. Both the above
    D. A hormone

21. Coenzyme A contains the following vitamin:
    A. Thiamine
    B. Pantothenic acid
    C. Vitamin B_6
    D. Folic acid

22. Coenzyme required for transamination is:
    A. NAD^+
    B. Thiamine pyrophosphate
    C. FMN
    D. Pyridoxal phosphate

23. **Enzyme increases the rate of reaction by:**
    A. Decreasing the energy of activation
    B. Increasing the energy of activation
    C. Increasing the free energy change of the reaction
    D. Decreasing the free energy change of the reaction
24. **Normal level of SGOT (AST) and SGPT (ALT) at 37° C is:**
    A. 0–50 IU/L
    B. 0–80 IU/L
    C. 60–180 IU/L
    D. 100–250 IU/L
25. **Acid phosphate level in serum is elevated in:**
    A. Acute pancreatitis
    B. Osteomalacia
    C. Prostatic carcinoma
    D. Obstructive jaundice
26. **The diagnostic enzyme in muscular dystrophy is:**
    A. Lipase
    B. Alkaline phosphatase
    C. Lactate dehydrogenase A(LDH)
    D. Creatine phosphokinase (CPK)/creatine kinase (CK)
27. **All the enzymes are increased in myocardial infarction *except*:**
    A. Alkaline phosphatase
    B. LDH
    C. CPK
    D. SGOT (AST)
28. **Which of the following enzymes in serum is specifically elevated in alcoholism?**
    A. SGPT (ALT)
    B. SGOT (AST)
    C. γ–glutamyl transpeptidase (γ-GT)
    D. Acid phosphatase
29. **Serum amylase is highly raised in:**
    A. Diabetes mellitus
    B. Acute pancreatitis
    C. Bone disorders
    D. Liver disorders
30. **The group transferring coenzyme is:**
    A. Coenzyme A
    B. NAD^+
    C. NADP
    D. FAD
31. **Creatine kinase is found in:**
    A. Myocardium
    B. Brain
    C. Muscles
    D. All of the above
32. **Following myocardial infarction, the last serum enzyme to return to normal is:**
    A. Creatine kinase
    B. GOT
    C. LDH
    D. GPT
33. **The following serum enzyme rises in viral hepatitis:**
    A. LDH
    B. GPT
    C. GOT
    D. All of the above

34. The following serum enzyme rises in myocardial infarction:
    A. Creatine kinase
    B. GOT
    C. LDH
    D. All of the above
35. Following myocardial infarction the earliest serum enzyme to rise is:
    A. Creatine kinase
    B. GOT
    C. GPT
    D. LDH
36. Enzymes, which contain lightly bound metal ions are called:
    A. Coenzyme
    B. Metalloenzyme
    C. Metal-activated enzyme
    D. Activated metal enzyme
37. Enzymes increase the rate of reaction by:
    A. Increasing the free energy rate of activation
    B. Decreasing the free energy of activation
    C. Charging the equilibrium constant of the reaction
    D. Increasing the free energy change of reaction
38. The group transferring coenzyme is:
    A. CoA
    B. NAD+
    C. NADP
    D. FAD

ANSWERS

6. (B)	7. (C)	8. (D)	9. (D)	10. (D)
11. (D)	12. (A)	13. (C)	14. (D)	15. (C)
16. (A)	17. (B)	18. (B)	19. (D)	20. (B)
21. (B)	22. (D)	23. (A)	24. (A)	25. (C)
26. (D)	27. (B)	28. (C)	29. (B)	30. (A)
31. (D)	32. (C)	33. (D)	34. (D)	35. (A)
36. (B)	37. (B)	38. (A)		

9
CHAPTER

Digestion and Absorption

DIGESTIVE FLUIDS

All foodstuffs except water, inorganic salts, vitamins and non-saccharides are hydrolysed into smaller molecules in the digestive tract before absorption from the intestines. The hydrolysis is accomplished by the enzymes of digestive fluids namely saliva, gastric juice, pancreatic juice and the intestinal juices.

Salivary Digestion

Saliva provides α-amylase (also known as ptyalin). The flow is stimulated by the sight, smell, taste and even thought of food. Besides water (99.5%), saliva includes a food lubricant called nucin (a glycoprotein) and an enzyme, α-amylase. This enzyme catalyses the partial hydrolysis of starch to dextrins and maltose and it works best at the pH of saliva in the range 5.8–7.1. Proteins and lipids pass through the mouth unchanged.

Gastric Juice

Gastric juice starts the digestion of proteins with pepsin. When food reaches the stomach, the cells of the gastric glands are stimulated by hormones to release the fluids that combine to give gastric juice. One kind of gastric gland secretes mucin, which coats the stomach to protect it against its own digestive enzymes and its acid. Mucin, is continuously produced and only slowly digested. When the protection of the stomach is hindered, part of the stomach itself could be digested leading to ulcers.

Another gastric gland secretes hydrochloric acid (pH 1–2) about a million times more acidic than blood. The acid coagulates proteins and activates the enzyme protease. Protein coagulation retains the protein in the stomach longer for exposure to the protease. Hydrochloric acid (HCl) denatures proteins making their internal peptide bonds more accessible to subsequent hydrolysis by proteases, which provides an acid environment for the action of pepsin.

The third gastric gland secretes the zymogen pepsinogen. Pepsinogen is changed into pepsin and protease, by the action of hydrochloric acid and traces of pepsin. The optimum pH is 1.0–1.5, which is found in the stomach fluid. Pepsin catalyses the only important digestive work in the stomach, namely the hydrolysis of some of the peptide bonds of proteins to make short polypeptides.

Adult gastric juice also has a lipase, but it does not start its work until it arrives in the higher pH medium of upper intestinal tract. The gastric juice of infants is less acidic than adults. To compensate for the protein coagulating work normally done by the acid, infant gastric juice contains rennin, a powerful protein coagulator. Because the pH of an infant's gastric is higher than that in adult, its lipase gets an early start on lipid digestion.

The churning and digesting activities in the stomach produce a liquid mixture called chyme. This is released in portions through the pyloric valve into the duodenum, the first 12 inches of the upper intestinal tract.

Pancreatic Juice

Pancreatic juice furnishes several zymogens and enzymes. As soon as the chyme appears in the duodenum, hormones are released that circulate to the pancreas and induce this organ to release two juices. One is dilute sodium bicarbonate, which neutralizes the acid in the chyme. The other is usually called pancreatic juice and it carries enzymes or zymogens involved in the digestion of practically everything in food. It contributes an α-amylase similar to that present in saliva, a lipase, nucleases and zymogens for protein digestion enzymes.

The conversion of the proteolytic zymogens to active enzymes begin with the enzyme called enteropeptidase released from cells that line the duodenum when chyme arrives. It catalyses the formation of trypsin from its zymogen, trypsinogen.

$$\text{Trypsinogen} \xrightarrow{\textit{Enteropeptidase}} \text{Trypsin}$$

Trypsin then catalyses the change of other zymogen into active enzymes.

$$\text{Procarboxypeptidase} \xrightarrow{\textit{Trypsin}} \text{Carboxypeptidase}$$

$$\text{Chymotrypsinogen} \xrightarrow{\textit{Trypsin}} \text{Chymotrypsin}$$

$$\text{Proelastase} \xrightarrow{\textit{Trypsin}} \text{Elastase}$$

Trypsin, chymotrypsin and elastase catalyse the hydrolysis of large polypeptides to smaller ones. Carboxypeptidase working from C-terminal ends of small peptides, carries the action further to amino acids and dipeptides or tripeptides.

Intestinal Juice

Intestinal juice contains the following enzymes:
1. Disaccharidase.
2. Peptidase.
3. Polynucleotidase.
4. Nucleosidase.
5. Enterokinase.
6. Phosphatase.
7. Lecithinase.

Disaccharidase: They are enzymes to hydrolyse disaccharides. They attack the glucosidic linkage of the disaccharides to convert them to the corresponding monosaccharides. For example:
   a. Maltase splits maltose into 2 molecules of glucose.
   b. Sucrase splits sucrose into glucose and fructose.
   c. Lactase splits lactose into glucose and galactose.

Peptidase: These are enzymes hydrolysing peptide chains. There are two main types of peptidases:
   a. Aminopeptidases act on the peptide linkage of terminal amino acids, possessing a free amino group.
   b. Tripeptidases and dipeptidases split tripeptides and dipeptides into their individual amino acids.

Polynucleotidase: It hydrolyses and splits the nucleotide into phosphoric acid and nucleoside.

Nucleosidase: It splits nucleosides into their nitrogenous bases and sugars.

Enterokinase: This enzyme is secreted by the duodenal and mucosal cells. It converts trypsinogen to trypsin. It does not have any direct digestive action.

Phosphatase: Enzyme phosphatase present in the intestinal juice, splits the phosphate from organic phosphate derivatives, such as glycerophosphate and hexose phosphate.

Lecithinase: Intestinal juice contains the lecithinase, which splits lecithins to yield fatty acids, glycerol, phosphoric acid and choline.

DIGESTION OF CARBOHYDRATES

In the mouth

Saliva contains salivary amylase (ptyalin), which catalyzes the hydrolysis of starch into maltose. However, this enzyme becomes inactive at a pH below 4, so that its activity ceases when it is mixed with the contents of the stomach where the pH falls to 1.5. Salivary amylase does not serve a very important function in digestion because the food does not remain in the mouth long enough for any appreciable hydrolysis to take place. Some hydrolysis of carbohydrates catalyzed by salivary amylase may take place in the stomach before the food is thoroughly mixed, but this is of little importance because there are intestinal enzymes capable of hydrolyzing starch and maltose. The principal function of saliva is to lubricate and moisten the food, so that it can be easily swallowed.

In the Stomach

The stomach contains no carbohydrates. So, no digestion of carbohydrates takes place there except for that catalyzed by salivary amylase. The activity of the salivary amylase ceases as soon as it becomes mixed with the acid contents of the stomach.

In the Small Intestine

The major digestion of carbohydrates takes place in the small intestine through the action of enzyme pancreatic amylase that catalyzes the hydrolysis of starch and dextrins into maltose. The maltose thus produced is hydrolyzed to glucose through the activity of the enzyme maltase from the intestinal mucosal cells. The optimum pH of pancreatic amylase is 7.1. The intestinal mucosal cells also contain the enzymes sucrose and lactose, which catalyze the hydrolysis of sucrose and lactose respectively.

$$(C_6H_{10}O_5)_n + nH_2O \xrightarrow{\text{Pancreatic amylase}} nC_6H_{22}O_{11}$$
Starch → Maltose

$$C_{12}H_{22}O_{11} + H_2O \xrightarrow{\text{Maltase}} 2C_6H_{12}O_6$$
Maltose → Glucose

If a monosaccharide such as glucose is eaten, digestion is not necessary because the monosaccharide is already in its simplest form and can undergo absorption into blood stream. Many adults cannot digest milk because they lack mucosal lactase. Such adults show milk intolerance with symptoms of abdominal cramps, bloating and diarrhea.

DIGESTION OF FATS

In the Mouth

A lingual lipase secreted by the dorsal surface of the tongue acts on the triglycerides particularly of the type found in milk. Lingual lipase has a pH range of 2.0–7.5 with optimum pH 4.0–4.5, so that it can continue its activity even at the low pH of the stomach.

In the Stomach

Although, gastric lipase is present, very little digestion of fat takes place because the pH of the stomach (1–2) is far below the optimum pH of that enzyme (7–8). Also fats must be emulsified before they can be digested by lipase and there is no mechanism for emulsification of fats in the stomach. In infants, whose stomach pH is higher, fat hydrolysis of milk takes place in the stomach.

In the Small Intestine

In the small intestine, the pancreatic lipase catalyzes the hydrolysis of fats into fatty acids and glycerol. This action is aided by bile salts, which emulsify the fats, so that they can be acted upon readily by pancreatic lipase.

$$\text{Fat + water} \xrightarrow{\textit{Pancreatic lipase}} \text{Fatty acids + glycerol}$$

DIGESTION OF PROTEINS

In the Mouth

As the saliva contains no enzymes for the hydrolysis of proteins, no digestion of protein takes place in the mouth.

In the Stomach

Precursor enzyme pepsinogen is converted to pepsin when it is mixed with the HCl of the stomach. Pepsin catalyzes the hydrolysis of proteins to polypeptides.

$$\text{Protein + Water} \xrightarrow{Pepsin} \text{Polypeptides}$$

In the Small Intestine

In the small intestine, the zymogen, trypsinogen from the pancreatic juice is changed into trypsin by the intestinal enzyme enterokinase. Trypsin in turn changes chymotrypsinogen, another pancreatic zymogen into chymotrypsin. Both trypsin and chymotrypsin catalyze the hydrolysis of protein, proteoses and peptones to polypeptides. The optimum pH of trypsin and chymotrypsin is 8–9.

The intestine enzymes aminopeptidase and dipeptidase catalyze the hydrolysis of polypeptides and dipeptides to amino acids. Carboxypeptidase, an enzyme of pancreatic juice, also catalyzes the hydrolysis of polypeptides to amino acids. Carboxypeptidase contains the element zinc (Zn).

Proelastase from pancreatic juice is converted to elastase by trypsin; elastase acts on protein and polypeptides to convert them into polypeptides and dipeptides respectively.

ABSORPTION OF CARBOHYDRATES

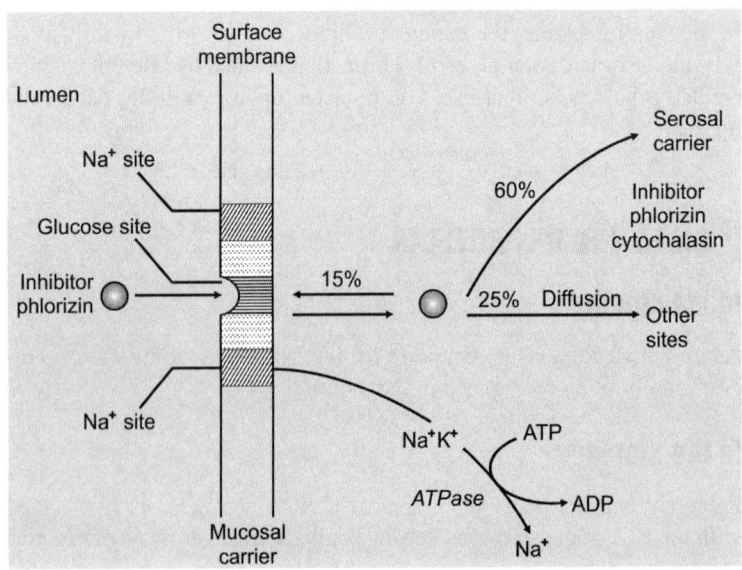

Fig. 9.1: Active transport of glucose

Active Transport of Glucose or Galactose by the Intestinal Epithelial Cells

Two mechanisms are responsible for the absorption of monosaccharides.
1. Active transport against a concentration gradient.
2. Simple diffusion.

Glucose and galactose are transported by active transport mechanism accomplished by a Na^+ symport system. The membrane carrier has binding sites for both Na^+ and sugar (Fig. 9.1). The molecular configuration that seem necessary for active transport are the –OH on carbon-2 should have the same configuration as in glucose, a pyranose ring should be present and a methyl or substituted methyl group should be present on carbon-5.

When the concentrations of glucose or galactose are very high in the lumen as immediately after a meal, the system accomplishes transport of sugar down its concentration gradient into the cell. When the luminal concentration of monosaccharide falls, the system performs up hill or active transport into cell. The driving force for this active transport is provided by the Na^+/K^+ pump at the basolateral membrane of the epithelial cell, which pumps Na^+ out of the cell, thus maintaining the Na^+ gradient. Thus, as Na^+ moves into the cell down its concentration gradient the coupled transport monosaccharide against its concentration gradient is able to occur. The carrier is an integral membrane protein that binds and transports two Na^+ ions for each sugar molecule. Its glucose site can be blocked by the glycoside phlorizin. Inhibitors of Na^+,K^+-ATPase system such as ouabain also block glucose absorption because of the resultant inability of the epithelial cell to transfer Na^+ from its serosal side to the plasma. Since, ouabain causes intracellular $[Na^+]$ to rise equilibrium with $[Na^+]$ on the mucosal side of the cell, the Na^+ gradient is abolished and transport of glucose becomes impossible.

Once inside the cell several routes of exit are possible for glucose. About 15% is carried back to the lumen by the transport system: 25% diffuses passively through the basal membrane of the cell. The remainder (60%) is transported out of the cell by a distinct carrier system at the serosal surface. This carrier is distinguished by its specific inhibition by phlorizin and cytochalasin B.

The transport system is so efficient that it under physiological circumstances such as glucose never accumulates within the intestinal epithelial cells. The overall process of carbohydrate digestion and absorption is so efficient that ordinarily all dietary carbohydrate has been absorbed by the time, the ingested material reaches the lower jejunum.

Fructose is absorbed by facilitated diffusion on a membrane carrier. The system moves the sugar from high concentrations in the lumen to low concentration within the cell and cannot accomplish uphill.

ABSORPTION OF LIPIDS

Main products of lipase action, i.e. fatty acids and monoacylglycerols are solubilized by incorporation into mixed micelles with conjugated bile salts. The micelles markedly increase the rate of delivery of the fatty acids and monoacylglyerols to the intestinal mucosa, which represents the absorptive surface. Since, these products are rapidly esterified to triacylglycerols within the mucosal cell, their concentration at the inner surface of the intestinal cell membrane is very low. Thus, fatty acids and monoacylglycerols leave the surface of the intestinal cell and being lipid soluble, passively diffuse across the membranes of the epithelial cells down their concentration gradients. This process of absorption of free fatty acids and monoacylglycerols is largely completed in the upper jejunum. The conjugated bile salts are reabsorbed in the ileum where they are actively transported and enter the enterohepatic circulation.

The products of the digestion of medium chain triacylglycerols (C_8–C_{12}) are water soluble and they do not require micellar solubilization and are directly absorbed into the intestinal cell.

The free glycerol released in the intestinal lumen is not reutilized, but passes directly to the portal vien. All long chain fatty acids absorbed by intestinal wall mucosal cells are utilized to form triacylglycerols. The enzymes involved in the process are in the endoplasmic reticulum. In the first reaction, the fatty acids are transformed to their corresponding acyl-CoA derivatives by acyl-CoA synthetase. Then, monoacylglycerol react with one molecule of fatty acyl-CoA to give diacylglycerol, catalyzed by monoacylglycerol transacylase. Finally, in the presence of diacylglycerol transacylase, diacylglycerol reacts with one molecule of acyl-CoA to give triacylglycerol.

An alternate and minor pathway for triacylglycerol resynthesis involves fatty acid esterification with phosphatidic acid, which in turn is derived from cellular glucose metabolism.

The final step in the absorption of the resynthesized triacylglycerols from the intestine are their incorporation into chylomicrons, which renders them water soluble, followed by secretion into the intestinal lymphatic drainage. Once secreted into the lymph, the chylomicrons enter the blood via the thoracic duct.

Cholesterol absorption also occurs in the small intestine. Cholesterol and its esters are sparingly soluble in water and are present in the lipid emulsion phase of the intestinal contents. Cholesterol esters are hydrolyzed by pancreatic esterases and the free cholesterol is incorporated into mixed micelles with bile salts. Cholesterol crosses the intestinal membrane and after absorption cholesterol is largely reesterified within the mucosal cell and incorporated within chylomicrons before secretion into the lymph.

ABSORPTION OF PROTEINS

End products of hydrolysis of proteins are amino acids. Absorption of amino acids occurs chiefly in the small intestine and is an active enzyme requiring process resembling the active transport of glucose. There are six or more specific transport systems for amino acids being carried into the bloodstream:
1. A system for small neutral amino acids, such as glycine.
2. A system for large neutral amnio acids, such as phenyl alanine.
3. A system of basic amino acids, such as lysine.
4. A system for acidic amino acids, such as aspartic acid.
5. A system for protein.
6. A system for very small peptides.

Amino acids compete with one another for absorption via a particular pathway. Thus, high levels of leucine lower the absorption of isoleucine and valine.

Occasionally, proteins also escape digestion and are absorbed directly into the blood. This occurs more often in the very young, since the permeability of their intestinal mucosa is greater, allowing the passage of antibodies of colostral milk. This passage of protein into blood may be sufficient to cause immunological sensitization and related food allergies.

The L-amino acids are absorbed more rapidly than D isomers and pass through the capillaries of the villi directly into the bloodstream, which carries them to the tissues to be used to build or replace tissue. The amino acids are also oxidized to furnish energy. Although, the body can store carbohydrates and fat, it cannot store protein.

ABSORPTION OF VITAMINS

Most vitamins are absorbed in the upper small intestine. The fat-soluble vitamins (A, D, E and K) need fat and bile salts to be absorbed. Taking a multivitamin capsule with water does not provide the fat necessary for the absorption of fat-soluble vitamins. Vitamin B_{12} absorption depends on its binding to an intrinsic factor produced in the stomach. This complex along with calcium ions finds acceptor sites in the lower small intestine.

BILE PIGMENTS: BILIVERDIN AND BILIRUBIN

When red blood cells (RBCs) die, the hemoglobin is liberated and the heme is separated from the globin. The body removes the iron from heme and reuses it. The heme with iron removed becomes bilirubin. Biliverdin is reduced in the reticuloendothelial cells of the liver, spleen and bone narrow to form biliverdin, the main bile pigment excreted into bile by the liver. In the intestines, some bilirubin is converted into stercobilinogen and stercobilin, a pigment that gives feces its characteristic yellow-brown color. Some bilirubin is absorbed into the bloodstream and comes to the liver where it is converted into urobilinogen and then to urobilin, which appears in the urine giving that fluid its characteristic color. Reactions are as below:

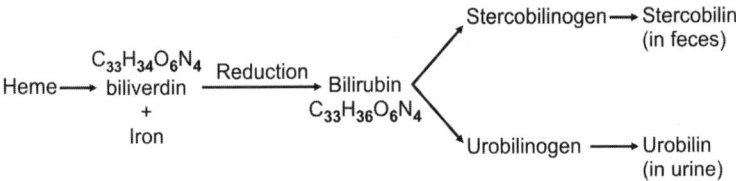

Biliverdin, bilirubin and urobilinogen are the bile pigments. If the bile duct is blocked, bile pigments remain in the bloodstream producing jaundice. When the bile duct is blocked, no bile pigment can enter the intestine and the feces will appear clay colored or nearly colorless.

Bilirubin is an orange-yellow pigment in the bile, whereas biliverdin is a green bile pigment, the oxidized form of bilirubin. Their presence in urine is detected by:

1. Gmelin's test.
2. Fouchet's test.

Bilirubin in the bile is reduced by bacteria in the intestine to urobilinogen (stercobilinogen). The greater part of the urobilinogen is reabsorbed and brought again in blood to the liver.

Bile

Fresh human bile is a clear golden yellow liquid formed and secreted by the liver. It is slightly viscous and tastes bitter. It has a pH 7.5–8.5.

About 500–700 mL of bile are secreted daily by the liver. A part of it, about 500 mL, is stored in the gallbladder, where it is concentrated and periodically discharged into small intestines. The bile in the gallbladder is more viscous and has a greenish tinge because of the presence of bile pigments. During digestion, the gallbladder contracts to supply bile to the intestines, via the common bile duct. The bile mixes with the pancreatic juice and helps to emulsify the water insoluble fatty materials and thus greatly increase the exposure to water and lipase. Triacylglycerols are hydrolyzed to fatty acids, glycerol and some monoacylglycerols.

Normally, bile is excreted by the liver into small intestine and eventually end up in the feces. The presence of bile in urine indicates obstruction to the flow of bile to the intestines. Bile in the urine is indicated by a greenish-brown color. Bile in the urine is also indicated by the presence of yellow foam, when urine is shaken.

Bile Salts

Sodium and potassium glycolate, and sodium and potassium taurocholate are both bile salts derived from cholic acid. They have the ability to lower the surface tension and increase surface area, thus aiding in the emulsification of fats. They also increase the effectiveness of pancreatic lipase in its digestive action on emulsified fats.

In addition, bile salts aid the absorption of fatty acids through the walls of the intestine. After absorption of these fatty acids, the bile salts are removed and carried back by portal circulation to the liver, where they are again returned to the bile. Bile salts also stimulate intestinal motility. Bile salts keep cholesterol in solution form.

The bile salts also assist in the absorption of the fat-soluble vitamins (A, D, E and K) from the digestive tract into blood. This work reabsorbs some bile pigments some of which eventually leave the body through urine. Presence of bile salts in the urine is tested by Hay's sulfur powder test.

QUESTIONS

1. **Name any four digestive enzymes. How are proteins digested and absorbed?**
2. **How is starch digested and absorbed?**

MULTIPLE CHOICE QUESTIONS

3. Pancreatic amylase digests starch and glycogen to:
   A. Isomaltose   B. Dextrin
   C. Maltose   D. All of the above
4. Carbohydrates are mainly absorbed from:
   A. Jejunum   B. Stomach
   C. Duodenum   D. Ileum
5. Which sugar is absorbed at the fastest rate from the small intestine?
   A. Fructose   B. Glucose
   C. Galactose   D. Ribose
6. The active transport of glucose is inhibited by:
   A. Ouabain   B. Phlorizin
   C. Both of the above   D. Digitonin
7. Which of the following hormones increases the absorption of glucose from gastrointestinal (GI) tract?
   A. Insulin   B. Glucagon
   C. ADH   D. Thyroid hormones
8. Which enzyme is involved in lipid digestion?
   A. Elastase   B. Lactase
   C. Lipase   D. Lactate dehydrogenase
9. Digestion of triglycerides requires:
   A. Bile salts   B. Bile pigments
   C. Intrinsic factor   D. Bile acids
10. Absorption of fats occurs mainly in:
    A. Stomach   B. Duodenum
    C. Jejunum   D. Ileum
11. Majority of absorbed fat appears in the form of:
    A. VLDL   B. LDL
    C. HDL   D. Chylomicrons
12. Milk protein is digested in the stomach by:
    A. Trypsin   B. Remin
    C. Rennin   D. HCl
13. The site of intestinal absorption of amino acid is:
    A. Jejunum   B. Stomach
    C. Ileum   D. Duodenum
14. Free L-amino acids are absorbed across the intestinal mucosa by:
    A. Sodium-dependent active transport B. Facilitated diffusion
    C. Passive diffusion   D. Osmosis

15. Pancreatic amylase is most active in the range:
    A. pH 1.8–2.2
    B. pH 4.0–5.0
    C. pH 6.2–7.2
    D. pH 8.0–9.0
16. Trypsin shows its optimum activity at:
    A. pH 1.8
    B. pH 4.0
    C. pH 8.9
    D. pH 7.5
17. The optimum pH for pepsin action:
    A. Between pH 1.5–2.2
    B. pH 4.0
    C. Between pH 7.0–7.1
    D. pH 7.5
18. Pancreatic juice contains the precursors of all of the following *except:*
    A. Trypsin
    B. Chymotrypsin
    C. Carboxypeptidase
    D. Aminopeptidase

ANSWERS

3. (D)	4. (A)	5. (C)	6. (C)	7. (D)
8. (C)	9. (A)	10. (C)	11. (D)	12. (C)
13. (A)	14. (A)	15. (C)	16. (C)	17. (A)
18. (D)				

CHAPTER 10

Basic Concepts of Metabolism

DEFINITION OF METABOLISM

Catabolic pathways (reactions) break down complex molecules such as proteins, polysaccharides and lipids to a few simple molecules like CO_2, NH_3 and H_2O. Anabolic pathways (reactions) form complex end products from simple precursors. Smaller molecules are used to synthesize big and complex molecules by anabolic reactions.

Anabolic and catabolic reactions are collectively called metabolic reactions. Metabolism is the total chemical changes taking place in the cell.

SOURCE OF ENERGY

Where does a muscle get its energy to contract? Where does the body get the energy necessary to synthesize protein, to send nerve impulses, to perform countless other functions?

The energy necessary for body functions comes from certain high-energy compounds that yield a large amount of energy on hydrolysis. The key compound of this type is adenosine triphosphate (ATP), hydrolysis of ATP to adenosine diphosphate (ADP) and inorganic phosphate, liberates about 7,600 cal/mol. This hydrolysis breaks one of the two high energy bonds designated by ~ in the structure.

However, the supply of ATP in the body is limited. There must be some mechanism for regulating this high-energy compound so that it will be available for continued use. Body changes ADP back to ATP by adding a high-energy phosphate group to ADP. This process is called phosphorylation.

[Structural formula of ATP: adenine–ribose–triphosphate]

The formula for ATP can be abbreviated as:

Adenosine—O—P(=O)(OH)—O~P(=O)(OH)—O~P(=O)(OH)—OH or A—P~P~P

[Structural formula of ADP: adenine–ribose–diphosphate]

The formula for ADP can be abbreviated as:

Adenosine—O—P(=O)(OH)~O~P(=O)(OH)—OH or A—P~P

BIOLOGICAL OXIDATION

Substrate molecules are oxidized by removal of hydrogen by dehydrogenases. The reduced dehydrogenases are then reoxidized by a group of respiratory catalysts known as catachrome system or electron transport or respiratory chain. Oxidation is loss (of electrons), reduction is gain (of electrons) and mnemonics **OIL RIG**.

Electron Transport (Respiratory) Chain

Biological oxidation consists of a series of reactions, which passes electrons to oxygen in a stepwise fashion. Each of these involves the loss of two electrons by the original organic compound and these electrons are passed to oxygen indirectly.

Energy rich molecules such as glucose or fatty acids are metabolized by a series of oxidation reactions ultimately leading to CO_2 and water. The metabolic intermediates of these reactions donate electrons to specialized coenzymes, nicotinamide adenine dinucleotide (NAD^+) and flavin adenine dinucleotide (FAD) to form the energy-rich reduced coenzymes, NADH and $FADH_2$. These reduced coenzymes, in turn donate a pair of electrons to a specialized set of electron carriers, collectively called electron transport chain or respiratory chain.

Each carrier of the electron transport chain can receive electrons from an electron donor and can subsequently donate electrons to the next carrier in the chain, ultimately to combine with oxygen and protons to form water. This requirement for oxygen makes the electron transport process, the respiratory chain, which accounts for the greatest portion of the body's utilization of oxygen.

As electrons are passed down the electron transport chain, they lose much of their free energy. Part of this free energy can be captured and stored by the production of ATP from ADP and Pi (Fig. 10.1).

The process by which ADP is phosphorylated to ATP as a result of reactions of electron transport system is called oxidative phosphorylation. The process is limited to mitochondrion. Various oxidations occur in other parts of the cell, which liberate only heat without producing any ATP.

The electron transport chain is present in the inner mitochondrial membrane and is the final common pathway by which electrons derived from different fuels of the

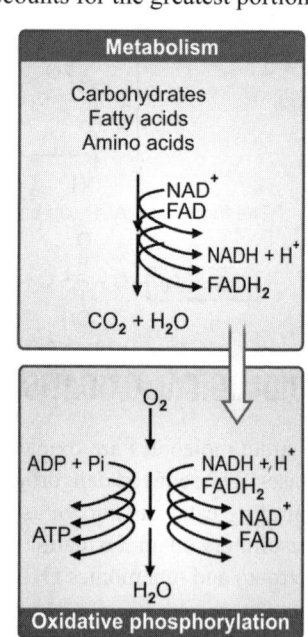

Fig. 10.1: Coenzymes in metabolism

body flow to oxygen. Electron transport and ATP synthesis by oxidative phosphorylation proceed continuously in all the cells of the body that contain mitochondria.

Major Electron Carriers

A wide variety of dehydrogenases participate in the oxidation of metabolic fuels (carbohydrates, lipids and proteins). Most of these enzymes use either NAD^+ or FAD as electron acceptors. The major carrier of electrons in reductive biosynthetic reactions is NADPH.

1. NAD^+ is the electron acceptor in reactions involving oxidations of hydroxylated carbon atom. NAD^+ accepts a hydride ion H^- (two electrons and a proton) to form NADH and the hydroxyl group is oxidized to carbonyl group.

$$R-\underset{H}{\underset{|}{\overset{OH}{\overset{|}{C}}}}-COOH + NAD^+ \longrightarrow R-\overset{O}{\overset{\|}{C}}-COOH + NADH + H^+$$

Reduction of NAD^+ to NADH

2. FAD is electron acceptor in reactions involving the oxidation of two adjacent atoms, resulting in the formation of a carbon-carbon double bond. A hydrogen atom is removed from each carbon atom and is transferred to FAD to form $FADH_2$.

$$R-\underset{H\;H}{\underset{|\;\;|}{\overset{H\;H}{\overset{|\;\;|}{C-C}}}}-R^1 + FAD \longrightarrow R-\underset{H\;H}{\underset{|\;\;|}{\overset{O}{\overset{\|}{C=C}}}}-R^1 + FADH_2$$

Reduction of FAD to $FADH_2$

3. NADPH is the major source of reducing power for biosynthetic pathways. In contrast to NADH which is generated and used primarily in the mitochondria, most of the NADPH is formed and used in the extra-mitochondrial reactions.

In a Nutshell

1. Electron acceptors = NAD^+, FAD.
2. Electron donors = NADH, NADPH.

Extraction of Energy from Metabolic Fuels

Energy is extracted from food via oxidation, resulting in the end products CO_2 and water. This occurs in four stages (Fig. 10.2).

In the stage I, metabolic fuels (carbohydrates, lipid and proteins) are hydrolyzed to their monomeric building blocks namely, glucose, fatty acids and amino acids.

In the stage II, the building blocks are degraded by various pathways to a common metabolic intermediate, acetyl-CoA. Most of the energy contained in the metabolic fuels are conserved in the chemical bonds (electrons) of acetyl-CoA.

In the stage III, the citric acid cycle oxidizes acetyl-CoA to CO_2 and the electron pairs present in the carbon-carbon and carbon-hydrogen bonds are transferred to electron carriers NADH and $FADH_2$.

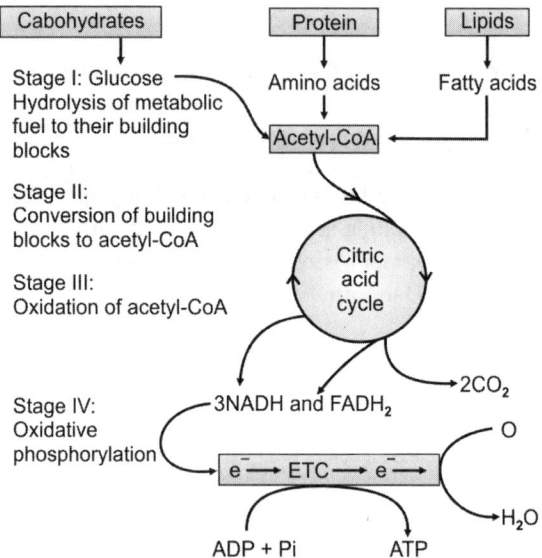

Fig. 10.2: Extraction of energy from metabolic fuels
(ETC, electron transport chain)

The stage IV is the extraction of energy from oxidative phosphorylation, when the energy in electron pairs of NADH and $FADH_2$ is released via ETC and is used to synthesize ATP.

BIOMEDICAL IMPORTANCE OF METABOLISM

1. The concept of metabolism provides a sound understanding of many diseases.
2. The variations and adaptations due to starvation, exercise, pregnancy and lactation are included in normal metabolism.
3. Abnormal metabolism results from nutritional deficiency, enzyme deficiency and excessive secretion of hormones.
4. Diabetes mellitus is an example of a disease caused by abnormal metabolism.

Carbohydrate Metabolism

1. Pyruvate and lactate are formed in the mammalian cells as a result of oxidation of glucose by glycolysis.
2. In the absence of oxygen, glycolysis occurs in the cytoplasm of the cells producing lactate only.
3. Under aerobic conditions pyruvate is metabolized to acetyl-CoA, which enters citric acid cycle for complete oxidation to CO_2 and H_2O.
4. Glucose also takes part in other metabolic processes:
   a. It is converted to glycogen for storage particularly in liver and skeletal muscles.
   b. The hexose monophosphate (HMP) shunt or the pentose phosphate pathway arriving from intermediates of glycolysis is a source of reducing equivalents (2H) for biosynthesis of fatty acids, cholesterol, etc. and is a source of ribose, which is required for nucleic acid formation.
   c. Triose phosphate of glycolysis is a source of glycerol of fat.
   d. Pyruvate and intermediates of TCA cycle form amino acids and cholesterol, the precursor of all steroid hormones in the body.

Lipid Metabolism

1. The long chain fatty acids are synthesized from acetyl-CoA derived from carbohydrates or from dietary lipids.
2. In the tissues, fatty acids are oxidized to acetyl-CoA or esterified to acylglycerol to form fat, which is the main calorie reserve of the body.
3. Acyl-CoA formed by the β-oxidation has the following significant roles in the body:

a. It liberates CO_2 and H_2O and also yields high energy. Therefore during oxidation of fatty acids by β-oxidation, for their complete oxidation, more energy is formed.
   b. It is a source of cholesterol biosynthesis.
   c. In liver it forms ketone bodies, which are alternate water-soluble tissue fuels. These fuels become important sources of energy under certain conditions like starvation.

Amino Acid Metabolism

1. Amino acids are required for protein synthesis.
2. The essential amino acids must be supplied in diet, since they are not synthesized by the tissues.
3. Diet can supplement the non-essential amino acids, which are also formed from the intermediates of citric acid cycle by transamination.
4. Excess amino nitrogen as a result of deamination gives the following products:
   a. CO_2 and H_2O via citric acid cycle.
   b. Glucose by gluconeogenesis.
   c. Ketone bodies.
5. Amino acids are precursors of many other important compounds like purines, pyrimidines and hormones such as epinephrines and thyroxine.

Inter-relationship in the Metabolism of Proteins, Lipids and Carbohydrates

Glucose is converted into glycerol through triosephosphate and acetyl-CoA through pyruvate. Acetyl-CoA helps the formation of fatty acids with malonyl-CoA. Glycerol and fatty acids combine to form triacylglycerol (neutral fat). The ketoacids in TCA cycle are converted into amino acids by transamination.

Fat is oxidized to form acetyl-CoA, which enters the citric acid cycle. Malate of citric acid cycle is permeable to pass through the mitochondrial membrane into cytosol where it is converted ultimately to glucose by gluconeogenesis. Fatty acids with odd number of carbon atoms also enter citric acid cycle being converted to propionate. Protein is hydrolyzed to amino acids.

Basic Concepts of Metabolism

QUESTIONS

1. How is energy extracted from food?
2. Define anabolism, catabolism and metabolism.
3. Write short notes on:
   A. Oxidative phosphorylation.
   B. Major electron carriers.
   C. Respiratory chain.

MULTIPLE CHOICE QUESTIONS

4. All the following statements regarding metabolism are correct *except:*
   A. It consists of anabolism (synthesis) and catabolism (degradation)
   B. It can be studied by in vitro and in vivo methods
   C. During anabolism, energy is liberated
   D. It indicates the sequence of chemical reactions undergone by the food from ingestion to excretion of metabolites
5. All the following in vivo methods are used to study metabolism *except:*
   A. Studies with purified vaccines
   B. Use of radioactive isotopes
   C. Respiratory exchange experiment
   D. Organ perfusion technique
6. Major methods to separate and purify biomolecules is:
   A. Salt fractionation
   B. Gel filtration
   C. Ultracentrifugation
   D. All of the above
7. Radioactive isotope used to study carbohydrate metabolism:
   A. 131 I_2
   B. 14 C
   C. 24 C
   D. 59 Fe
8. Radioactive isotope study thyroid function in:
   A. 14 C
   B. 131 I
   C. 32 P
   D. 45 Ca
9. Oxidation in defined as the following *except:*
   A. Loss of electron
   B. Loss of hydrogen
   C. Addition of oxygen
   D. Gain of electron
10. Oxidoreductases involved in biological oxidation are all of the following *except:*
    A. Dehydrogenases
    B. Hydroperoxidases
    C. Transaminases
    D. Oxygenases

11. **The sequence of enzymes and electron carries for the transport of reducing equivalent from substrates to molecular oxygen:**
    A. Ornithine cycle
    B. Cori cycle
    C. Respiratory chain
    D. γ-glutamyl
12. **The respiratory chain (electrotransport chain) is located in:**
    A. Nucleus
    B. Ribosomes
    C. Lysosomes
    D. Mitochondria
13. **All of the following electron carriers are components of the electron transport chain** *except:*
    A. $NADP^+$
    B. NAD^+
    C. FAD
    D. Coenzyme Q
14. **When the substrate enters the respiratory chain through NAD linked dehydrogenase the ATP yield is:**
    A. 4
    B. 3
    C. 5
    D. 6
15. **Number of ATP molecules produced when reducing equivalents entering ETC through FAD-linked dehydrogenase is:**
    A. 2
    B. 3
    C. 5
    D. 6
16. **The energy currency of the cell is:**
    A. GRP
    B. ATP
    C. ADP
    D. Glucose
17. **Cytochromes are enzymes, which function as electron transfer agent in:**
    A. Transamination
    B. Hydrolysis
    C. Conjugation reaction
    D. Oxidation and reduction
18. **Oxidation phosphorylation is a process for:**
    A. Phosphorylation of glucose
    B. Generating creatine phosphate
    C. Generating ATP
    D. Utilizing ATP
19. **All of the following are concerned with mechanism of oxidative phosphorylation** *except:*
    A. Conformational coupling hypothesis
    B. Chemiosmotic theory
    C. Chemical coupling hypothesis
    D. Beer-Lambert law

ANSWERS

4. (C)	5. (A)	6. (D)	7. (B)	8. (B)	
9. (D)	10. (C)	11. (C)	12. (D)	13. (A)	
14. (B)	15. (A)	16. (B)	17. (D)	18. (C)	
19. (D)					

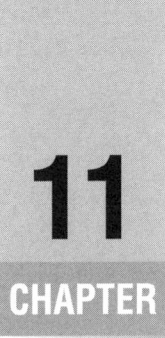

11 CHAPTER

Metabolism of Carbohydrates

Carbohydrate metabolism is basically the metabolism of glucose and substances related to glucose. Carbohydrates supply more than 50% of the energy requirements of the body.

FATE OF GLUCOSE AFTER ABSORPTION

In the liver, glucose undergoes a variety of chemical changes depending upon the physiological need of the body.
1. When there is physiological demand for energy, glucose may be oxidized completely to CO_2, water and energy (glycolysis and citric acid cycle).
2. Excess glucose may be converted to glycogen and deposited in liver, muscle and tissues (glycogenesis).
3. To maintain the blood glucose level liver glycogen is reconverted to glucose, which enters the blood (glycogenolysis).
4. Excess glucose after conversion to glycogen may be converted to fatty acids and stored as triglycerides in the fat depots.
5. In muscle contraction, only partial degradation (glucosis) may take place resulting in the formation of lactic acid, which is largely disposed off by the liver.
6. Small amounts of glucose may be utilized for the synthesis of ribose and deoxyribose for the synthesis of nucleic acids.

INTERMEDIARY METABOLISM OF CARBOHYDRATES

The metabolism of carbohydrate may be subdivided in the following categories.

Glycogenesis: The synthesis of glycogen from glucose.

Glycogenolysis: Breakdown of liver and muscle glycogen (hydrolysis of glycogen into glucose).

Glycolysis: The oxidation of glucose or glycogen to pyruvate by Embden-Meyerhof pathway.

Hexose monophosphate shunt: This is an alternate aerobic pathway to the Embden-Meyerhof pathway for oxidation of glucose.

Oxidation of pyruvate to acetyl-CoA: The necessary step prior to the entry of the products of glycolysis into the citric acid cycle.

Gluconeogenesis: Formation of glucose or glycogen from non-carbohydrate sources.

Transport of Glucose to Cells: Facilitated Transport

Glucose cannot directly diffuse into the cell, but enters by one of the two transport mechanisms. In first mechanism, the facilitated (active) transport is mediated by a family of at least five glucose transporters in the cell membrane designated GLUT1 to GLUT5.

Glycolysis—Embden-Meyerhof Pathway

Glycolysis is the central pathway of glucose metabolism. It occurs in the cytosol of all cells. Glycolysis is defined as the pathway that converts glucose to pyruvate (Fig. 11.1).

The glycolytic pathway is employed by all tissues for the breakdown of glucose to provide energy (in the form of ATP) and intermediates for other metabolic pathways. Carbohydrate metabolism is the metabolism of glucose because all sugars (whether arising from the diet or from catabolic reactions in the body) ultimately can be converted into glucose.

Reactions of Glycolysis

The conversion of glucose to pyruvate can be summarized as follows:

Glucose 6-phosphate + 2 ADP $\longrightarrow$ 2 Pyruvic acid + 2 ATP
(from glycogen or glucose)   (pyruvate)

The ATP formed is utilized for muscle contraction. As ATP is used it is converted to ADP and then must be regenerated. Over 90% of energy is the RBCs is produced by glycolysis.

Net production of ATP = 6 + 4 – 2 = 8 (in aerobic glycolysis).
= 4 – 2 = 2 (in anaerobic glycolysis).

Aerobic Glycolysis

Pyruvate is the end product of glycolysis in cells with mitochondria and an adequate supply of oxygen. This series of 10 reactions is called aerobic glycolysis because oxygen is required to reoxidize the NADH formed during the oxidation of glyceraldehyde 3-phosphate. Aerobic glycolysis is followed by the oxidative decarboxylation of pyruvate to acetyl-CoA, the fuel for citric acid cycle.

Net production of ATP in aerobic glycolysis is $6 + 4 - 2 = 8$.

Anaerobic Glycolysis

Alternatively, the pyruvate can be reduced by NADH to form lactate. This conversion of glucose to lactate is called anaerobic (short supply of oxygen) glycolysis because there is no net formation of NADH and therefore it can occur in the absence of oxygen. Anaerobic glycolysis allows the continued production of ATP in tissues that lack mitochondria (e.g. RBCs).

Net production of ATP in anaerobic glycolysis is $4 - 2 = 2$.

GLYCOLYSIS

All the enzymes of Embden-Meyerhof pathway are present in the cytosol. The 10 steps of glycolysis are:

1. *Phosphorylation of glucose:* Glucose enters the glycolytic pathway by the phosphorylation to glucose 6-phosphate. It takes place in all tissues, but mainly in the liver and muscles.
2. *Isomerism of glucose 6-phosphate:* Glucose 6-phosphate to fructose-6-phosphate by the enzyme phosphoglucose isomerase.
3. *Phosphorylation of fructose 6-phosphate:* Fructose 6-phosphate is changed to 1,6-biphosphate by the action of enzyme phosphofructokinase. ATP is converted to ADP during this reaction.
4. *Cleavage of fructose 1,6-diphosphate:* Enzyme aldolase cleaves fructose 1,6-biphosphate to two three-carbon compounds, glyceraldehyde 3-phosphate and dihydroxyacetone phosphate.
5. *Isomerization of dihydroxyacetone phosphate:* Dihydroxyacetone phosphate is converted to glyceraldehyde 3-phosphate by the action of the enzyme phosphotriose isomerase. This isomerization results in the production of two molecules of glyceraldehyde 3-phosphate from the cleavage products of fructose 1,6-biphosphate.
6. *Oxidation of glyceraldehyde 3-phosphate:* The conversion of glyceraldehyde 3-phosphate to 1,3-biphosphoglycerate by glyceralde-

hyde-3-phosphate dehydrogenase is the first oxidation-reduction reaction of glycolysis. During this reaction, NAD^+ is reduced to $NADH + H^+$. Because there is only a limited amount of NAD^+ in the cell, the NADH formed must be reoxidized to NAD^+ for glycolysis to continue. Two major mechanisms for oxidizing NADH are:
  a. The NADH-linked conversion of pyruvate to lactate.
  b. Oxidation via respiratory system (aerobic).
7. *Formation of ATP from 1,3-diphosphoglycerate:* 1,3-diphosphoglycerate is changed to 3-phosphoglycerate by the action of enzyme phosphoglycerokinase. In this reaction two ADPs (one each for 3 carbon compound) are changed to two ATPs, which replaces the two ATPs consumed in the earlier formation of glucose 6-phosphate and fructose 1,6-biphosphate.
8. *Shift of the phosphate group from carbon 3* to carbon 2,3-phosphoglycerate is changed to 2-phosphoglycerate by the action of the enzyme phosphoglyceromutase.
9. *Dehydration of 2-phosphoglycerate:* 2-phosphoglycerate is changed to phosphoenolpyruvate by the action of enzyme enolase.
10. *Formation of pyruvate:* The phosphoenolpyruvate is changed to pyruvate by the action of enzyme pyruvic kinase. During this reaction, two ADPs are changed to ATPs (one for each 3-carbon compounds).

The sequence of reactions involved in glycolysis is summarized below.

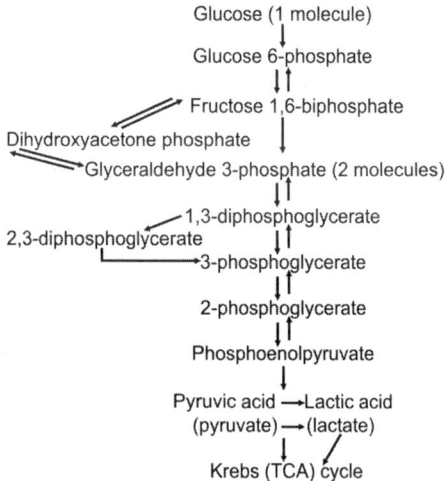

Fig. 11.1: Glycolysis—Embden-Meyerhof pathway

Reduction of Pyruvate to Lactate

Pyruvate is changed to lactate through the enzyme lactic dehydrogenase. At the same time, NADH + H$^+$ are changed to NAD$^+$ (Fig. 11.2).

The formation of lactate is the major steps for pyruvate in RBCs, lens and cornea of the eye, kidneys, medulla, tears and leukocytes.

Energy Production in Glycolysis

The net gain of ATP molecules during glycolysis is eight (Table 11.1).

TRICARBOXYLIC ACID CYCLE (KREBS CYCLE/CITRIC ACID CYCLE)

Unlike glycolysis, which takes place in the cytoplasm, the tricarboxylic acid (TCA) cycle (Fig. 11.3) occurs within the mitochondria. Erythrocytes differ from most other human cells in that they lack mitochondria, and cannot therefore use TCA cycle.

The TCA cycle also called citric acid or Krebs cycle is so named because several of its intermediates have three carboxyl groups; citrate, cis-aconitate and isocitrate. The remaining six intermediates are dicarboxylic acids.

The TCA cycle is the final common pathway of oxidation (the metabolism) of carbohydrates, fatty acids and proteins (amino acids) through which acetyl-CoA is completely oxidized to CO_2 and finally water. Although its primary function is energy production, it also provides intermediates to synthesize the amino acids and porphyrins.

TABLE 11.1: ATP molecules gain in aerobic glycolysis

Sl No	Reactions— aerobic phase	ATP used	ATP formed
1.	Glucose + ATP → Glucose 6-phosphate	1	
2.	Fructose 6-phosphate + ATP → Fructose 1,6-biphosphates	1	
3.	Reoxidation of 2 (NADH + H$^+$) formed in reaction catalyzed by glyceraldehyde 3-phosphate dehydrogenase, in the respiratory chain (aerobic phase)		6
4.	2 (1,3-diphosphoglyceric acid) to 2 (3-phosphoglyceric acid)		2
5.	2 (phosphoenolpyruvic acid) to 2 (enol pyruvic acid)		2
		2	10

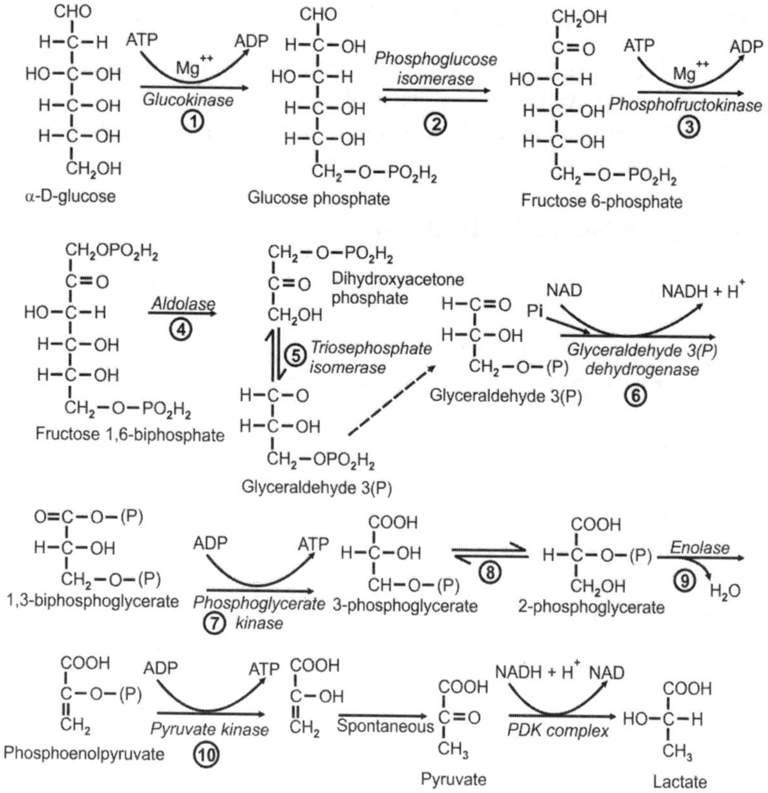

Fig. 11.2: Glycolysis

The aerobic sequence converts the pyruvic acid and lactic acids (from anaerobic glycolysis) into CO_2, H_2O and energy although a series of 8 reactions called citric acid cycle or Krebs cycle. The cycle uses oxygen transported to the cells by hemoglobin; hence the term aerobic. The cycle takes place in the mitochondria, the 'powerhouse' of the cell.

The first step in the aerobic process is the formation of acetyl-CoA (active acetate) form pyruvic acid. Hence, acetyl-CoA is the, acetyl derivative of coenzyme A and is the converting substance in the metabolism of carbohydrates, lipids and fats. Acetyl-CoA becomes the fuel for Kerbs cycle.

Acetyl-CoA reacts with oxaloacetic acid and goes through the eight steps of Kerbs cycle. At the end of the cycle, oxaloacetic acid is regenerated and picks up another molecule of acetyl-CoA to carry it through the cycle.

Metabolism of Carbohydrates

During the cycle acetyl-CoA is oxidized to CO_2 and at the same time NADH and $FADH_2$ are produced. These enter into the electron transport chain that functions in the inner membranes of the mitochondria. The overall reaction of the Krebs cycle can be summarized in the following equation:

$$\text{Acetyl-CoA} + 3NAD^+ + FAD + GDP + Pi + 2H_2O \longrightarrow$$
$$+$$
$$CoA + 2CO_2 + 3NADH + 3H^+ + FADH_2 + GTP + 2H_2O$$

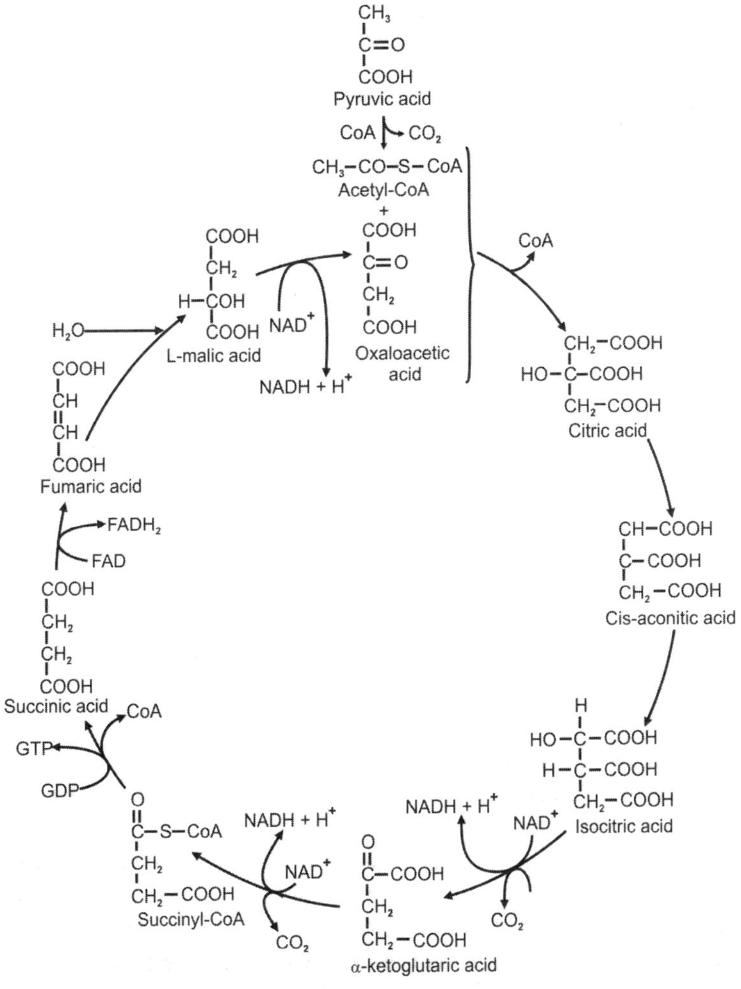

Fig. 11.3: Citric acid cycle

Two C atoms enter the cycle as acetyl-CoA and leave as CO_2. Four pairs of electrons are transferred during each turn of the cycle, three pairs of electrons for reducing NAD^+ to $NADH + H^+$ and one pair for reducing FAD to $FADH_2$.

EIGHT STEPS IN CITRIC ACID CYCLE

1. Synthesis of citric acid from acetyl-CoA and oxaloacetic acid.
2. Isomerization of citric acid to isocitric acid.
3. Oxidation and decarboxylation of isocitric acid yielding the first NADH molecule produced in the cycle and first release of CO_2.
4. Oxidative decarboxylation of α-ketoglutaric acid: The mechanism of this oxidative decaboxylation is similar to that used for conversion of pyruvic acid to acetyl-CoA. The reaction releases the second CO_2 and produces the second NADH in the cycle.
5. Cleavage of succinyl-CoA: Succinate thiokinase cleaves the high-energy thioester bond of succinyl-CoA. The reaction is coupled to phosphorylation of GDP to GTP. The energy content of GTP is same as that of ATP and the 2 molecules are interchangeable.
6. Oxidation of succinic acid: Succinic acid is oxidized to fumaric acid by succinate dehydrogenase producing the reduced coenzyme $FADH_2$. FAD rather than NAD^+ is the electron acceptor because the reducing power of succinic acid is not sufficient to reduce NAD^+.
7. Hydrolysis of fumaric acid to produce malic acid.
8. Oxidation of malic acid to oxaloacetic acid. This reaction produces the third and final NADH of the cycle. Steps 6, 7 and 8 are for the regeneration of oxaloacetic acid.

Citric Acid Cycle: Summary

Acetyl-CoA is joined by oxaloacetate to form citrate. Citrate loses 2 molecules of CO_2 stepwise and in the last step of the cycle oxaloacetate is regenerated for initiating a new cycle by reaction with another molecule of acetyl-CoA. In the citric acid cycle 2 molecules of CO_2 are formed as end product. During the oxidation of acetate to CO_2 some coenzyme molecules are reduced. The reduced coenzyme molecules are oxidized (regenerated) via a series of reactions, which involve the transfer of hydrogen atoms from acetate and other intermediates to oxygen. Such series of oxidation-reduction reactions are known as electron transport chain. Thus the electron transport chain produces most of ATPs formed in the oxidation of glucose.

Citric Acid Cycle: The Common Pathway

Citric acid is the common pathway for the metabolism of carbohydrates, fats and proteins since it provides the complete oxidation of acetyl-CoA to CO_2 and water (Fig. 11.4).

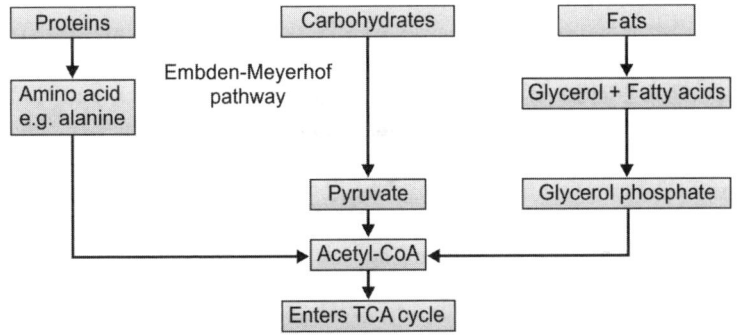

Fig. 11.4: Citric acid cycle as a common pathway

ENERGETICS

Energy Production in Glycolysis and TCA Cycle

From the lowest to the highest forms of life, ATP is universally used as the principal carrier of energy for bodily functions. It is the chief means used by the body to trap energy available by oxidation. Virtually all biochemical energetics comes down to the synthesis and use of ATP.

Almost any energy-demanding activity of the body consumes ATP. An adult human being at rest consumes about 40 kg of ATP per day. Muscle contract can be written as a chemical reaction of ATP changing to adenosine diphosphate and inorganic phosphate (Pi).

ATPs Generated in TCA Cycle

If ATP release from pyruvic acid is considered then there are six sites at which energy is generated. If acetyl-CoA is considered only five sites of energy generation are left. These sites are as follows.
   Conversion of:
1. Pyruvic acid to acetyl-CoA, 1 NADH   = 3 ATP
2. Isocitric acid to α-ketoglutaric acid, 1 NADH = 3 ATP
3. α-ketoglutaric acid to succinyl-CoA, 1 NADH   = 3 ATP

4. Succinyl-CoA to succinic acid, 1 GTP   = 1 ATP
5. Succinic acid to fumaric acid, 1 FADH$_2$ = 2 ATP
6. Malic acid to oxaloacetic acid, 1 NADH   = 3 ATP
                                    Total   15 ATP

Net ATP produced per glucose molecule = 15 × 2 = 30
Total ATP per glucose (aerobic oxidation) = 30 + 8 = 38.

When 1 molecule of glucose is broken down, 38 molecules of ATP are produced (30 from citric acid cycle and 8 from glycolysis).

When 1 mole of glucose (180 g) is converted into CO_2 and H_2O, 2,868 kJ of energy is released. This energy is enough to produce 100 ATP molecules. However, in cells only 38 molecules of ATP are produced on the oxidation of 1 molecule of glucose. Thus the efficiency of energy conversion is only 38%. This is more than any man-made device designed for energy utilization. The rest 62% of energy is liberated as heat and is utilized to maintain the body temperature.

Glycolysis and Krebs cycle: To get maximum available energy from glucose, it has to be oxidized completely to CO_2 and H_2O.

The pyruvic acid or lactic acid produced by the muscle and liver is oxidized to acetyl-CoA, which combines with a molecule of oxaloacetate

Relaxed muscle + ATP ⟶ Contracted muscle + ADP + Pi

to form citric acid. During the citric acid cycle, the acetyl-CoA is oxidized to CO_2 and H_2O with the production of large amounts of energy and oxaloacetate molecule is regenerated.

Hexose Monophosphate Shunt and Uronic Acid Pathway

Glucose is also metabolized through certain other pathways, which are not so important for energy production, but are extremely important as synthetic pathways for a number of substances. HMP pathway and the uronic acid pathway are of this category.

Uronic Acid Pathway

Uronic acid pathway is another alternative pathway for oxidation of glucose. It provides D-gluconic acid, which is used for the synthesis of glucose.

Hexose monophosphate shunt/HMP shunt is an alternate pathway for oxidation of glucose. It is not meant for energy and ATP is not produced. This pathway provides NADPH, which is used for reductive synthesis of pentoses, which is used for nucleic acid synthesis. This pathway operates only in certain special tissues like liver, adipose tissue, lactating mammary gland, lens of the eye, adrenal cortex, gonads, etc.

It is a multicyclic process, 3 molecules of glucose 6-phosphate enter the cycle, producing 3 molecules of CO_2 and 3 molecules of 5 carbon residues to give 2 molecule of glucose 6-phosphate and 1 molecule of glyceraldehyde 3-phosphate.

$NADP^+$ is used as hydrogen acceptor and not NAD^+ and CO_2 is produced in this pathway, which is not produced in glycolysis.

BLOOD SUGAR LEVEL AND ITS CLINICAL SIGNIFICANCE

Normal Value

The range of normal fasting or postabsorptive blood glucose taken at least 13 hours after last meal as per glucoseoxidase method is 70–100 mg%.

The concentration of glucose in the blood is the net result of two processes, which are explained in this Chapter in Homeostasis part.

Abnormalities in Blood Glucose Level

Increase in blood glucose level above normal is hyperglycemia and decrease is hypoglycemia.

Causes of Hyperglycemia

1. Diabetes mellitus in which fasting blood sugar may vary from normal to 500 mg% and more, depending on the severity of the disease.
2. Hyperactivity of the thyroid, pituitary and adrenal glands.
3. In pancreatitis and carcinoma of pancreas.
4. Sepsis and in many infectious diseases.
5. Emotional stress.

Causes of Hypoglycemia

The blood glucose in this condition is below 40 mg%.
1. Overdosage of insulin in the treatment of diabetes mellitus.
2. Hypoactivity of thyroid, hypopituitarism and hypoadrenalism.
3. Severe liver diseases.
4. In childhood, an idiopathic hypoglycemia, due to sensitivity to the amino acid leucine.
5. In glycogen storage diseases like von Gierke disease, liver phosphorylase disease; due to impaired ability to produce glucose from glycogen.

Glycosuria: Although normal urine contains virtually no sugar under certain circumstances, glucose or other sugars may be excreted in urine, e.g. glycosuria, fructosuria, galactosuria.

Diabetes Mellitus

Diabetes mellitus is a metabolic disease due to absolute or relative insulin deficiency. The word mellitus is related to sugar, as the urine of the patient contains sugar. The disease causes loss of weight as the body mass is syphoned off through urine.

Diabetes mellitus is a common condition. About 10% of the total population and about 1/5 of persons above age of 50 suffer from this disease. It is a major cause of morbidity and mortality. The disease may be classified into two clinical types:
1. 'Juvenile' onset diabetes. Now called type I insulin-dependent diabetes mellitus (IDDM).
2. Maturity onset diabetes called type II non-insulin-dependent diabetes mellitus (NIDDM).

Causes

1. Disorder of carbohydrate metabolism, cause of which is deficiency or diminished effectiveness of insulin resulting in hyperglycemia and glycosuria.

2. Heredity: In both types of diabetes, familial tendency is noted. Genetic factors are more important in those who develop after 40 years.
3. Autoimmunity: Insulin-dependent juvenile type may be an autoimmune disorder and has been found to coexist with other autoimmune disorders.
4. Infections: Certain virus infections may precipitate juvenile type.
5. Obesity: Majority of middle-aged maturity onset diabetes is caused by obesity. Stress like pregnancy may also precipitate the disease.
6. Diet: Over eating and under activity are also predisposing factors in elderly/middle-aged maturity onset diabetes.
7. Insulin antagonism: In maturity onset diabetes, the deficiency of insulin is relative and glucose-induced insulin secretion may be greater and more prolonged than normal. The relative deficiency may be due to insulin antagonism.

Clinical Features and Biochemical Correlations

Large amounts of glucose may be excreted in the urine (may be 90–100 g/day in some cases). When the blood glucose level exceeds the renal threshold of 180 mg%, glucose is excreted in urine. Due to osmotic effect, more water accompanies the glucose in the urine (polyuria). To compensate for this loss of water, the thirst center is activated and more water is taken (polydipsia). The loss and ineffective use of glucose leads to breakdown of fat and protein and this leads to loss of weight. To compensate for the loss of glucose and protein, patient will take more food (polyphagia).

Oral Glucose Tolerance Test

Glucose tolerance test (GTT) is a standard test that determines the ability of a person to metabolize a given load of glucose.
Carbohydrates tolerance: The ability of the body to utilize carbohydrates may be ascertained by measuring its carbohydrates tolerance. It is indicated by the nature of blood glucose curve following the administration of glucose.

The test is normally carried out in the morning after a night's fast but if necessary it may be done 4–5 hours after the last food was taken.

Blood is taken for the determination of the fasting blood sugar and a specimen of urine is collected. 50 g of glucose is dissolved in about 100–150 mL of water and are then given. Blood for the estimation of blood sugar is drawn at half hourly intervals for 2½ hours after the glucose has been consumed. Urine specimens are collected at the intervals soon after blood is taken. The blood sugar estimation is carried out and a graph is plotted with sugar in mg against time in hours (Fig. 11.5).

Explanation and Significance of a Normal Curve

1. A sharp rise to a peak, averaging about 50% above the fasting level within 30–60 minutes. Extent of the rise varies considerably from person-to-person, but maximum should not exceed 160–180 mg% in normal subjects.
   Reason: Rise is due to glucose directly absorbed from the intestine, which temporarily exceeds the capacity of the liver and tissues to remove it. As the blood glucose concentration increases, regulatory mechanisms come into play.
2. A sharp fall to approximately the fasting level at the end of 1½–2 hours.
   Reason: Glucose now leaves the circulation faster than it is entering.
3. Hypoglycemic dip: Continuing fall to a slightly subfasting (10–15 mg% lower than fasting value) at 2 hours and subsequent rise to fasting level at 2½–3 hours.
   Reason: The hypoglycemic dip is due to 'inertia' of the regulatory mechanisms. The decreased output of glucose by liver and increased utilization induced by the rising blood glucose are not reversed as rapidly as the blood sugar falls.

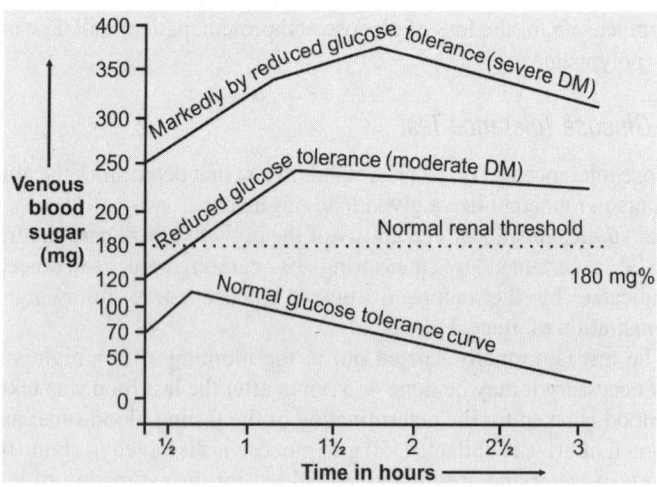

Fig. 11.5: Glucose tolerance test

Diabetic Type of GTC

1. Fasting blood glucose is definitely raised. 110 mg% or more.
2. The highest value is usually reached after 1–1½ hours.
3. The highest value exceeds the normal renal threshold of 180 mg%.
4. Urine samples always contain glucose except in some chronic diabetes or nephritis, which may have raised renal threshold.
5. The blood glucose does not return to the fasting level within 2½ hours. This is the most characteristic feature of the true diabetes mellitus.

REGULATION (HOMEOSTASIS) OF BLOOD GLUCOSE LEVEL

The maintenance of blood sugar level at:
  FBS = 70–100 mg%
  RBS = 80–120 mg%
PPBS = 100–140 mg% under all conditions is known as homeostasis of blood sugar level. It is regulated by hormonal and nervous factors.

The blood sugar level is maintained by two factors (Fig. 11.6).
1. Factors adding glucose to blood.
2. Factors that remove glucose from blood.

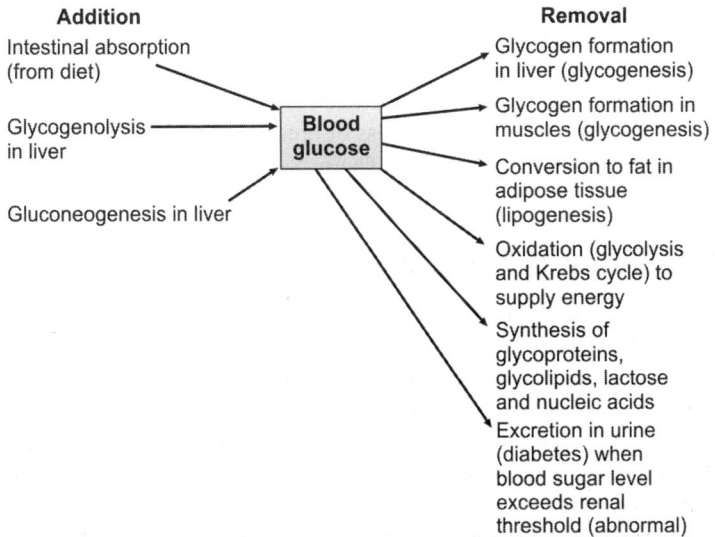

Fig. 11.6: Homeostasis

Glycogenesis (Glycogen Synthesis)

Liver and muscle cells can convert glucose to glycogen by a series of steps called glycogenesis (glycogen creation). The liver holds 70–110 g of glycogen (5% of its weight) and the muscles taken as a whole, contain 170–250 g.

The initial step of glycogenesis is the conversion of glucose-6-P to glucose1-P by phosphoglucomutase. Next, glucose-1-P reacts with uridine triphosphate (UTP) to create UDP-glucose.

$$\text{Glucose 6-P} \xrightarrow{Mg^{++}} \text{Glucose 1-P}$$

$$\text{Glucose 1-P} + \text{UTP} \longrightarrow \text{UDP-glucose} + \text{Protein phosphatase 1}$$

Glycogen synthase then adds this bound glucose in α-1-4 linkage to the glycogen polymer, liberating UDP.

$$\text{UDP-glucose} - (\text{glucose})_n \longrightarrow (\text{glucose})_{n+1} + \text{UDP}$$

In this manner addition of glucose molecules takes place up to eight units. Now a second enzyme called the branching enzyme acts by establishing connection between the 1st and the 6th carbon atoms of the amylose chains and a glycogen molecule is formed ultimately.

Glycogenolysis

When muscles need glucose, they take it back out of glycogen. When the blood needs glucose as the blood sugar has dropped too much, the liver hydrolyzes as much of its glycogen reserves as needed and puts the glucose into circulation. The process of breakdown of liver glycogen to glucose is called glycogenolysis. The process is controlled by several hormones.

Blood Glucose in Postabsorptive State

The postabsorptive state or fasting state is the condition obtaining 12–14 hours after the last meal. There is no intestinal absorption at this time. At the same time, it is not prolonged starvation, which itself leads to several abnormalities in metabolism. The condition of a subject (patient) between 8 AM and 10 AM, if he had his dinner the previous evening at 8 PM and has eaten nothing, thereafter in the night or morning, is said to be postabsorptive.

Under these conditions, the only source of glucose to blood is from liver glycogen. At rest, the tissues of an adult man will be utilizing almost

200 mg% glucose per minute by taking up the glucose from blood. This much will be added by the liver. The glycogen concentration of the liver averages 5% of its weight. Thus an adult liver weighing 1,800 g can store about 90 g of glycogen, which can supply at the rate of 200 mg%/minute for only 7–8 hours.

The skeletal muscles (about 28 kg in an adult male) has a glycogen content of 1% and can hold 280 g of glycogen. This can indirectly supply glucose and blood lactose and liver glycogen for almost 24 hours. But blood sugar levels are maintained fairly constant during long periods of starvation by gluconeogenesis from non-carbohydrates sources such as amino acids and fatty acids.

Gluconeogenesis: The formation of glucose or glycogen from non-carbohydrates sources is called gluconeogenesis. During periods of prolonged starvation when no carbohydrate is available from food, it is by gluconeogenesis that the liver maintains a continuous supply of glucose for the metabolism of brain, erythrocytes and for anaerobic metabolism of skeletal muscles. Glyconeogenesis occurs mainly in the liver and kidneys.

Glycogenic amino acids, lactates pyruvic, glycerol and propionic acid can form glucose. The mechanism involved are essentially the reversal of Krebs cycle and glycolysis.

ROLE OF HORMONES IN THE HOMEOSTASIS OF BLOOD SUGAR LEVEL

Hormones play a very important role in regulating the blood glucose levels. There are two sets of hormones, which are involved in blood glucose regulation and these two sets of hormones show opposite actions to each other.
1. Insulin causes a fall in blood glucose levels (hypoglycemic in nature).
2. The hormones of the second group raise the level (hyperglycemic in nature).

Such hormones are glucagon, glucocorticoids, growth hormone, adrenocorticotropic hormone (ACTH) and thyroxine. Thus, all these are antagonistic to insulin (diabetogenic hormones).

Insulin

This hormone of the β-cells of the islets of Langerhans lowers the blood sugar concentration. Shortly after a meal, there is postprandial (after

meal) hyperglycemia. The β-cells of the islets of Langerhans of pancreas sense this hyperglycemia and release insulin. The hormone enhances the uptake of glucose by tissues probably by enhancing the transport of glucose across the cell membrane. Insulin acts as a key that 'unlocks' the 'door' on cell surface to allow glucose to enter the cell. Insulin decreases the blood glucose level in the following ways:
1. It increases the uptake of glucose by muscle and adipose tissue.
2. Increases glycogenesis, glycolysis and HMP shunt pathway.
3. It inhibits gluconeogenesis and glycogenolysis.
4. It increases the synthesis of protein.
5. It inhibits catabolism of proteins and lipid thus insulin is an anabolic hormone.

Glucagon

This hormone is secreted from α-cells of pancreas in response to hypoglycemia. It increases blood glucose level by:
1. Increasing glycogenolysis and gluconeogenesis in the liver.
2. Decreasing glycolysis and glycogenesis.

Epinephrine

Epinephrine (adrenaline) is secreted by the adrenal medulla in response to any form of stress, hypoglycemia, emotions like fear, anger, joy, sorrow, etc. It increases blood glucose level by:
1. Promoting glycogenolysis in the liver and muscles.
2. Enhancing gluconeogenesis.
3. Inhibiting insulin secretion.
4. Decreasing glycolysis and increasing lipolysis in adipose cell (release of glycerol).

Glucocorticoids

Cortisol is the major glucocorticoid from adrenal cortex and has a hyperglycemic effect by:
1. Increasing gluconeogenesis.
2. Increasing protein breakdown in muscle and liberating amino acids for gluconeogenesis.
3. Inhibiting insulin stimulated uptake of glucose by tissues.
4. Inhibiting glycogenesis.
5. Increasing glycogenolysis.

Growth Hormone

This is secreted from a anterior pituitary in response to hypoglycemia. It increases blood glucose level by:
1. Decreasing the uptake of glucose by muscle and its utilization for glycolysis.
2. Promoting the release of fatty acids from adipose tissue into blood thus inhibiting glucose utilization.

Adrenocorticotropic hormone (ACTH) are also secreted from anterior pituitary and acts similar to growth hormone to increase blood glucose level. They increase gluconeogenesis in the liver. They also increase protein breakdown in tissues and make amino acids available to liver for gluconeogenesis. They also decrease the uptake of glucose by tissues. The overall affect is an increase in the blood sugar level.

Thyroid Hormone (Thyroxine)

Thyroxine is produced from the thyroid gland and is diabetogenic. It increases blood sugar by:
1. Increasing intestinal absorption of glucose.
2. Increasing hepatic glycogenolysis.
3. Increasing glycogenolysis in the liver.

Anything which lowers insulin activity or raises the activity of other hormones will produce hyperglycemia and glycosuria, a condition known as diabetes.

QUESTIONS AND ANSWERS

1. **Can muscle glycogen be a source of blood glucose?**
   Ans: No, as it lacks the enzyme glucose 6-phosphate.

2. **What is galactosemia?**
   Ans: Excretion of galactose in urine due to the deficiency of enzyme galactose 1-phosphate uridyl transferase leads to a condition known as galactosemia.

3. **What is true glucose?**
   Ans: True glucose means only glucose, without taking into account the presence of any other reducing substance in the blood.

4. **How will you estimate true glucose?**
   Ans: By glucose oxidase method.

5. **What are the conditions in which blood sugar level is low?**
   Ans: A. Overdosage of insulin in the treatment of diabetes.
      B. Hypothyroidism.
      C. Addison's disease.
6. **What are the conditions in which blood sugar level is raised?**
   Ans: A. Diabetes mellitus.
      B. Hyperthyroidism.
      C. Hyperadrenalism.
      D. Hyperpituitarism.
      E. Thyrotoxicosis.
7. **What is the normal blood sugar level?**
   Ans: 80–100 mg%.
8. **What is the kidney threshold of glucose?**
   Ans: 180 mg%.
9. **What is the hormone which regulate blood sugar level?**
   Ans: Insulin.
10. **What are the functions of insulin?**
    Ans: A. Insulin promotes the entry of glucose in all the tissues of the body except liver.
       B. It helps in glycogenesis.
       C. It prevents glycogenolysis.
       D. It inhibits gluconeogenic enzymes.
11. **What are the hormones which keep the blood sugar level high?**
    Ans: A. Glucagon.
       B. Epinephrine.
       C. Adrenal cortex hormones.
       D. Growth hormones and ACTH.
       E. Thyroid hormone.
12. **Why cannot insulin be given orally?**
    Ans: Insulin is a polypeptide and is digested by the enzymes of the digestive system into amino acids before it reaches the blood. Hence it cannot be given orally.
13. **What is renal glycosuria?**
    Ans: As a result of low kidney threshold, glucose appears in the urine. Blood sugar level remains normal.
14. **What is the abnormality in the urine sample of diabetic patient and starving patient?**
    Ans: In a diabetic patient, urine will show the presence of glucose and ketone bodies. In starving patient only ketone bodies will be present.

15. **What are the different reducing sugars that appear in the urine and under what conditions?**
    Ans: A. Glucose appears in the urine in renal glucosuria and diabetes mellitus.
    B. Lactose: During later stages of pregnancy and lactation.
    C. Galactose: In galactosuria due to the deficiency of the enzyme galactose 1-phosphate uridyl transferase. This condition is encountered in children.
    D. Fructose: Due to consumption of lots of fruits containing fructose such as grapes, plums and cherry.
    E. Pentoses: Due to consumption of lots of fruits containing pentoses. Also in congenital abnormality to metabolize L-xylulose.

16. **What is glycolysis?**
    Ans: The breakdown of glucose to pyruvic acid or lactic acid is called glycolysis.

17. **Which is the regulatory enzyme in glycogenolysis?**
    Ans: Phosphofructokinase (PFK).

18. **What is the ATP yield in glycolysis under an aerobic condition?**
    Ans: 8 ATP per molecule of glucose metabolized.

19. **What is the ATP yield under aerobic conditions?**
    Ans: 38 ATP per molecule of glucose metabolized, i.e. glycolysis 8 ATP and TCA cycle 30 ATP.

20. **How many ATP are formed in the TCA cycle?**
    A. From acetyl-CoA
    Ans: 12 ATP.
    B. From pyruvate
    Ans: 15 ATP.

21. **Why is citric acid cycle considered the common pathway for carbohydrate, fat and protein metabolism?**
    Ans: Acetyl-CoA comes from all the three metabolism, which are:
    a. Carbohydrate metabolism: Glycolysis.
    b. Fat metabolism: β-oxidation.
    c. Protein metabolism: Transamination.
    Citric acid cycle provides the complete oxidation of acetyl-CoA to CO_2 and water and hence is the common pathway for all the above three metabolisms.

22. **What is oxidative decarboxylation?**
    Ans: Oxidation accompanied by decarboxylation.

23. **What is the oxidative decarboxylation product of pyruvic acid?**
    Ans: Pyruvic acid $\xrightarrow[-2H, -CO_2]{\text{Oxidative decarboxylation}}$ Acetyl-CoA

24. **What is the enzyme for the above oxidative decarboxylation reaction?**
    Ans: Enzyme involved is pyruvate dehydrogenase complex consisting of three enzymes:
    A. Pyruvate dehydrogenase.
    B. Dihydrolipoyl transacetylase.
    C. Dihydrolipoyl dehydrogenase.
25. **What are the cofactors of the above reaction?**
    Ans: A. Thiamine pyrophosphate (TPP).
    B. Lipoic acid.
    C. Coenzyme A (CoASH).
    D. Flavin adenine dinucleotide (FAD).
    E. Nicotinamide adenine dinucleotide (NAD).
    F. Mg^{++} ions.
26. **What is β-oxidation?**
    Ans: Oxidation taking place at β-carbon atom, which is then oxidized to carboxyl group.
27. **Where does β-oxidation take place?**
    Ans: Mitochondria.
28. Describe briefly two mechanisms of blood sugar level.
29. What is the normal fasting level of blood glucose? Discuss the factors controlling the blood glucose level.
30. Write short notes on:
    A. Insulin.
    B. Glucose tolerance test (GTT).
31. Define and give examples of anabolism and catabolism.
32. How many grams of glucose would be necessary to supply 2,500 kcal?
33. List the starting material and end product(s) of each of the following:
    A. Glycolysis.
    B. Krebs cycle.
    C. Glycogenolysis.
    D. Glycogenesis.
    E. Electron transport.

MULTIPLE CHOICE QUESTIONS

34. **The glycolytic pathway is located in:**
    A. Mitochondria   B. Cytosol
    C. Microsomes   D. Nucleus
35. **The end product of aerobic glycolysis is:**
    A. Acetyl-CoA   B. Lactate
    C. Pyruvate   D. CO_2 and H_2O

36. **Glycolysis is always anaerobic in:**
    A. Liver
    B. Brain
    C. Kidneys
    D. Erythrocytes
37. **In glycolysis, glucose is degraded to give:**
    A. 4 molecules of pyruvate
    B. 2 molecules of acetate
    C. 2 molecules of pyruvate
    D. 4 molecules of acetate
38. **Glucose is the only source of energy for:**
    A. Myocardium
    B. Kidneys
    C. Erythrocytes
    D. Thrombocytes
39. **Complete outdating of 1 molecule glucose into CO_2 and H_2O yields:**
    A. 8 ATP equivalents
    B. 15 ATP equivalents
    C. 30 ATP equivalents
    D. 38 ATP equivalents
40. **Each turn of citric acid cycle produces:**
    A. 2 NADH + $FADH_2$ + 2 GTP
    B. 3 NADH + 1 ATP + 1 GTP
    C. 4 NADH + 2 ATP + 2 GTP
    D. 3 NADH + 2 ATP + 1 GTP
41. **The cofactor required by hexokinase is:**
    A. Fe^{++}
    B. Mn^{++}
    C. Mg^{++}
    D. Zn^{++}
42. **Glycogenesis is increased by:**
    A. Glucagon
    B. Insulin
    C. Epinephrine
    D. cAMP
43. **Glucose 3-phosphate for the synthesis of triglycerides in adipose tissue is derived from:**
    A. Glucose
    B. Phosphatidic acid
    C. Diacylglycerol
    D. Glycerol
44. **Gluconeogenesis takes place in:**
    A. Adipose tissue
    B. Muscles
    C. Kidneys
    D. Brain
45. **Glyconeogenesis is decreased by:**
    A. Glucagon
    B. Epinephrine
    C. Insulin
    D. Glucocorticoids
46. **Hexose monophosphate shunt provides:**
    A. Glucose 1-phosphate for glycogen synthesis
    B. Glycerol 3-phosphate for triglyceride synthesis
    C. NADPH for fatty acid synthesis
    D. Glucuronic acid for mucopolysaccharide synthesis
47. **Substrate for invertase is:**
    A. Lactose
    B. Maltose
    C. Sucrose
    D. Dextrin
48. **Between meals, blood glucose level can be maintained by:**
    A. Glycogenolysis in the liver
    B. Glycogenolysis in muscles
    C. Both of the above
    D. None of the above

49. The enzyme which splits a 6 carbon compound into two 3 carbon compounds in glycolysis is:
   A. Phosphotriose isomerase   B. Enolase
   C. Phosphoglycerate mutase   D. Aldolase

50. Glucagon can affect the rate of glycogenesis and glycogenolysis in:
   A. Liver and skeletal muscles B. Liver and heart muscles
   C. Liver   D. Skeletal and heart muscles

51. Blood glucose level is increased by all of the following *except:*
   A. Glucagon   B. Glucocorticoids
   C. Insulin   D. Epinephrine

52. The complete oxidation of glucose occurs in:
   A. Glycolysis   B. HMP shunt
   C. TCA cycle   D. Glycolysis and TCA cycle

53. Glycogenesis is a process by which glycogen is synthesized from:
   A. Pyruvic acid   B. Lactic acid
   C. Glycerol   D. Glucose

54. Glucose tolerance decreases in the following condition:
   A. Hyperthyroidism   B. Diabetes mellitus
   C. Hyperadrenalism   D. Hyperthyroidism

ANSWERS

34. (B)	35. (C)	36. (D)	37. (C)	38. (C)
39. (D)	40. (A)	41. (C)	42. (B)	43. (A)
44. (C)	45. (C)	46. (C)	47. (C)	48. (A)
49. (D)	50. (B)	51. (C)	52. (D)	53. (D)
54. (D)				

12 CHAPTER

Metabolism of Lipids

Atherosclerosis, the deposition of lipid plaques on the lining of arteries is a leading cause of death. Because of the association between atherosclerosis and hyperlipoproteinemia (elevated serum lipoproteins), an extensive campaign of medical research has been launched to study lipid metabolism.

PLASMA LIPIDS

In mammals, principal lipids that have metabolic significance are: triacylglycerol (TAG) also called neutral fats (NFs), phospholipids, steroids, mainly cholesterol, together with products of their metabolism such as long chain fatty acids (free fatty acids), glycerol and ketone bodies.

Extraction of plasma lipids with a suitable lipid solvent and subsequent separation of the extract into various classes of lipids, show the presence of equal quantities of:
1. Triacylglycerol (TAG).
2. Phospholipids (PL).
3. Cholesterol and much smaller fraction of non-esterified long chain fatty acid (NEFA) or free fatty acid (FFA).

Much of the carbohydrates of the diet is converted to fat, before it is utilized for the purpose of energy. Its calorific value is more than double (9.3 kcal/g) that of carbohydrates and proteins and therefore fat is the most concentrated form in which potential energy is stored in the body.

A minimal amount of fat is essential in the diet to provide an adequate supply of certain polyunsaturated FAs (the essential FAs) and of fat-soluble vitamins. Besides being a carrier of these essential compounds, dietary fat is necessary for their efficient absorption from the gastrointestinal tract.

Transportation of Plasma Lipids

Fats are insoluble in water and hydrophobic. To transport them in blood, the most insoluble lipids are associated with more polar ones, such as phospholipids and then combining them with cholesterol and protein to form a hydrophilic lipoprotein complex. Thus the triglycerides derived from intestinal absorption of fat or from the liver are transported in the blood as chylomicrons and very low-density lipoproteins (VLDL). Fat is released from adipose tissues in the form of FFAs and carried in unesterified state in the plasma as an albumin FFA complex.

DIGESTION AND ABSORPTION OF LIPIDS

No digestion of lipids occurs in the mouth or stomach because:
1. The amount of lipase present in saliva and gastric juice is insignificant.
2. There is no mechanism for emulsifying fatty materials in this region.
3. The pH of gastric juice is not conducive for lipid digestion.

The major site of lipid digestion is the small intestine. The main requisites are—pancreatic lipase and bile salts. Bile salts derived from bile, lower the surface tension and emulsify fats, dissolve FAs and water insoluble soaps. The alkaline content of the pancreatic biliary secretions neutralizes and shifts the pH of the food material to the alkaline side for the action by the pancreatic lipase. The lipase hydrolyses the triglycerides to 40% FFAs and glycerol, 50%–57% monoglycerides and diglycerides. 3%–10% is absorbed as triglycerides.

The 2-monoglycerides produced as intermediates are converted to 1-monoglycerides by an enzyme isomerase, which is then digested by lipase to glycerol and FFAs. Of the four products of triglyceride hydrolysis namely FFAs, glycerol, monoglycerides and diglycerides, FFAs and glycerol are easily absorbed as they are water soluble and are then carried away by blood.

Higher FAs, monoglycerides and diglycerides are absorbed with the help of bile salts in the form of water-soluble aggregates. Inside the intestinal epithelial cell, 1-monotriglycerides are hydrolyzed by intracellular lipases to give FAs and glycerol, whereas diglycerides are used for triglyceride synthesis.

Higher FAs are largely utilized for the triglycerides synthesis inside the intestinal epithelial cells and are carried as chylomicrons, which are hydrophobic. Water-soluble triglycerides are covered with a layer of hydrophilic phospholipids, free and esterified cholesterol and some proteins.

LIPID METABOLISM

Most of the energy in fats is contained in the long hydrocarbon chains of FAs. They are the main energy reserve of the body producing 43.62 kJ/g on oxidation, much more than that generated by the oxidation of carbohydrates or proteins (16.8 kJ/g). The FA are oxidized in mitochondria of liver cells and skeletal muscles. During this process, two carbon fragments are removed sequentially to generate acetyl-CoA, which enters the citric acid cycle for production of adenosine triphosphate (ATP) as described in the previous chapter. Palmitic acid, a C-16 FA produces 129 molecules of ATP.

$$\text{Lipids} \xrightarrow{\text{Hydrolysis}} \text{Fatty acids} + \text{Glycerol} \xrightarrow{\beta\text{-oxidation}} \text{Acetyl-CoA} \xrightarrow{\text{Citric acid cycle}} \text{ATP}$$

Lipolysis

Lipolysis is defined as triglyceride hydrolysis, liberates FAs from their main storage depots. Lipolysis begins with the intestinal hydrolysis of dietary triglycerides by pancreatic lipase. Once absorbed into the intestinal mucosa, the resultant FFAs, glycerol and monosaccharides are resynthesized into triglycerides, which combine with lesser amount of protein, phospholipid and cholesterol to form chylomicrons. Plasma lipoprotein lipase, hydrolysis triglycerides in the chylomicrons into FFA and glycerol. Adipose tissue contains a hormone sensitive lipase that hydrolyses its triglycerides.

The glycerol released in lipolysis travels to the liver, where it is phosphorylated to glycerol-3-P. For every 2 moles of glycerol-3-P, 1 mole of glucose can be synthesized in gluconeogenesis. Glycerol-3-P also serves as a precursor to triglyceride synthesis.

Oxidation of Fatty Acids

Large proportions of the absorbed fat is temporarily stored in the liver, which is also the main site for the oxidation and synthesis of FAs.

β-oxidation of Fatty Acids

As the principal route for catabolizing FAs, oxidation occurs in the mitochondria, the intracellular 'power house'. β-oxidation is so named because it oxidizes the β-carbon atom of a FAs to a β-keto acid with sequential removal of two carbon fragment acetyl-CoA.

Alpha-oxidation of FAs occurs in the human brain. The rare inherited absence of an enzyme required for α-oxidation causes Refsum's disease. α-oxidation of FAs is a minor pathway that is found in the liver.

The β-oxidation basically consists of four reactions that can be summarized as follows:

1. $-CH_2-CH_2- + FAD \xrightarrow{\text{Dehydrogenation}} -CH=CH- + FADH_2$

2. $-CH=CH- + H_2O \xrightarrow{\text{Hydrolysis}} -\underset{OH}{\underset{|}{CH}}-CH_2-$

3. $-\underset{OH}{\underset{|}{CH}}-CH_2- + NAD \xrightarrow{\text{Dehydrogenation}} -\underset{O}{\overset{\parallel}{C}}-CH_2- + NADH+H^+$

4. $-\underset{O}{\overset{\parallel}{C}}-CH_2- + CoASH \xrightarrow[\text{CoASH}]{\text{Cleavage by}} -\underset{\substack{\text{Fatty acyl-}\\\text{CoA}}}{\underset{O}{\overset{\parallel}{C}}-S-CoA} + \underset{\substack{\text{Acetyl-}\\\text{CoA}}}{CH_3-CoA}$

The pathway of β-oxidation begins as acyl-CoA dehydrogenase oxidises the FAs (Fig. 12.1) to create a trans double bond between the α- and β-carbon atoms, thereby reducing FAD to $FADH_2$.

This monoenoic is named enoyl-CoA. A hydratase then hydrolyses (hydrates) this double bond yielding β-hydroxyacyl-CoA. A second dehydrogenase oxidises this β-hydroxy group to a β-keto group, creating β-ketoacyl-CoA, and reducing NAD^+ to NADH. Finally, a thiolase uses SH binding of CoASH to cleave the bond between α- and β-carbon atoms liberating acetyl-CoA. The remaining fatty acyl-CoA with two less carbon atoms than the original, can then re-enter β-oxidation cycle.

ENERGETICS

Each passage through β-oxidation removes two carbon atoms from the FAs as acetyl-CoA and produces one molecule of $FADH_2$ and 1 mole NADH, which yield 5 moles of ATP under reoxidation to FAD and NAD^+ in the electron transport chain (2 moles ATP per mole of $FADH_2$ oxidized and 3 moles ATP per mole of NADH oxidized). The complete β-oxidation of palmitic acid ($C_{15}H_{31}COOH$) on completion of β-oxidation produces 8 acetyl-CoA. Transport of electrons in the respiratory chain from reduced $FADH_2$ and NADH in each cycle produces 5 high-energy phosphate bonds. Hence 7 cycles (7 acetyl-CoA) = 7 × 5 = 35 ATP.

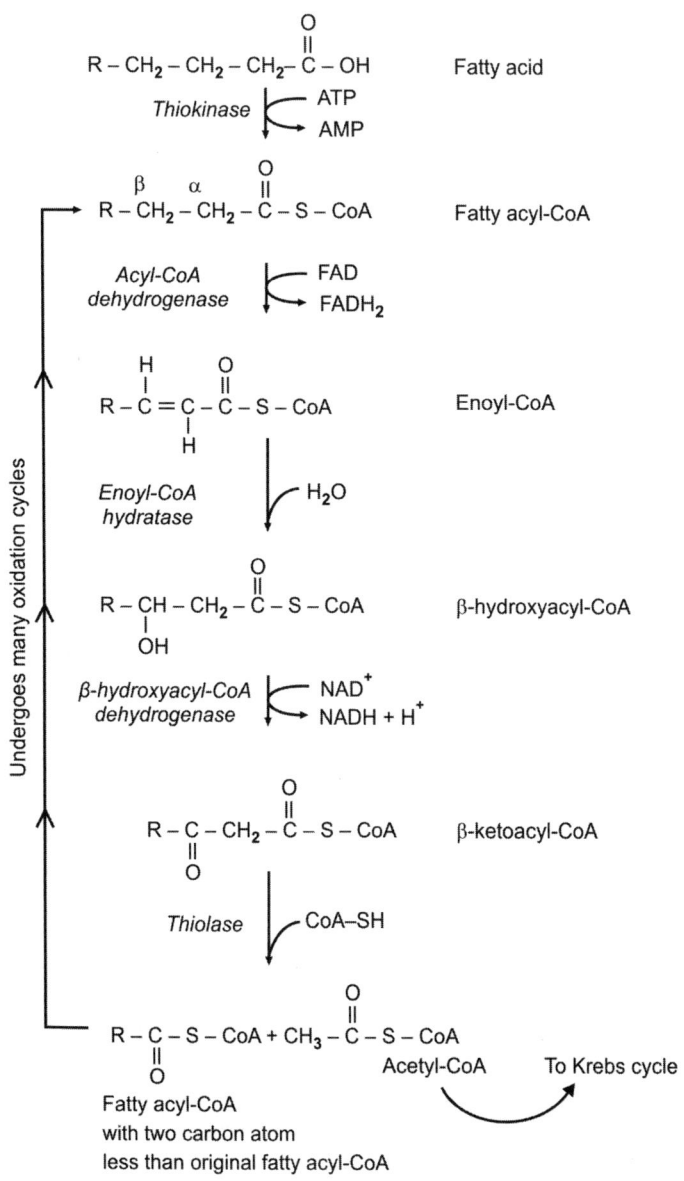

Fig. 12.1: Acetyl-CoA synthesis

Total 8 molecules of acetyl-CoA, when oxidized in TCA cycle will produce 12 × 8 = 96 ATP.
Total high-energy phosphate bonds produced = 131.
In initial activation of FA, ATP utilized = 2.
Hence net ATP produced from 1 mole of palmitic acid is (131 − 2) = 129. Energy production = 129 × 7.6 = 980 kcal/mol of palmitic acid.
Calorie value of palmitic acid (Bomb calorimeter) = 2,340 kcal/mol. Hence, efficiency:

$$\frac{980}{2,340} \times 100 = 41\% \text{ of the total energy of combustion of FA.}$$

The remaining energy is used as heat by the body.

Metabolism of Adipose Tissue

The adipose tissue serves as a storage site for excess fat as well as reserve store of energy, that can be mobilized when needed. It is a storage depot for fats under well fed conditions and reserve source under conditions of starvation.

The triglycerides stored in the adipose tissue are not inert. They undergo daily turnover with new TAG molecules being synthesized and a definite fraction being broken down.

The triglyceride stores in adipose tissue are continually undergoing lipolysis (hydrolysis) and esterification. These two processes are not the forward and reverse phases of the same reaction, but are entirely different pathways involving different reactants and enzymes.

The resultant of these two processes determines the size of the FFAs pool in adipose tissue, which in turn is the source and determinant of the level of FFA circulating in the plasma.

Under well fed conditions, active lipogenesis occurs in the adipose tissue. The dietary FAs transported by the chylomicrons and the endogenously synthesized triglycerides brought by VLDL from liver are both taken up by adipose tissue and esterified and stored as TAG. The lipoprotein molecules are broken down by the lipoprotein lipase present on the capillary wall. The glycerol phosphate used for esterification is derived from glycolysis. The pyruvate formed in the adipose tissue by glycolysis may be oxidatively decarboxylated to acetyl-CoA and used for FAs synthesis. The citrate from the mitochondria reaches the cytoplasm and gets hydrolysed to acetyl-CoA and oxaloacetate. The hexose monophosphate shunt is also active in adipose tissue to provide sufficient reducing power in the form of NADPH for FAs synthesis.

Thus, it is seen that in the well fed conditions, the adipose tissue stores excess calories as TAG and takes up the dietary TAG. The process of glycogenesis by adipose tissue is favored by insulin by increasing the activity of several of the enzymes involved (See section on 'Lipid Metabolism').

The metabolic pattern totally changes under conditions of fasting. TAG from adipose tissue is mobilized under the effects of hormones, glucagon and epinephrine, that are lipolytic. The intracellular hormone sensitive lipase of the adipose tissue is activated by the cAMP-mediated activation cascade. The phosphorylated form of the enzyme is active which acts on TAG and liberates FAs. These FAs are transported by plasma bound to albumin and taken up by tissues like skeletal muscle, heart muscle and liver and used as an alternative source of fuel.

Fatty Liver and Lipotropic Factors

Fatty liver refers to the disposition of excess triglycerides in the liver cells in excess of 5% of the weight of liver. The liver is able to take up FAs from bloodstream and esterify it into TAG. These triglycerides along with endogenously synthesized by the liver is incorporated into VLDL and secreted from the liver. The balance between the storage of TAG in adipose tissue and liver is delicate and can revert to a net transfer of FAs to the liver resulting in accumulation of TAG in liver.

The net accumulation of fat in liver (Fig. 12.2) is mainly due to three reasons:
1. The hepatic uptake of FAs from the bloodstream is dependent on their concentration in blood.
2. The liver has only a limited capacity to dispose off the FAs by oxidation.
3. The capacity of the liver to secret VLDL is also limited.

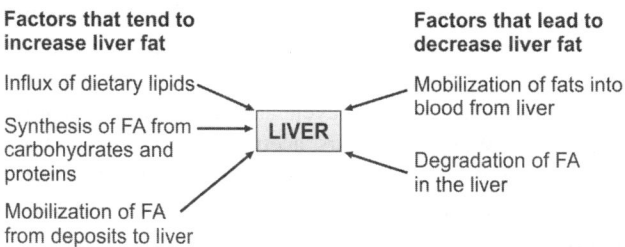

Fig. 12.2: Factors influencing accumulation of liver fat

Causes of Fatty Liver

1. Increased mobilization of fats from depots to liver. This type of fatty liver is known as physiological fatty liver. This occurs in:
   a. Diabetes mellitus.
   b. Starvation.
   c. Carbohydrate deprivation.
2. Impaired utilization of fat in the liver and impaired transport of fat from liver. This type is called pathological fatty liver. In this there is a metabolic blockage in the synthesis of VLDL. It may be due to:
   a. Deficiency of FAs.
   b. Deficiency of choline.
   c. Deficiency of pyridoxine, inositol, vitamin E and pantothenic acid.
   d. Poisoning by CCl_4, ethionamide.
   e. Alcoholism.

Lipotropic Agents

Agents such as choline, methionine, betaine and inositol effect removal of fat from the liver and thus prevent accumulation of fat in liver cells. Such substances, which prevent accumulation of fat in liver are called lipotropic agents.

Ketone Body Metabolism

Acetoacetic acid, β-hydroxybutyric acid and acetone are classified as ketone bodies, acetone bodies or ketones. The process of their formation is known as ketogenesis. Ketone bodies are produced in the liver. They are acidic and detected by Rothera's test.

Ketogenesis

In a diabetic patient, in starvation, or in any situation, in which carbohydrate metabolism is restricted, the body utilizes oxaloacetate to produce glucose for brain and muscles. This reduces the amount of oxaloacetate available for Krebs cycle and acetyl-CoA cannot be properly metabolized. When this occurs, acetyl-CoA is changed into acetoacetyl-CoA, which is converted into acetoacetic acid in the liver by the enzyme deacylase. Acetoacetic acid may be changed into acetone and β-hydroxybutyric acid.

The ketone bodies pass into the bloodstream in very small amounts under the normal circumstances. The total ketone bodies concentration in blood is normally, below 1 mg/100 mL of blood and the average excretion in urine in 24 hours is less than 125 mg. Normally the ketone bodies are carried in the bloodstream, mainly to the kidneys and muscles, where acetoacetic acid is oxidized after conversion to acetoacetyl-CoA. The latter is then cleaved by thiolase, when 2 moles of acetyl-CoA are formed. Then it enters the tricarboxylic acid (citric acid) cycle. This process of oxidation of ketone bodies is called ketolysis and is an alternate source of energy for the peripheral tissues.

Ketosis

When the rate of ketogenesis in the liver exceeds the rate of ketolysis in the periphery, the concentration of ketone bodies in the blood increases resulting in ketonemia. At this stage, ketone bodies are excreted in detectable quantity in the urine. This is ketonuria—when ketonuria and ketonemia are marked, acetone which is volatile escapes in the exhaled air giving rise to acetone smell in the breath. Ketonemia, ketonuria and the acetone odor of the breath together is ketosis. If ketosis is severe, acidosis will set in and this is accompanied by excretion of large amounts of water to carry the ketone bodies. At this stage, the patient becomes profoundly acidotic and passes into comatose stage.

Two main causes of ketosis are starvation and diabetes mellitus. In starvation, there is deprivation of carbohydrates and in diabetes, carbohydrates are not efficiently utilized. The person survives on his/her own stores of glycogen in the liver for energy. When this is depleted, energy is derived by the breakdown of fats in the body. The accelerated fat metabolism leads to the formation of large amounts of acetyl-CoA and ketone bodies giving rise to ketosis and ketonuria.

Biosynthesis of Cholesterol

Normal adult synthesizes about 1–1.5 g of cholesterol per day. Liver is the main site of cholesterol biosynthesis, but intestines (intestinal mucosa) is also an important site. Other tissues, where cholesterol synthesis takes place are skin, adrenal cortex, testes and aorta. The cholesterol biosynthesis takes place in the extramitochondrial compartment of the cell (Fig. 12.3).

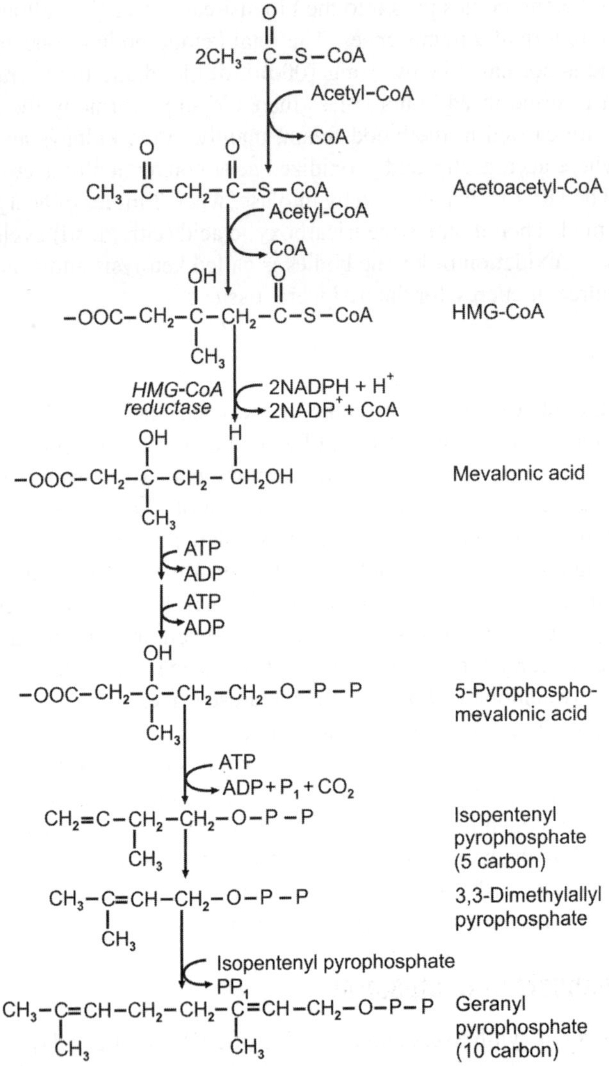

$$2CH_3-\overset{O}{\underset{\|}{C}}-S-CoA$$

↓ ⤴ Acetyl-CoA
↴ CoA

$$CH_3-\overset{O}{\underset{\|}{C}}-CH_2-\overset{O}{\underset{\|}{C}}-S-CoA \qquad \text{Acetoacetyl-CoA}$$

↓ ⤴ Acetyl-CoA
↴ CoA

$$^-OOC-CH_2-\underset{\underset{CH_3}{|}}{\overset{\overset{OH}{|}}{C}}-CH_2-\overset{O}{\underset{\|}{C}}-S-CoA \qquad \text{HMG-CoA}$$

HMG-CoA reductase ⤴ 2NADPH + H$^+$
↴ 2NADP$^+$ + CoA

$$^-OOC-CH_2-\underset{\underset{CH_3}{|}}{\overset{\overset{OH}{|}}{C}}-CH_2-\overset{H}{\underset{|}{C}}H_2OH \qquad \text{Mevalonic acid}$$

⤴ ATP
↴ ADP
⤴ ATP
↴ ADP

$$^-OOC-CH_2-\underset{\underset{CH_3}{|}}{\overset{\overset{OH}{|}}{C}}-CH_2-CH_2-O-P-P \qquad \text{5-Pyrophospho-mevalonic acid}$$

⤴ ATP
↴ ADP + P$_i$ + CO$_2$

$$CH_2=\underset{\underset{CH_3}{|}}{C}-CH_2-CH_2-O-P-P \qquad \begin{array}{l}\text{Isopentenyl}\\\text{pyrophosphate}\\\text{(5 carbon)}\end{array}$$

↓

$$CH_3-\underset{\underset{CH_3}{|}}{C}=CH-CH_2-O-P-P \qquad \begin{array}{l}\text{3,3-Dimethylallyl}\\\text{pyrophosphate}\end{array}$$

⤴ Isopentenyl pyrophosphate
↴ PP$_i$

$$CH_3-\underset{\underset{CH_3}{|}}{C}=CH-CH_2-CH_2-\underset{\underset{CH_3}{|}}{C}=CH-CH_2-O-P-P \qquad \begin{array}{l}\text{Geranyl}\\\text{pyrophosphate}\\\text{(10 carbon)}\end{array}$$

Contd...

Contd...

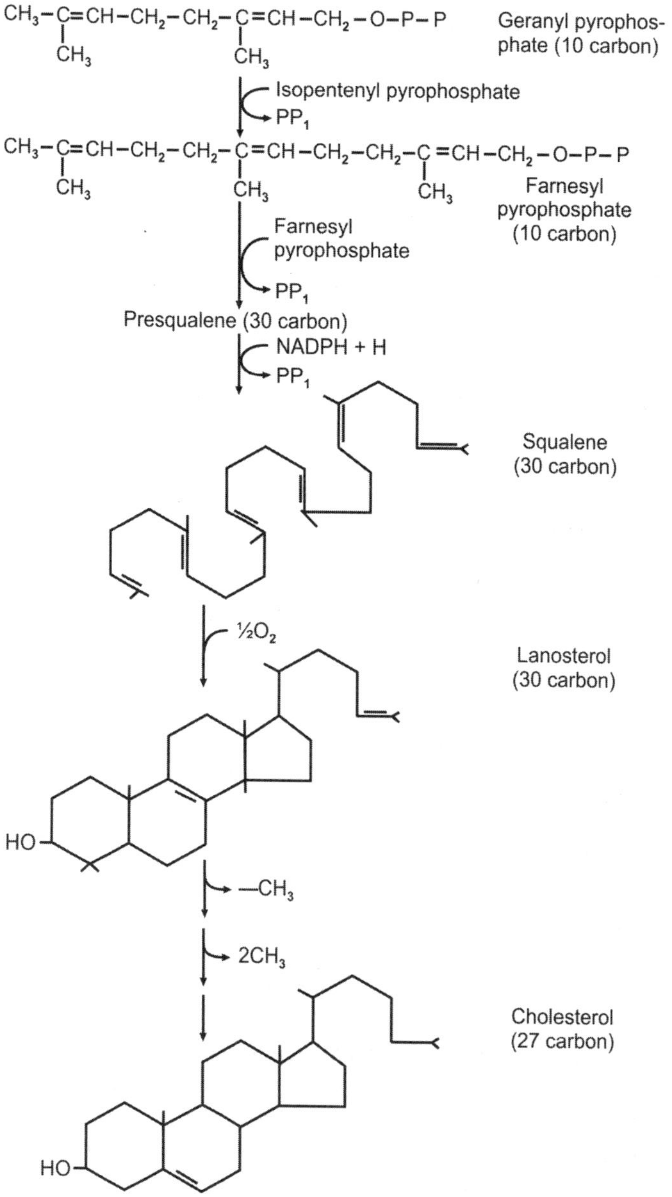

$$CH_3-\underset{CH_3}{C}=CH-CH_2-CH_2-\underset{CH_3}{C}=CH-CH_2-O-P-P \quad \text{Geranyl pyrophosphate (10 carbon)}$$

↓ ⤹ Isopentenyl pyrophosphate
↘ PP_1

$$CH_3-\underset{CH_3}{C}=CH-CH_2-CH_2-\underset{CH_3}{C}=CH-CH_2-CH_2-\underset{CH_3}{C}=CH-CH_2-O-P-P$$

Farnesyl pyrophosphate (10 carbon)

↓ ⤹ Farnesyl pyrophosphate
↘ PP_1

Presqualene (30 carbon)

↓ ⤹ NADPH + H
↘ PP_1

Squalene (30 carbon)

↓ ⤹ ½O_2

Lanosterol (30 carbon)

↓ ↦ —CH_3

↓ ↦ 2CH_3

Cholesterol (27 carbon)

Fig. 12.3: Cholesterol biosynthetic pathway

The sources of all the carbon atoms in cholesterol is acetyl-CoA. Acetyl-CoA is the fundamental or building block unit of cholesterol synthesis.

Synthesis of cholesterol takes place in various stages (details are given in Figures 12.1 and 12.2).

1. Formation of mevalonate from acetyl-CoA via HMG-CoA.
2. Three successive phosphorylation followed by decarboxylation to give isoprene units, mainly isopentenyl pyrophosphate.
3. Condensation of six isoprene units to give C-30 terpene, i.e. squalene.
4. Cyclization of squalene to lanosterol.
5. Conversion of lanosterol to cholesterol.

Cholesterol is transported in the blood as lipoproteins. Humans have two sources of cholesterol: dietary cholesterol and synthesis from acetate. The greater the dietary intake of cholesterol, the lower the rate of cholesterol biosynthesis in the liver and adrenal cortex. Although cholesterol itself has no calorific value in foods, its presence in the diet spares the energy necessary to synthesize cholesterol.

QUESTIONS AND ANSWERS

1. **How is fat digested and absorbed?**
2. **Describe the β-oxidation of fatty acids. Mention how many 129 ATPs are released on complete oxidation of palmitic acid?**
3. **How are fatty acids synthesized in the body?**
4. **What are ketone bodies?**
   Ans: A. Acetoacetic acid.
        B. β-hydroxybutyric acid.
        C. Acetone.
5. **What is the nature of ketone bodies?**
   Ans: Ketone bodies are acidic.
6. **Who is the net producer of ketone bodies?**
   Ans: The liver.
7. **Can liver utilize the ketone bodies. If not why?**
   Ans: Liver cannot utilize ketone bodies because the activating enzyme for ketone bodies utilization is absent in the liver.
8. **What are the tissues, which prefer ketone bodies for utilization?**
   Ans: Extrahepatic tissues prefer ketone bodies for utilization because they possess the activating enzymes.

9. **How are the ketone bodies formed?**
   Ans: Ketone bodies are formed as intermediate break down products of fat metabolism. If carbohydrate metabolism is defective, more fat breaks down for energy purposes. Hence more ketone bodies are formed.
10. **What is fatty liver? What are its causes?**
    Ans: Fatty liver refers to the deposition of excess of triglycerides in the liver cells.
11. **What are the lipotropic agents? Name them.**
    Ans: They are agents such as choline, methionine, betaine and inositol, which help removal of fat from the liver.

MULTIPLE CHOICE QUESTIONS

12. **β-oxidation of fatty acids require all the following coenzymes *except*:**
    A. CoA B. FAD
    C. NAD D. NADP
13. **The following can be oxidized by β-oxidation pathway:**
    A. Saturated fatty acids B. Monounsaturated fatty acid
    C. Polyunsaturated fatty acid D. All of the above
14. **Ketone bodies are synthesized in:**
    A. Adipose tissue B. Muscles
    C. Brain D. Liver
15. **All of the following statements about the ketone bodies are true *except*:**
    A. Their synthesis increases in diabetes mellitus
    B. They are synthesized in mitochondria
    C. They can deplete the alkali reserve
    D. They can be oxidized in the liver
16. **Net generation of energy on complete oxidation of palmitic acid is:**
    A. 129 ATP equivalents B. 131 ATP equivalents
    C. 146 ATP equivalents D. 148 ATP equivalents
17. **Net ATP production on complete oxidation of stearic acid in:**
    A. 129 B. 131
    C. 146 D. 148
18. **Histamine is formed from histidine by:**
    A. Deamination B. Dehydrogenation
    C. Decarboxylation D. Carboxylation
19. **Following are the ketone bodies *except*:**
    A. Acetoacetate B. Acetone
    C. Oxaloacetate D. β-hydroxybutyrate

20. **Ketone bodies production is more in starvation because of:**
    A. Availability of more glucose for oxidation
    B. Availability of more fatty acids for oxidation
    C. Availability of less glycerol and oxaloacetate
    D. Availability of more CoA
21. **In β-oxidation of fatty acids, coenzymes required are:**
    A. NAD and NADP
    B. FAD and NAD
    C. FAD and FMN
    D. $FADH_2$ and $NADH^+H^+$
22. **Fatty liver is due to:**
    A. Overmobilization of fat from liver to fat depot
    B. Undermobilization of fat from tissues to fat depot
    C. Over feeding of fat
    D. All of the above
23. **Serum triglycerides are contributed by all the following** *except:*
    A. Dietary fat
    B. Fat synthesized in the body
    C. Fat retained by kidneys
    D. Fat synthesized from glucose
24. **Conditions and agents that cause fatty liver include:**
    A. Alcoholism
    B. High-fat diet
    C. Deficiency of lipotropic factors
    D. All the above
25. **Bile facilitates action of lipase by:**
    A. Emulsification
    B. Saponification
    C. Inhibition of emulsification
    D. Inhibition of soap formation
26. **Cholesterol is transported from liver to adipose tissue by:**
    A. Chylomicrons
    B. VLDL
    C. LDL
    D. HDL
27. **Diet having a high ratio of polyunsaturated, saturated fatty acid can cause:**
    A. Increase in serum glycerides
    B. Decrease in serum cholesterol
    C. Decrease in serum HDL
    D. Skin lesions
28. **VLDL remnants can be converted into:**
    A. VLDL
    B. LDL
    C. HDL
    D. Chylomicrons
29. **HDL is synthesized in:**
    A. Adipose tissue
    B. Liver
    C. Intestine
    D. All of the above
30. **Pancreatic lipase requires for its acton:**
    A. Colipase
    B. Bile salts
    C. Phospholipids
    D. All of the above
31. **Lipogenesis is decreased in all the following** *except:*
    A. Restricted calorie intake
    B. High-fat intake
    C. Deficiency of insulin
    D. High-carbohydrates intake

32. **Plasma becomes milky:**
    A. Due to high level of HDL
    B. Due to high level of LDL
    C. During fasting
    D. After a meal

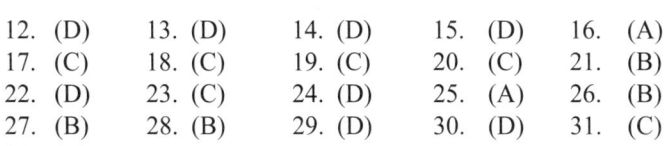

ANSWERS

12. (D)	13. (D)	14. (D)	15. (D)	16. (A)
17. (C)	18. (C)	19. (C)	20. (C)	21. (B)
22. (D)	23. (C)	24. (D)	25. (A)	26. (B)
27. (B)	28. (B)	29. (D)	30. (D)	31. (C)
32. (D)				

13 CHAPTER
Metabolism of Proteins

DIGESTION OF PROTEINS BY ENZYMES

Role of Enzyme

Different dietary proteins are sources of 20 amino acids. Proteins are hydrolyzed to their constituent amino acids by the action of the following enzymes.
Pepsin: Converts proteins to proteoses and peptones.
Trypsin: Cleaves peptide bonds involving carboxyl groups of arginine and lysine.
Chymotrypsin: Cleaves peptide bonds involving carbonyl groups of phenylalanine, tyrosine and tryptophan.
Carboxypeptidases: Cleaves proteins and peptides from the carbonyl end.
Aminopeptidases: Cleaves proteins and peptides from the amino end.
Dipeptidases: Cleaves dipeptides.

Absorption

Amino acids present in dietary proteins are in L-form. The L-form of amino acids are absorbed much faster than the D-form. All amino acids are absorbed by active process. Active process requires adenosine triphosphate (ATP), pyridoxal phosphate, Mn^{2+}, Na^+ and K^+.

Metabolic Pool

Amino acids from blood diffuse in the body fluids and reach all the tissue cells, where they are taken up by tissues by active transportation process. At the same time, most of the tissue proteins undergo disintegration constantly and release their amino acid content to the blood stream. This is the endogenous source of amino acids. They mix with the exogenous amino acids derived from food and build up the reservoir of amino acids called metabolic pool of amino acids (Fig. 13.1).

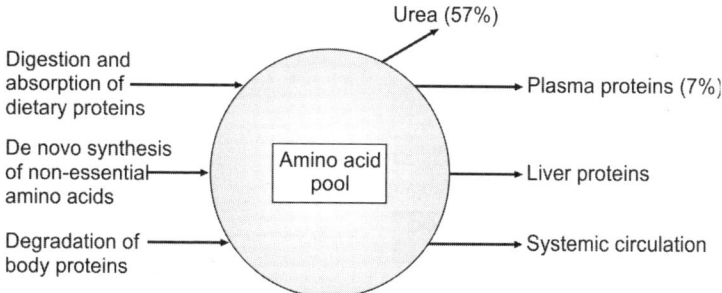

Fig. 13.1: Metabolic pool of amino acids

Nitrogen Balance

In a healthy adult maintaining a constant weight, the intake of nitrogen in food (mainly as dietary proteins) will be balanced by an excretion of an equal amount of nitrogen in urine (in the form of urea, uric acid, creatinine and amino acids) and in feces as unabsorbed nitrogen; hence in this individual the nitrogen is balanced. An individual whose intake of nitrogen is greater than the output, has a positive nitrogen balance. In growing period and during convalescence from illness, the body puts on weight and nitrogen intake will be more than output since some of the nitrogen is retained as tissue proteins.

An individual whose intake of nitrogen is less than the output has a negative nitrogen balance. In old age, during illness and starvation, weight is lost resulting in negative nitrogen balance.

Nitrogen balance is determined by subtracting fecal and urinary nitrogen from ingested nitrogen.

GENERAL PATHWAY OF PROTEIN METABOLISM

The general pathway of protein metabolism is shown in Figure 13.2. The amino acids from the 'pool' are utilized for two purposes as shown in Table 13.1.

Metabolism of Amino Acids (Breakdown)

Alpha-NH_2 group of amino acids, derived either from the diet or breakdown of tissue proteins is converted first to NH_3 and then to urea and is excreted in the urine.

Formation of NH_3 and urea can be discussed under the following heads:
- Transamination
- Oxidative deamination
- Decarboxylation
- Formation of urea.

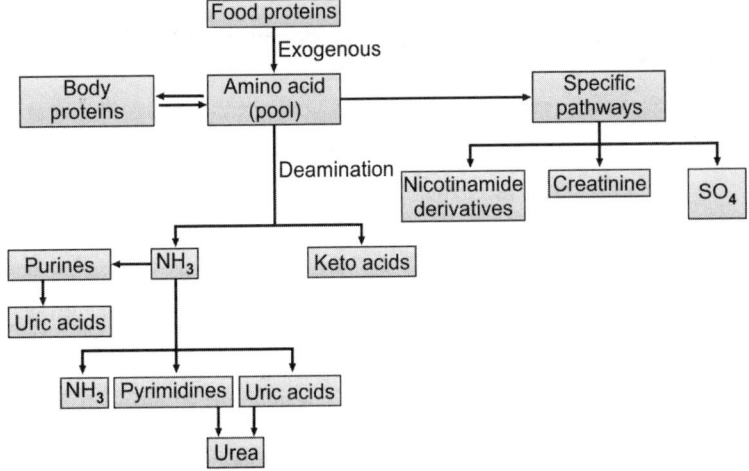

Fig. 13.2: General scheme of the pathway of proteins and amino acid metabolism

Transamination

Transamination is a reversible reaction in which α-NH_2 group of one amino acid is transferred to a α-keto acid resulting in the formation of a new amino acid and a keto acid. The general reaction is represented as:

TABLE 13.1: Features of anabolism and catabolism	
Anabolic phase (synthesis)	*Catabolic phase* (breakdown)
Protein biosynthesis, tissue proteins, blood proteins, enzymes, hormones	Transamination
	Oxidative deamination
Synthesis of non-protein nitrogen substances like creatinine, purines, pyrimidines, glutathione and choline	Decarboxylation
	Utilization of nitrogen residue Glutamine synthesis Urea cycle

Metabolism of Proteins

$$\underset{\substack{\text{Donor} \\ \alpha\text{-amino acid}}}{\overset{R_1}{\underset{\text{COOH}}{H-C-NH_2}}} + \underset{\substack{\text{Recipient} \\ \alpha\text{-keto acid}}}{\overset{R_2}{\underset{\text{COOH}}{C=O}}} \rightleftharpoons \underset{\substack{\text{New} \\ \alpha\text{-keto acid}}}{\overset{R_1}{\underset{\text{COOH}}{C=O}}} + \underset{\substack{\text{New} \\ \alpha\text{-amino acid}}}{\overset{R_2}{\underset{\text{COOH}}{C-NH_2}}}$$

By transamination, the body can synthesize any non-essential amino acid, it needs. The body can control the concentrations of non-essential amino acids by converting excess amino acids to needed acids by transamination.

The transaminases require pyridoxal phosphate as the coenzyme. The pyridoxal phosphate acts as a carrier of amino group from amino acid to keto group as represented below:

R_1 amino acid ⟶ Pyridoxal phosphate ⟶ R_2 amino acid
R_2 keto acid ⟵ Pyridoxamine phosphate ⟵ R_2 keto acid

Transaminases are present practically in all the tissues. The most abundant are the glutamate oxaloacetate transaminase (GOT) or aspartate transaminase (AST) and glutamate pyruvate transaminase (GPT) or alanine transaminase (ALT). AST is predominant in the heart. AST levels are increased in cardiac infarction and cirrhosis of the liver ALT levels are raised in liver diseases infective hepatitis. Determination of the concentration of AST and ALT in serum is used to assess the degree of cardiac and liver damages. For example,

$$\underset{\substack{\text{Glutamic acid} \\ (\alpha\text{-amino acid})}}{\overset{\text{COOH}}{\underset{\text{COOH}}{\overset{(CH_2)_2}{\underset{\text{HC}-NH_2}{|}}}}} + \underset{\substack{\text{Oxaloacetic acid} \\ (\alpha\text{-keto acid})}}{\overset{\text{COOH}}{\underset{\text{COOH}}{\overset{CH_2}{\underset{C=O}{|}}}}} \xrightarrow{\text{SGOT/AST}} \underset{\substack{\alpha\text{-ketoglutaric acid} \\ (\alpha\text{-keto acid})}}{\overset{\text{COOH}}{\underset{\text{COOH}}{\overset{(CH_2)_2}{\underset{C=O}{|}}}}} + \underset{\substack{\text{Aspartic acid} \\ (\alpha\text{-amino acid})}}{\overset{\text{COOH}}{\underset{\text{COOH}}{\overset{CH_2}{\underset{H-C-CH_2}{|}}}}}$$

$$\underset{\substack{\text{Glutamic acid} \\ (\alpha\text{-amino acid})}}{\overset{\text{COOH}}{\underset{\text{COOH}}{\overset{(CH_2)_2}{\underset{\text{HC}-NH_2}{|}}}}} + \underset{\substack{\text{Pyruvic acid} \\ (\alpha\text{-keto acid})}}{\overset{\text{CH}_3}{\underset{\text{COOH}}{\overset{|}{\underset{C=O}{|}}}}} \xrightarrow{\text{SGPT/AST}} \underset{\substack{\alpha\text{-ketoglutaric acid} \\ (\alpha\text{-keto acid})}}{\overset{\text{COOH}}{\underset{\text{COOH}}{\overset{(CH_2)_2}{\underset{C=O}{|}}}}} + \underset{\substack{\text{Alanine} \\ (\alpha\text{-amino acid})}}{\overset{\text{CH}_3}{\underset{\text{COOH}}{\overset{|}{\underset{C-NH_2}{|}}}}}$$

Decarboxylation

Amino acids are decarboxylated to give the corresponding amines. The enzyme is decarboxylase with pyridoxal phosphate as coenzyme. Decarboxylation of amino acids gives rise to some of the biologically active amines.

Histidine	→ Histamine (powerful vasodilator)
Tyrosine	→ Tyramine (increases blood pressure)
Glutamic acid	→ α-aminobutyric acid (stimulates neuronal activity)
Tryptophan	→ Tryptamine
5-hydroxytryptophan	→ 5-hydroxytryptamine
Arginine	→ Agmatine (in bacteria only)

Oxidative Deamination

Oxidative deamination involves the removal of α-amino group of amino acids to produce their keto acids. The enzyme is amino acid oxidase. The amino acid is first dehydrogenated by the flavoprotein of the enzyme, α-amino acid oxidase forming an α-amino acid. In the next step, water molecule is added spontaneously and decomposes to the corresponding α-keto acid with the loss of α-imino nitrogen as NH_3.

$$CH_3-\underset{\underset{NH_2}{|}}{CH}-COOH \xrightarrow{\text{Amino acid oxidase}} CH_3-\underset{\underset{O}{\|}}{C}-COOH + NH_3 \uparrow$$

Alanine (α-amino acid) → Pyruvic acid (α-keto acid)

UREA SYNTHESIS

Urea cycle is also known as Krebs-Henseleit cycle or ornithine cycle (fromation and disposal of NH_3 in the liver). Urea is the chief end product of amino acid metabolism and it is synthesized in the liver. Increase in the dietary protein is followed by increase in urine urea. A normal healthy adult excretes 2–30 g of urea per day. The normal blood urea level is 15–35 mg/100 mL.

The deamination of amino acids produces ammonia, which is toxic. By Krebs-Henseleit cycle, it is converted to urea, a non-toxic compound which is transported via the blood to the kidneys and excreted in urine. Krebs and Henseleit have elucidated the following five steps of urea synthesis, i.e. five sequential enzymatic reactions taking place in the liver:

1. Synthesis of carbamoyl phosphate, an unstable intermediate.
2. Synthesis of citrulline.
3. Synthesis of argininosuccinic acid.
4. Cleavage of argininosuccinic acid to produce arginine.
5. Cleavage of arginine to form ornithine and urea.

Used cycle can be summarized as:

$$2NH_3 + CO_2 \xrightarrow{Enzymes} O=C{\overset{NH_2}{\underset{NH_2}{}}} + H_2O$$

Step 1: Synthesis of Carbamoyl Phosphate, an Unstable Intermediate

The biosynthesis of urea begins with the condensation of CO_2, NH_3 and ATP to form carbamoyl phosphate, a rection catalyzed by mitochondrial carbamoyl phosphate synthase. The enzyme requires biotin and N-acetyl-glutamic acid (ACA) as coenzymes. Lack of this enzyme produces a very serious disorder hyperammonemia.

$$NH_3 + CO_2 + H_2O + 2ATP \xrightarrow[Mg^{2+}, biotin, AGA]{Carbamoyl\ phosphate\ synthase} H_2N-\overset{O}{\underset{}{C}}-O-\overset{O}{\underset{OH}{P}}-OH$$

Carbamoyl phosphate
+ 2ADP + Pi

Step 2: Synthesis of Citrulline

Carbamoyl phosphate donates its carbamoyl group to ornithine to form citrulline and release phosphate in a reaction catalyzed by ornithine transcarbamoylase. Lack of this enzyme will produce a different type of hyperammonemia.

$$H_2N-\overset{O}{C}-O-\overset{O}{\underset{OH}{P}}-OH + \underset{\text{Ornithine}}{\begin{array}{c}NH_2\\|\\CH_2\\|\\CH_2\\|\\H-C-NH_2\\|\\COOH\end{array}} \xrightarrow{\text{Ornithine transcarbamylase}} \underset{\text{Citrulline}}{\begin{array}{c}NH_2\\|\\C=O\\|\\NH\\|\\CH_2\\|\\(CH_2)_2\\|\\H-C-NH_2\\|\\COOH\end{array}}$$

Step 3: Synthesis of Argininosuccinic Acid

Citrulline and aspartic acid (derived from transmination of aspartic acid) combine to form argininosuccinic acid. The reaction is catalyzed by enzyme argininosuccinate synthase.

$$\underset{\text{Citrulline}}{\begin{array}{c} CH_2-NH-\overset{\overset{O}{\|}}{C}-NH_2 \\ | \\ (CH_2)_2 \\ | \\ H-C-NH_2 \\ | \\ COOH \end{array}} + \underset{\text{Aspartic acid}}{\begin{array}{c} COOH \\ | \\ H_2N-CH \\ | \\ CH_2 \\ | \\ COOH \end{array}} \underset{Mg^{2+}}{\overset{ATP \quad AMP}{\rightleftharpoons}} \underset{\text{Argininosuccinic acid}}{\begin{array}{c} CH_2-HN-\overset{\overset{NH}{\|}}{C}-NH-\overset{COOH}{\underset{|}{CH}} \\ | \qquad\qquad\qquad\qquad CH_2 \\ (CH_2)_2 \qquad\qquad\qquad | \\ | \qquad\qquad\qquad\qquad COOH \\ H-C-NH_2 \\ | \\ COOH \end{array}}$$

Step 4: Cleavage of Argininosuccinic Acid to Produce Arginine

Cleavage of argininosuccinic acid by enzyme argininosuccinase yields arginine and fumaric acid. Some fumaric acid may be converted back to aspartic acid and some enters the Krebs cycle.

$$\underset{\text{Argininosuccinic acid}}{\begin{array}{c} \overset{NH}{\underset{\|}{C}}-NH-\overset{COOH}{\underset{|}{CH}} \\ | \qquad\qquad CH_2 \\ NH \qquad\qquad | \\ | \qquad\qquad COOH \\ CH_2 \\ | \\ (CH_2)_2 \\ | \\ H-C-NH_2 \\ | \\ COOH \end{array}} \xrightarrow{\textit{Argininosuccinase}} \underset{\text{Arginine}}{\begin{array}{c} \overset{NH}{\underset{\|}{C}}-NH_2 \\ | \\ NH \\ | \\ CH_2 \\ | \\ (CH_2)_2 \\ | \\ H-C-NH_2 \\ | \\ COOH \end{array}} + \underset{\text{Fumaric acid}}{\begin{array}{c} COOH \\ | \\ C-NH_2 \\ \| \\ CH \\ | \\ COOH \end{array}}$$

Step 5: Cleavage of Arginine to form Ornithine and Urea

Enzyme arginase splits arginine into urea and ornithine.

$$\underset{\text{Arginine}}{\begin{array}{c} \overset{HN}{\underset{\|}{C}}-NH_2 \\ | \\ NH \\ | \\ CH_2 \\ | \\ (CH_2)_2 \\ | \\ H-C-NH_2 \\ | \\ COOH \end{array}} + H_2O \xrightarrow{\textit{Arginase}} \underset{\text{Urea}}{\begin{array}{c} NH_2 \\ | \\ C=O \\ | \\ NH_2 \end{array}} + \underset{\text{Ornithine}}{\begin{array}{c} NH_2 \\ | \\ (CH_2)_3 \\ | \\ H-C-NH_2 \\ | \\ COOH \end{array}}$$

Ornithine, so formed again enters in the urea cycle at the second step to continue the cycle. Urea is absorbed by the blood, brought to kidneys and excreted in urine.

This is a catalytic process. The enzymes are located partly in the mitochondria for first two steps and partly for next three steps in the cytoplasm. One molecule of NH_3 and one molecule of CO_2 are converted to one molecule of urea for each turn of the cycle and ornithine is regenerated at the end. The overall process in each turn of the cycle requires 3 molecules of ATP (Fig. 13.3).

Significance of Urea Cycle: Detoxification of NH_3

Major biological role of this pathway is the detoxification of NH_3. Toxic ammonia is converted into a non-toxic substance urea and excreted in urine. The urea cycle occurs predominantly in the liver, although it also exists in the brain and kidneys. Ammonia is also used up in the formation of glutamine and for amination of α-keto acid to form α-amino acid.

Urea synthesis is not an independent process, but is connected with vital metabolic reactions in the body. Synthesis of urea is important because of its integration with the citric acid cycle, which serves as the source of supply of aspartate. Also the fumerate derived from argininosuccinate integrates with the citric acid cycle.

Uremia: This is a pathological clinical state, when blood urea increases above 50 mg%. Acute uremia is associated with anuria (suppression of excretion of urine).

Metabolic Disorders of Urea Cycle

For each enzyme of the urea cycle, there is a rare inherited deficiency disorder that is almost always fatal in infancy. The urea concentration is extremely low in affected individuals.

Hyperammonemia gives rise to mental retardation. Any defect of urea cycle enzymes gives elevated levels of ammonia. It is because of increased level of ammonia in the blood.

METABOLISM OF GLUTAMIC ACID

It is α-aminoglutaric acid. Glutamic acid plays an important role in the metabolism of amino acids. It is generated during transmination reactions.

```
COOH
|
CH₂
|
CH₂
|
CH – NH₂
|
COOH
```
Glutamic acid

Most amino acids transfer their amino group to α-ketoglutaric acid to form glutamic acid.

Amino acid + α-ketoglutarate $\xrightarrow{Aminotransferase}$ α-keto acid + Glutamic acid

Glutamic acid is also formed during the metabolism of other amino acids such as histidine, proline and arginine.

Glutamic acid can react with a molecule of NH_3 in presence of ATP, to form glutamine.

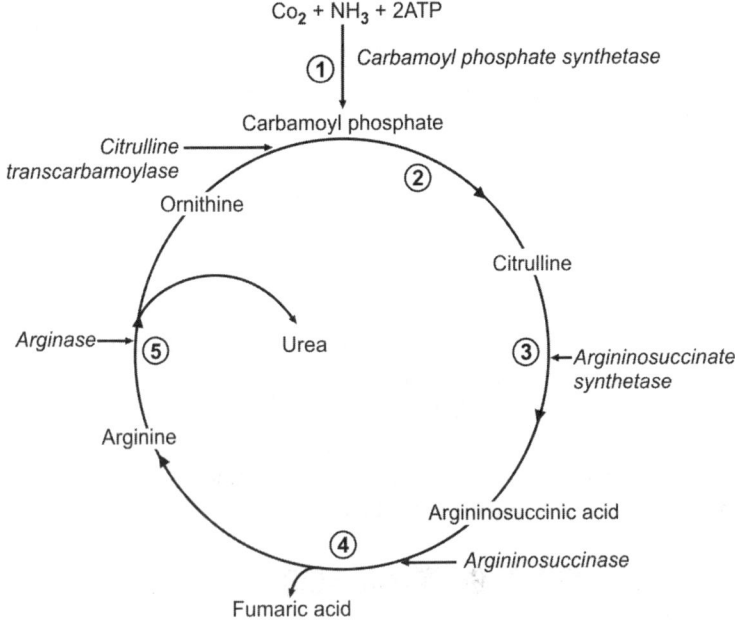

Fig. 13.3: Urea cycle

Metabolism of Proteins

```
COOH                            COOH
|                               |
CH – NH₂                        CH – NH₂
|          Glutamine synthase   |
CH₂    + NH₃ ⟶                  CH₂
|           ATP   ADT + Pi      |
CH₂                             CH₂
|                               |
COOH                            C=O
                                |
                                NH₂
Glutamic acid                   Glutamine
```

The formation of glutamine from glutamic acid in the brain and intestine is of significance in the disposal of NH_3, from the intestinal tract in a non-toxic form. It helps to change ammonia into a non-toxic form.

QUESTIONS

1. How are the proteins digested and absorbed in the body?
2. Describe the urea cycle in detail.
3. Give the methods of deamination of amino acids. What is the fate of liberated ammonia?
4. Describe the importance of transamination in amino acid metabolism.
5. Discuss the formation and disposal of ammonia in the liver.
6. Describe the metabolic pathways available for the detoxification of ammonia in the body.

MULTIPLE CHOICE QUESTIONS

7. Positive nitrogen balance is seen in:
    A. Starvation
    B. Wasting diseases
    C. Growing age
    D. Intestinal malabsorption
8. Alanine can be synthesized from:
    A. Glutamate and α-ketoglutarate
    B. Pyruvate and glutamate
    C. Pyruvate and α-ketoglutarate
    D. Aspartate and α-ketoglutarate
9. During catabolism of amino acids their amino groups are transferred mainly to:
    A. Pyruvate
    B. Oxaloacetate
    C. α-ketoglutarate
    D. Ornithine
10. The organ, which is extremely sensitive to ammonia toxicity is:
    A. Liver
    B. Brain
    C. Kidneys
    D. Heart

11. **Immediate detoxification of ammonia is done in the brain by fixing it in the form of:**
    A. Glutamine
    B. Alanine
    C. Aspartate
    D. Asparagine

12. **The major site of urea synthesis is:**
    A. Brain
    B. Kidneys
    C. Liver
    D. Muscles

13. **The carbon atoms of urea are provided by:**
    A. CO_2
    B. Aspartate
    C. Ornithine
    D. None of the above

14. **Some amino acids are considered non-essential for man because:**
    A. They are not required for protein synthesis
    B. They do not form any biologically important compound
    C. They can be synthesized in the body
    D. They are formed from essential amino acids

15. **Some amino acids are considered essential for man because:**
    A. Their half lives are very long
    B. They cannot be synthesized in the human body
    C. They can form other non-essential amino acids
    D. Besides proteins, they form other specialized compounds

16. **Pancreatic juice contains proteolytic enzymes *except*:**
    A. Pepsin
    B. Trypsin
    C. Chymotrypsin
    D. Carboxypeptidase

17. **Gastric juice contains proteolytic enzymes *except*:**
    A. Pepsin
    B. Trypsin
    C. Rennin
    D. Gelatinase

18. **Following proteolytic enzymes are absent in adults:**
    A. Pepsin
    B. Elastase and collagenase
    C. Rennin
    D. Trypsin and chymotrypsin

19. **Positive nitrogen balance is seen in all *except*:**
    A. Convalescence
    B. Fever
    C. Growth
    D. Pregnancy

20. **Negative nitrogen balance means:**
    A. Nitrogen intakes is more than excretion
    B. Nitrogen excretion is more than intake
    C. Nitrogen intake and excretion are the same
    D. Nitrogen excretion is less than intake

21. **The α-amino acids are absorbed from the intestine by:**
    A. Active transport
    B. Endocytosis
    C. Facilitated diffusion
    D. Passive diffusion

22. Transamination requires the following enzymes:
    A. Coenzyme A
    B. Pyridoxal phosphate
    C. TPP
    D. Nicotinamide
23. Urea is produced in the body because:
    A. It is stored in the liver
    B. It is used for synthetic purpose
    C. It is used for non-synthetic purpose
    D. It is for detoxify ammonia
24. Urea synthesis involves all the following *except:*
    A. Transferase
    B. Synthase
    C. Lyase
    D. Oxidase
25. Fate of ammonia is:
    A. Urea synthesis
    B. Sythesis of amino acids
    C. Glutamine formation
    D. All of the above
26. Normal concentration of urea in blood is:
    A. 20–40 mg%
    B. 25–45 mg%
    C. 20–60 µg%
    D. 30–50 mg%
27. Urea synthesis requires the following *except:*
    A. Ammonia
    B. CO_2
    C. Aspartate
    D. NAD^+
28. In liver failure, serum ammonia concentration is increased due to:
    A. Decreased ammonia excretion
    B. Increased protein articulation
    C. Inefficient urea synthesis
    D. Decreased glutamine synthesis
29. Urea cycle is associated with TCA in the following respects:
    A. For the synthesis of arginine
    B. For the synthesis of citrulline
    C. For the synthesis of ornithine
    D. For the conversion of fumarate to aspartate
30. Creatine phosphate is high energy compound because:
    A. It is equal to ATP
    B. It gives less than 7.3 kcal energy
    C. It gives more than 7.3 kcal energy
    D. It gives less than 10.3 kcal energy
31. Amino acids involved in creatinine formation are:
    A. Glycine, arginine and methionine
    B. Glycine, arginine and cysteine
    C. Glycine, cysteine and glutamine
    D. Glycine, arginine and glutamic acid
32. Choline is synthesized from:
    A. Cysteine
    B. Cytosine
    C. Methionine
    D. Arginine

33. The substance from which ammonia is produced by the kidney is:
    A. Glycine
    B. Alanine
    C. Valine
    D. Phenylalanine
34. Most of the amino acids are metabolized in:
    A. Kidneys
    B. Liver
    C. Heart
    D. Intestine
35. The urea cycle spans two cellular compartments, which are:
    A. Cytosol and vacuole
    B. Cytosol and endoplasmic reticulum
    C. Cytosol and mitochondria
    D. Cytosol and nucleus
36. The reaction in which α-amino group is transferred to the α-carbon atom of α-ketoglutarate is called:
    A. Decarboxylation
    B. Transamination
    C. Deamination
    D. Hydroxylation
37. Milk protein is digested in the stomach by:
    A. Trypsin
    B. Revin
    C. Rennin
    D. DHCL
38. All the following are catabolic pathway of amino acids *except:*
    A. Acetylation
    B. Transacylation
    C. Transamination
    D. Deamination
39. Which coenzyme is required for the removal of the amino group?
    A. NAD$^+$
    B. Pyridoxal phosphate
    C. FAD$^+$
    D. Thiamine
40. Which amino acid is not involved in urea cycle?
    A. Arginine
    B. Aspartic acid
    C. Glycine
    D. Ornithine
41. The link between TCA cycle and urea cycle is through:
    A. Citrate
    B. Pyruvate
    C. Fumaric acid
    D. Malate
42. Phenyl ketonuria (PKU) is characterized by:
    A. Urine becoming dark on standing
    B. Urine with a mousy odor
    C. Urine with smell of burnt sugar
    D. Increased tyrosine lent in urine

ANSWERS

7. (C)	8. (B)	9. (D)	10. (B)	11. (A)
12. (C)	13. (A)	14. (C)	15. (B)	16. (A)
17. (D)	18. (C)	19. (B)	20. (B)	21. (A)
22. (B)	23. (D)	24. (A)	25. (A)	26. (A)
27. (D)	28. (C)	29. (A)	30. (A)	31. (A)
32. (C)	33. (A)	34. (B)	35. (C)	36. (B)
37. (C)	38. (A)	39. (B)	40. (D)	41. (C)
42. (B)				

14 CHAPTER

Immunochemistry

IMMUNITY

Immunity is the ability of the body to resist invasion by microorganisms and influence of toxins that cause tissue damage.

Types

1. Innate immunity:
   a. Non-specific.
   b. Specific.
2. Acquired immunity:
   a. Active.
   b. Passive.

Antigen: This is a substance, which when introduced into the body, stimulate the production of antibody with which it specifically reacts.

Haptens: These are substances, which cannot induce antibody formation, but can react specifically with antibodies.

The smallest unit of antigenicity is known as antigenic determinant or epitope.

They are peptides or monosaccharide residues. They have a specific chemical structure, electrical charge and are capable of stimulating an antibody, which reacts at that site.

IMMUNE RESPONSE

The specific reactivity induced by an antigenic stimulus in a host is known as immune response.

The immune response is of two types:

1. Antibody-mediated immune (AMI) (humoral) response.
2. Cell-mediated immune (CMI) response.

ANTIBODY-MEDIATED IMMUNE (HUMORAL) RESPONSE

Antibody-mediated immune response provides defence against bacterial pathogens and viruses that invade through respiratory or gastrointestinal tract. It also prevents recurrence of viral infections. It participates in the pathogenesis of immediate hypersensitivity reactions.

The production of antibodies occurs in three steps:
1. Entry of antigen, its distribution in the tissue and contact with appropriate immunocompetent cells.
2. Processing of antigen by cells.
3. Secretion of antibody.

CELL-MEDIATED IMMUNE RESPONSE

Cell-mediated immune response is a type of specific immune response that does not involve antibody.

It is mediated by T lymphocytes. CMI provides protection against fungi, viruses and intracellular bacterial pathogen. It participates in graft-versus-host reaction. It provides immunity against cancer. CMI is provided by T lymphocytes and their products—lymphokines.
1. Monokines secreted by monocytes and macrophages help in CMI.
2. Lymphokines and monokines together constitute cytokines.
3. Cytokines are soluble products secreted by lymphocytes, macrophages, neutrophils and natural killer cells.

For further details, please refer to immunology in 'Medical Microbiology' book by Author.

MECHANISMS OF ANTIBODY PRODUCTION

There are two broad groups of theories of antibody formation:
1. Instructive theories.
2. Selective theories.

The instructive theories postulate that an immunocompetent cell (ICC) is capable of synthesizing antibodies of all specificity. The antigen instructs ICC to produce the complementary antibody. Selective theories, on the contrary, postulate that ICCs have only a restricted immunological range. The antigen selects the appropriate ICC to synthesize an antibody. The most accepted theory is 'clonal selection theory'.

Clonal Selection Theory

Clonal selection theory was proposed by Burnet (1957). The theory states that during fetal development a large number of clones of immunological competent cells (ICCs), bearing specific antibody patterns, are produced by a process of somatic mutation of ICCs against all possible antigens. Clones of cells with immunological reactivity with self-antigens are eliminated during embryonic life. Such clones are called 'forbidden clones'. Persistence of forbidden clones or their development in later life by somatic mutation leads to autoimmune processes. Each ICC is capable of reacting with one antigen or a small number of antigens. Contact with specific antigens leads to a cellular proliferation to form clones synthesizing the antibody. The conical selection theory is widely accepted.

MAJOR HISTOCOMPATIBILITY COMPLEX

The major histocompatibility complex (MHC) in humans is known as the human leukocyte antigen (HLA) complex.

Human Leukocyte Antigen Complex

Histocompatibility antigens mean cell surface antigens that evoke immune response to an incompatible host resulting in allograft rejection. These alloantigens are present on the surface of leukocytes in man and are called human leukocyte antigens (HLA) and the set of genes coding for them is called the HLA complex.

The HLA complex of genes are grouped in three classes:
1. *Class I MHC antigens (HLA-A, HLA-B, HLA-C):* The MHC class I antigens are present on the surface of all nucleated cells. They are involved in graft rejection and cell-mediated cytolysis.
2. *Class II MHC antigens (HLA-DR, HLA-DQ and HLA-DP):* They have a very limited distribution and are principally found on the surface of macrophages, monocytes, activated T lymphocytes (CD4) and B lymphocytes. They are primarily responsible for the graft-versus-host response.
3. *Class III MHC antigens:* Class III genes encode C2, C4 complement components of the classical pathway and properdin factor B of alternate pathway.

FREE RADICALS

Free radicals are atoms or molecules containing one or more unpaired electrons in their outer orbit. They are highly reactive species and have a tendency either to loose an electron, thereby acting like a reducing agent or gain an electron, thereby acting as oxidizing agents. Thus, they can initiate chain reaction by extracting an electron from a neighboring molecule to complete its own orbit.
1. The most important radicals are derived from molecular oxygen and contain oxides of nitrogen, especially nitric oxide.
2. These free radicals may act as signaling molecules in physiological and biochemical activities or may provide defence against invading microorganisms.
3. Failure of these protective mechanisms may lead to pathological conditions.
4. Oxygen-derived free radicals and related non-radical compound (H_2O_2) are referred to as reactive oxygen species (ROS).
5. Not all ROS are free radicals, e.g. singlet oxygen and hydrogen peroxide.

Formation of Reactive Oxygen Species

When the oxygen molecule (O_2) is introduced into a reducing environment, it may undergo a series of reactions leading to the formation of ROS. The reactive intermediates, which are formed usually remain tightly bound in the active sites of the enzymes, until the reaction is completed. Thus, free radicals usually have only a transient existence in the catalytic process. But occasionally, they may escape from the active site of the enzyme and lead to destructive effect.

Enzyme Reactions with Free Radicals as Byproducts

Various reactions occurring in cells depend on a supply of oxygen (dioxygen). In such type of reactions, free radicals are generated as byproducts. The enzyme catalyzing oxygen requiring reactions can be classified into:
♦ Oxidases
♦ Monooxygenases
♦ Dioxygenases.

Free radicals can be neutral, positively or negatively charged. To gain stability it removes electrons from neighboring molecules, thereby initiating chain reactions like lipid peroxidation, thereby causing immense tissue damage leading to cancer, cardiovascular diseases, cataract, ulcerative colitis, rheumatoid arthritis, Crohn's disease, e.g. superoxide anion (O_2), hydroxyl radical (OH).

ANTIOXIDANTS

Antioxidants are substances, which counteract the deleterious effect of free radical, e.g. enzymes like catalase, peroxidase, ceruloplasmin, etc. Vitamins like vitamin E, vitamin C, β-carotene, selenium, etc.

Oxidized LDL is a risk factor for atherosclerosis. Vitamin E prevents oxidation of LDL and thereby reduces atherosclerosis.

Action of Antioxidants

Different antioxidants act at different levels:
1. They may prevent the initiation of chain reactions by removing free radicals.
2. They may scavenge free radicals generated in chain reactions, thereby interrupting the chain sequence.
3. They may remove peroxides, thereby preventing further generation of ROS.
4. There are two main lines of defence against ROS:
   a. Enzymatic antioxidant system also called scavenger enzymes.
   b. Non-enzymatic (nutrient) antioxidant systems.

Vitamin E

1. The antioxidant property of vitamin E is most important and natural property, which prevents peroxidation of polyunsaturated fatty acids contained in cellular phospholipids by removal of free radicals such as OH; superoxide (O_2) anions.
2. Antioxidant action of tocopherols prevents the peroxidative effects of atmospheric pollutants like O_2, H_2O_2 and NO_2 on membrane lipids of bronchi, bronchioles and alveoli.
3. Antioxidant action of tocopherol protects selenide at their active sites of membrane proteins against free radicals.
4. Tocopherols prevent oxidation of vitamin A and carotenes, and reduce their wastage.

Vitamin C

1. Vitamin C, flavoprotein and carotenoids are able to regenerate vitamin E, which can act as antioxidant.
2. Vitamin C, β-carotene and flavoprotein are also able to reduce and detoxify oxygen intermediates in cells.

STRUCTURAL AND CONTRACTILE PROTEINS

Structural Proteins

Collagen

The major structural protein found in connective tissue is collagen (Greek word 'kolla' meaning substance to produce glue). It is the most abundant protein in the body. Almost 25%–30% of the total weight of protein in the body is by collagen. It is present in almost all organs and serves to hold together the cells in the tissues. It is the major fibrous element of tissues like bone, teeth, tendons, cartilage and blood vessels. The other connective tissue proteins that play a structural role are elastin and proteoglycans.

The immature collagen is soluble. The insoluble nature is unsuitable for carrying out structural studies. The basic structural unit of collagen is tropocollagen. The tropocollagen is made up of three polypeptide chains of the same size.

Collagen is synthesized by fibroblasts intracellularly. The polypeptide chains of collagen are synthesized in the form of large precursors called procollagen.

It is then secreted and extracellular procollagen is cleaved by specific peptidases to form procollagen. This removal of the peptides is important for the proper formation of triple helical rod-like structure of tropocollagen.

Elastin

Elastin is a protein found in the connective tissue and it is the major component of elastic fibers. The elastic fibers can stretch and then can resume their original length. They have high tensile strength. They are found in the ligaments as well as the walls of blood vessels, especially in large vessels like aorta.

Elastin has a distinct amino acid composition. One third of the residues are glycine. Proline is present in large amounts, so also alanine.

Hydroxyproline is present in small amounts, while hydroxylysine is absent. When elastin matures desmosine cross-links are formed from four lysine residues. Copper deficiency blocks the formation of aldehydes, which are essential for cross-linking.

Keratin

Keratin proteins are present in hair, nails and skin. They are also present in epidermal appendages like horn and hoof. The fibers present are called α-keratins and matrix as keratohyalin. The keratin fibrins are first formed, which aggregate into bundles. They mainly have the α-helical structure. The keratohyalins matrix has cystein-rich polypeptide chains, which are held together by disulfide bonds. The proportion of keratins vary depending on the degree of cross-linking and the number of disulfide bonds: The more the number of disulfide bonds, the harder the keratin is. In addition to the disulfide bonds, covalent bonds are also seen between lysine and glutamic acid residues of adjacent polypeptide chains, forming amide bonds.

The keratin present in the chain has more number of disulfide bonds, which give mechanical strength. On disrupting these bonds by reduction, the solubility increases, while the tensile strength decreases. This is used in artificial waving of hair.

Contractile Proteins

Actin and Myosin

Movement is an important property of life, especially of members of the animal kingdom. The organism may move as a whole (walking) or movement of cells may occur or it may occur at subcellular level. The function of movement is performed by contractile proteins, which convert chemical energy into mechanical energy. The important contractile proteins are actin and myosin in muscles.

The muscle fibrils are mainly proteins. These proteins are characterized by their elasticity or contractile power.

Myosin: It is the most abundant protein in muscle. It is a globulin, soluble in dilute salt solutions and insoluble in water. Myosin is composed of subunits of about 80 mm in length with molecular weight approximately 200,000.

Actin: It is a globulin, molecular weight 60,000, which binds one ATP per molecule. The immediate source of energy required for muscular contraction is derived by the hydrolysis of ATP to ADP.

MULTIPLE CHOICE QUESTIONS

1. During respiratory burst, all the following ROS are formed *except:*
   A. Superoxide
   B. Hydrogen peroxide
   C. Hydroxy radical
   D. Nitric acid
2. The main biological target for attack by free radicals is *except:*
   A. PUFA
   B. Protein
   C. DMA
   D. Glycosaminoglycan
3. All the following are antioxidant nutrients *except:*
   A. Vitamin E
   B. Vitamin C
   C. Carotenoid and flavonoid
   D. Phylloquinone
4. The minerals function as antioxidants *except:*
   A. Manganese
   B. Copper
   C. Zinc
   D. Iron
5. The following enzymes act as antioxidants *except:*
   A. Superoxide dismutase
   B. Lactate dehydrogenase
   C. Catalase
   D. Glutathione peroxidase
6. α-tocopherol prevents rancidity by virtue of this property:
   A. Antioxidant
   B. Oxidant
   C. Hydrogenation
   D. Phosphorylation
7. Free radicals are:
   A. Chemical species with unpaired electron
   B. Ion having both positive and negative charges
   C. Positively-charged ion
   D. Negatively-charged ion

ANSWERS

1. (D)   2. (D)   3. (D)   4. (D)   5. (B)
6. (A)   7. (A)

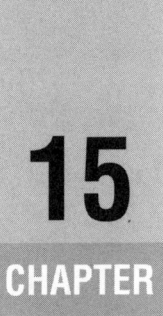

CHAPTER 15

Hormones: Outline Chemistry and Functions

INTRODUCTION

Hormones are chemicals produced by ductless glands and are transported by blood to target tissues to produce inhibitory or stimulatory effect in these tissues. Hormones are synthesized in the body unlike vitamins. The role of hormones is to provide communications between cells to regulate their development and coordinate various cellular activities. Since the communication among cells is done by hormones, they are called chemical messengers. Hormones present in the blood are bound to plasma protein fractions and transported along with them. For example, thyroxine and corticosteroids are bound to globulin; estrogens and androgens are bound to albumin.

Hormones are substances synthesized in the body in small quantities, but have a profound biochemical effect in the control and regulation of metabolic events and contribute in some cases to intercellular and intracellular communication.

Functions of hormones cover four major areas namely:
1. Reproduction.
2. Growth and development.
3. Maintenance of internal environment.
4. Energy production, utilization and storage.

Similarities with Enzymes

1. They act as body catalysts resembling enzymes in many respects.
2. They are required only in small quantities.
3. They are not used up in reactions.

Differences from Enzymes

1. They are produced in an organ other than the target tissues.
2. They are secreted in blood prior to use. Thus, the target levels of hormones can give some indication of endocrine gland activity and target organ exposure.
3. While all enzymes are proteins, only some hormones are proteins, a few are peptides. Some hormones are derived from amino acids, while some are steroids in nature.

Hormone Secretion

Hormones are secreted by specialized cells known as glands. Hormones are recognized by special structures called receptors located on the cell surface of the target cells. On receiving a chemical signal with the help of a hormone, the receptors trigger a cell response by bringing about particular changes in the properties of the cells.

The secretion of hormones is controlled by the anterior lobe of the pituitary gland. This gland is located at the base of the brain. These pituitary hormones are transported to other glands, such as adrenal cortex, thyroid and sex glands, etc. to stimulate the production of other hormones. Hormones are highly potent and so are produced in small quantities.

Hormone Secreting Glands

Major hormone secreting glands are:
1. Pituitary.
2. Thyroid.
3. Parathyroid.
4. Adrenal.
5. Pancreas.
6. Ovaries.
7. Testes.

CLASSIFICATION OF HORMONES

Hormones do not have any special structural feature in common. Chemically they belong to different classes of compounds.

Based on the Chemical Structure

Hormones can be classified into the following three major classes namely steroids, polypeptides and amino acid derivatives.
1. Steroid hormones: For example, adrenocorticosteroid hormones, androgens, estrogens and progesterone.
2. Peptide hormones: For example, insulin, glucagon, parathormone, calcitonin and pituitary hormones.
3. Amine hormones: These are derived from amino acid tyrosine. For example, epinephrine, norepinephrine and thyroid hormones.

Based on the Mode of Action

1. Hormones, which act by binding to their receptors on the plasma membrane, e.g. insulin.
2. Hormones, which act through the second messenger, cAMP, e.g. glucagon.
3. Hormones, which bind to high affinity receptor proteins in the cytosol move to the nucleolus as a complex, interact with chromatin there, increases the production of mRNA and thereby proteins, e.g. steroids.
4. Hormones, which straight away move to the nucleus and interact with specific receptor proteins in the nucleus and increase transcription and translation, e.g. triiodothyronine (T_3).
5. Hormones, which increase the extent of translation without increasing transcription, e.g. insulin, adrenocorticotropic hormone (ACTH).

FACTORS REGULATING HORMONE ACTION

Action of a hormone at a target organ is regulated by four factors:
1. Rate of synthesis and secretion of hormones.
2. In some cases, specific transport systems in plasma.
3. Hormone-specific receptors in target cell membranes, which differ from tissue to tissue.
4. Ultimate degradation of the hormone usually by the liver or kidneys.

Mode of Action of Hormones

1. Induction of enzyme synthesis at the nuclear level, e.g. thyroxine, steroid hormones.
2. Some hormones do not influence transcription, i.e. mRNA production.

3. Some hormones act at the level of the biomembranes first. They may have no activity in membrane free preparation.
4. Many hormones will be functionless, if cAMP does not serve them, hence cAMP is called the second messenger of those hormones, which are themselves first messengers.
5. Action through calcium. Many hormones discharges its function through calcium.

STEROID HORMONES

Steroid hormones are those which have a steroid nucleus. The steroid nucleus has a four ring network, consisting of three cyclohexane rings and one cyclopentane ring joined in a particular manner. In addition to hormones, the steroid is also present in vitamin D, drugs and bile acids.

Steroid nucleus　　　　　Cholesterol

If an alcoholic hydroxyl group is present in the steroid it is known as a sterol. Cholesterol is the most common sterol present in animals.

SEX HORMONES

Sex hormones are the important steroid hormones. In males, steroid hormones are synthesized in the testes and the adrenal cortex. Testosterone, dihydrotestosterone and androgens are the male sex hormones. During puberty, these stimulate the development of male sex characteristics. Estrogens are the female sex hormones, which are produced primarily in ovaries. Female sex hormones are responsible for the development of female sex characteristics during puberty.

Some other steroids such as cortisone, corticosterone and aldosterone affect metabolism, minerals and water balances. The deficiency of these hormones leads to loss of fluids, while an excess of these hormones causes an increase in blood pressure. Androgens and estrogens have significant effect on the anabolic systems. Androgens and estrogens are abused by athletes, weight-lifters and other sports persons to increase their muscle mass and strength. Such uses of anabolic steroids is now banned in competitive sports. Some female sex hormones, which are synthesized on a large scale are used as oral contraceptives.

Testosterone   Estriol

Androgens

Androgens are produced by testes.

Biochemical Effects

1. Influence protein metabolism: Anabolic effect on protein conservation and retention of nitrogen, thereby muscle growth and maintenance of muscle mass.
2. Mineral metabolism.
3. Carbohydrate metabolism.
4. Citric acid cycle and fatty acid synthesis are stimulated by androgens.

Estrogens

Ovarian hormones produced by the graafian follicles of the ovary. Responsible for the regulation of menstrual cycle as well as reproductive cycle.

Biochemical Effects

Estrogen stimulates the development, maturation and function of the female sex organs and thereby the secondary sex characteristics:
1. Proliferation of vaginal epithelium, endometrium.
2. Increases secretion of mucus by the cervical glands.
3. Growth of uterine tissue and mammary gland.

4. Reduces hyperlipidemia, hypercholesterolemia, prevents atherosclerosis.
5. Estrogen administration elevates calcium and phosphorus.

Progesterone

Secreted by corpus luteum during the later half of the menstrual cycle. Development of mammary luster and maintenance of uterus during gestation period.

PEPTIDE HORMONES

Insulin

Insulin is a protein hormone, secreted by the β-cells of the islets of Langerhans of pancreas. It has been isolated and prepared in the crystalline form. Crystalline insulin contains zinc (Zn). It has a molecular weight of 5,734.

Insulin molecule is composed of two polypeptide chains, the glycyl or 'A' chain and phenylalanine or 'B' chain containing a total of 51 amino acids. The glycyl chain is acidic and contains 21 amino acids. The phenylalanine chain is basic and contains 30 amino acids. Both the chains are held together by disulfide bridges.

The target tissues of insulin are the muscles, liver, adipose tissue and heart.

Insulin circulates in blood mostly along with β- and γ-globulin of plasma protein. The normal concentration of plasma insulin is 6–25 mIU per liter. Insulin promotes the entry of glucose in all tissues of the body except liver.

Metabolic Actions of Insulin

1. Lowering of blood glucose level.
2. Increase in the rate of oxidation of glucose in tissues.
3. Increasing glycogen formation in the liver and muscles.
4. Depressing gluconeogenesis.
5. Accelerating the rate of conversion of glucose to fat (lipogenesis).
6. Depressing ketogenesis.
7. Increasing protein synthesis.

Insulin is administered parenterally to reduce hyperglycemia in diabetes mellitus.

It brings down blood glucose level by increasing the oxidation of glucose and promoting glycogenesis in liver and muscles.

Insulin Deficiency: Diabetes Mellitus

- Due to inadequate insulin production
- Insulin not binding to the receptors
- Accelerated insulin destruction
- Insulin inhibitors and antagonists.

Diabetes Mellitus—Two Types

1. Type I: Real deficiency or shortage of insulin in the circulating plasma, 10%—juvenile IDDM (insulin-dependent diabetes mellitus), injection of insulin.
2. Type II: Because of resistance to the hormone due to lack of receptors or their decreased number in proportion to body size. 90%—NIDDM (non-insulin-dependent diabetes mellitus), no injection—by diet/oral hypoglycemic drugs enhance the action of receptor.

Glucagon

Glucagon is a hyperglycemic, glycogenolytic hormone. It is secreted by the α-cells of the islets of Langerhans in pancreas. It is a protein consisting of a straight polypeptide chain, which contains 29 amino acid residues. It has a MW of 3,485. Glucagon is very active when administered intravenously and has an effect opposite to that of insulin. The blood sugar rises immediately, reaches a peak in about 30 minutes and returns to the original level in 1 hour.

AMINE HORMONES

Amine hormones are water-soluble compounds having an amino group, e.g. adrenaline (epinephrine) and thyroid hormones.

Adrenaline

Adrenaline is needed to prepare people for emergency in several ways. Adrenaline increases the rate of heart beat, the heart output and blood pressure and thus prepares the cardiovascular system for emergency section. It stimulates the breakdown of liver glycogen into blood glucose, which is the fuel for anaerobic muscular work. These properties make adrenaline one of the most valuable drugs.

Thyroid and its Hormones

The normal adult thyroid gland weighs about 20 g. It contains protein thyroglobulin, which releases thyroid hormones into the blood of capillaries surrounding the cells. Main hormones secreted are tetraiodothyronine (T_4, thyroxine) and triiodothyronine (T_3).

$$HO-\underset{\underset{|}{5'}}{\overset{\overset{|}{3'}}{\bigcirc}}-O-\underset{\underset{|}{5}}{\overset{\overset{|}{3}}{\bigcirc}}-CH_2-\overset{NH_2}{\underset{|}{CH}}-COOH$$

3,5,3',5'-tetraiodothyronine (Thyroxine or T_4)

Biosynthesis and Secretion

The thyroid gland contains more than half of the total iodine content in the body. It has a remarkable capacity to concentrate iodide brought to it by the circulating blood.

Transport

The thyroid hormones are carried in plasma in combination with albumin and two specific plasma proteins.

One of them is the thyroxine-binding globulin (TBG) and the other thyroxine-binding prealbumin (TBPA).

A small amount is free thyroxine 0.05%, which is a metabolically active hormone.

Mechanism of Action

Two important functions—in growth and development of the body as well as having a stimulating effect on the total metabolism.

Calorigenic action: Stimulate most of the oxidation reactions and regulate the metabolic rates in the body.

Done by stimulation of enzymatic system—basal metabolic rate (BMR) low in hypothyroidism, increases in hyperthyroidism.

Carbohydrate metabolism: Thyroid hormones accelerate the rate of glucose oxidation, promote intestinal absorption of glucose and increase glycogenolysis in the liver.

Thyroxine (T_4)

Thyroxine secreted by thyroid gland has a MW of about 680,000. It is synthesized in thyroid gland from tyrosine. It is stored in the colloid of the thyroid follicles in the form of a glycoprotein called thyroglobulin, hydrolysis of which gives triiodothyronine and tetraiodothyronine (thyroxine). They are also abbreviated as T_3 and T_4. T_3 is 5–10 times biologically more active than T_4.

Metabolic Effects

Thyroxine produces a widespread enhancement of metabolism in almost all the tissues of the body as follows.

Calorigenic effect: Thyroxine increases the rate of energy exchange and oxygen consumption of all tissues except the thyroid gland itself. BMR increases.

Protein metabolism: In small physiological doses, thyroxine promotes protein anabolism, resulting in retention of nitrogen and positive nitrogen balance.

Carbohydrate metabolism: Effects as follows:
1. Increases the rate of intestinal absorption of glucose.
2. Hyperglycemia is associated with increased degradation of insulin.
3. Thyroxine enhances gluconeogenesis.
4. Glycolysis, Krebs cycle and HMP pathway are enhanced.

Lipid metabolism: Thyroxine increases the rate of oxidation of fats. It promotes liberation of free fatty acids from adipose tissues and raises the concentration of free fatty acids in blood.

Effect as Na^+/K^+-ATPase pump: Enhance the function of Na^+/K^+-ATPase pump thus increasing the ATP utilization.

Antithyroid Agents

1. Agents, which retard the synthesis of thyroid hormone, e.g. thiocyanate, thiocarbamide, sulfa drugs, perchlorate.
2. Synthetic analogues of the thyroxine 2',6'-diiodothyronine.
3. Deep X-ray therapy destroys the thyroid tissue and thus depresses the thyroid activity.
4. Cobalt chloride administration interferes with thyroid hormone synthesis and clinical myxedema and goiter may result.

5. Certain organic compounds are present in vegetables like cabbage and turnip, which act as natural goitrogens and depress thyroid activity. Present as goitrins in the raw foods and are destroyed on cooking.

Hypothyroidism

In child: Cretinism—slow growth, dwarfism, mental retardation, dry skin, scatty hair, saddled nose, puffy lips, vacant expression.

In adult: Myxedema—BMR and body temperature decreases. Sensitivity to cold, puffiness of face, anemia and reduction of physical and mental functions.

Hyperthyroidism

Increased activity accompanied by excessive secretion of the thyroid hormone occurs in Grave's disease (exophthalmic goiter) and toxic adenoma.

Nervousness, irritability, loss of weight, increased body temperature, increased appetite, protrusion of the eyeballs.

Goiter

Enlargement of thyroid gland caused by deficiency of iodine in the diet. Iodine enriched salt is now compulsory.

Parathyroid Glands and their Hormones

Closely associated with the thyroid gland as two pairs of small glands. Weight 50–300 mg. It produces a parathyroid hormone (PTH). Parathormone having a profound influence on calcium (Ca) and phosphate (P) metabolism. It maintains the serum Ca^{++} level within normal physiological limits.

Biochemical Effects

1. The serum calcium is raised, but serum phosphorus is lowered.
2. The excretion of both Ca and P is increased.
3. Ca from the bone gets mobilized and added to the serum.
4. The serum alkaline phosphatase activity is increased.

ADRENAL MEDULLA

Medullary portion releases two hormones—epinephrine and norepinephrine.

Epinephrine

Epinephrine is elaborated by the adrenal medulla as a result of sympathetic stimulation produced during fight, fright and flight, and in emergencies like cold, fatigue and shock.

Neural stimulation, fright, emotional conditions like anger, etc. are responsible for a quick release of catecholamine hormones.

Physiological and Biochemical Functions

1. Sympathomimetic function: Epinephrine cause a rise in BP due to arteriolar vasoconstriction particularly in the skin, mucous membrane and splanchnic viscera.
2. Arterioles of skeletal muscle undergo vasodilation. Overall effect is rise in BP, pulse rate, heart rate and cardiac output.

Norepinephrine

Rise in BP by increasing peripheral resistance. Overall vasoconstriction and has no effect on cardiac output.

Functions

Action on smooth muscle: Epinephrine dialates bronchial musculature, relaxes the musculature of the gastrointestinal tract and contracts the pyloric sphincter.

Effects on carbohydrate metabolism: Epinephrine promotes glycogenolysis in the muscle and liver. It produces an increase in blood lactic acid level and as well as blood glucose level. Norepinephrine has only 1/8 activity of epinephrine in glycogen breakdown.

Effects on lipid metabolism: Stimulates lypolysis in adipose tissues and releases free fatty acids into the blood.

PANCREATIC ISLET CELLS

1. Endocrine part—islets of Langerhans.
2. Islets cells are of 4 types: A, B, D and F cells
   - A cells—α-cells—produce glucagon
   - B cells—β-cells—insulin
   - D cells—somatostatin.

ADRENAL CORTEX

Although all the six steroid hormones are biosynthesized from cholesterol by the adrenal cortical tissues of man, only two of this, corticosterone and cortisol are released into the bloodstream with small amounts of aldosterone.

Biochemical Effects of Corticosteroids

1. Effects on metabolism: Corticosteroids exert a profound action on carbohydrate, lipid, nucleic acid and protein metabolisms.
2. Action on digestive secretion: Hydrochloric acid (HCl) production and pepsinogen secretion by the cells of the gastric mucosa are enhanced by cortisone.
3. Hematological changes.
4. Electrolyte and water metabolism: Regulate the concentration of Na^+ and K^+ in the extracellular fluid.
5. Bone and calcium metabolism.
6. Immune response and anti-inflammatory response.

GASTROINTESTINAL HORMONES

Gastrin

- By antral gastric mucosa
- Stimulates gastric secretion.

Secretin

Stimulates the pancreas to produce an increased volume of pancreatic juice.

Cholecystokinin

Stimulate the contraction of gallbladder enhancing the flow of bile into the duodenum.

HYPOTHALAMIC AND PITUITARY HORMONES

The hypothalamus produces two types of endocrine factors:
a. The hypothalamic neuropeptides.
b. The hypothalamic releasing factors.

It releases six hormones, which are called 'releasing factors'. Some stimulate the release of pituitary hormone, while a few inhibit their release. They are release-inhibiting hormones. Releasing factors exert a tonic control on the production and release of pituitary hormones.
1. Thyrotropin-releasing hormone (TRH)/TRF.
2. Corticotropin-releasing hormone (CRH)/CRF.
3. Growth hormone-releasing hormone (GHRH).
4. Growth hormone release-inhibiting hormone (GHRIH)/(somatostatin).
5. Gonadotropin-releasing hormone.
6. Prolactin release-inhibiting hormone.

Anterior Pituitary Hormones

The anterior pituitary hormones are mostly trophic in nature, stimulating the secretion of other hormones. There are three types of cells secreting hormones—acidophils, basophils and chromophobes. Secretion of all anterior pituitary hormones are under the control of hypothalamic releasing or inhibitory factors. The following six hormones are secreted by the anterior pituitary:
1. Growth hormone (GH) or somatotropin.
2. Thyroid-stimulating hormone (TSH).
3. Adrenocorticotropic hormone (ACTH).
4. Interstitial cell-stimulating hormone (ICSH).
5. Follicle-stimulating hormone (FSH).
6. Lactogenic hormone.

Growth Hormone or Somatotropin

Major effect of growth hormone is to stimulate growth. The effect of GH is mediated through somatomedin-C also known as insulin-like growth factor-1 (IGF-1). The growth of long bones and soft tissues is stimulated by this factor. The uptake of amino acids by cells is increased, with a resultant increase in the rate of protein synthesis. The anti-insulin effect causes lipolysis and hyperglycemia. The secretion of GH is stimulated by hypoglycemia and suppressed by hyperglycemia. The GHRH is the major secretory stimulant. Somatostatin inhibits secretion of GH. Somatostatin is secreted mainly by hypothalamus.

The abnormalities of GH secretion may have different manifestations depending on the age of onset. Excess secretion in children leads to gigantism and in adults acromegaly. GH-secreting tumor is often the cause and removal of the tumor leads to cessation of growth.

Adrenocorticotropic Hormone or Corticotropin

Adrenocorticotropic hormone (ACTH) is one of the pituitary hormones secreted as a large precursor molecule, which is cleaved to give several peptides each with important biological effect. The precursor or polypeptide is known as proopiomelanocortin (POMC). The secretion of POMC is under the control of CRF. The active ACTH is a polypeptide with 39 amino acids of which the N-terminal of 25 amino acids alone are required for biological activity. ACTH binds to specific receptors on the adrenal gland, then activates adenylyl cyclase as that cAMP level is raised. ACTH increases the synthesis of corticosteroids by the adrenal cortex and also stimulates their release from the gland. It also increases the transfer of cholesterol from plasma lipoproteins to fasciculata cells.

Thyroid-stimulating Hormone or Thyrotropic Hormone

Thyroid-stimulating hormone is produced by basophil cells of anterior pituitary and is glycoprotein in nature. Functions are as follows:
  a. The TSH stimulates the synthesis of thyroid hormones at all stages and on iodine uptake, organification and coupling.
  b. It enhances the release of stored thyroid hormones.
  c. It increases DNA content, RNA and translation of proteins, cell size.
  d. It stimulates glycolysis, TCA cycle, PPP and phospholipid synthesis.
  e. It activates adipose tissue lipase to enhance release of fatty acids (lipolysis).

QUESTION

1. **Short notes on:**
   A. Thyroxine, insulin.
   B. Gastrointestinal (GI) hormones.
   C. Thyroid hormones.
   D. Adrenal gland hormones.

MULTIPLE CHOICE QUESTIONS

2. **All the following are protein/peptide hormones *except*:**
   A. Oxytocin
   B. Insulin
   C. Epinephrine
   D. Glucagon

3. **A steroid hormone is:**
   A. Thyroxine
   B. Parathyroid hormone
   C. Oxytocin
   D. Cortisol

4. **Factors regulating hormone action are:**
   A. Rate of synthesis and secretion
   B. Hormone specific receptors
   C. Specific transport systems in plasma
   D. All of the above

5. **Which is a hormone derived from tyrosine?**
   A. Glucagon
   B. Thyroxine
   C. PABA
   D. Alloxan

6. **Insulin is secreted by:**
   A. α-cells of islets of Langerhans of pancreas
   B. Anterior lobe of pituitary gland
   C. α-cells of islets of Langerhans of pancreas
   D. β-cells of the islets of Langerhans of pancreas

7. **α-cells of islets of Langerhans of pancreas secrete:**
   A. Insulin
   B. Glucagon
   C. Oxytocin
   D. Gastrin

8. **Which hormone contains sulfur in its structure?**
   A. Glucagon
   B. Insulin
   C. LD
   D. Epinephrine

9. **All the following are hyperglycemic hormones *except*:**
   A. Epinephrine
   B. Thyroxine
   C. Insulin
   D. Glucagon

10. **The hormone whose deficiency causes diabetes mellitus is:**
    A. Glucagon
    B. Cortisol
    C. Epinephrine
    D. Insulin

11. **An example of a glucocorticoid:**
    A. Cortisol
    B. Aldosterone
    C. Glucagon
    D. Insulin

12. **Which of the following hormones is most important in regulating sodium and potassium balance?**
    A. Cortisol
    B. Estradiol
    C. Progesterone
    D. Aldosterone

13. **All steroid hormones are formed from:**
    A. Arachidonic acid
    B. Acetyl-CoA
    C. Glycine
    D. Cholesterol

14. **Epinephrine is synthesized from:**
    A. Tryptophan
    B. Tyrosine
    C. Glycine
    D. Arginine

15. **Diabetes insipidus occurs due to the abnormal secretion or action of:**
    A. Aldosterone
    B. Insulin
    C. ADH
    D. Oxytocin

ANSWERS

2. (C)	3. (D)	4. (D)	5. (B)	6. (D)
7. (A)	8. (B)	9. (C)	10. (D)	11. (A)
12. (D)	13. (C)	14. (B)	15. (C)	

16
CHAPTER

Blood Chemistry

CONSTITUENTS OF BLOOD

The chemical composition of blood is complex. It is an aqueous solution of ions and organic molecules, which also have suspended particles. Suspended particles in blood are red blood cells (erythrocytes), white blood cells (leukocytes) and platelets.

Blood without suspended particles is called blood plasma. Blood serum is obtained when fibrinogen, a particular protein, is removed from plasma. The major blood constituents are given in Table 16.1.

Clotting of Blood

1. When blood is drawn and allowed to clot, a clear liquid (serum) separates from the clotted blood. Plasma, on the other hand, separates from the cells only when blood is prevented from clotting.
2. The blood clot is formed by a protein (fibrinogen), which is present in the soluble form in the plasma and it is transformed to an insoluble network of fibrous material (fibrin, the substance of the blood clot) by the clotting mechanism.
3. The change of fibrinogen into fibrin is caused by thrombin, which in fluid blood occurs as prothrombin. The conversion of prothrombin to thrombin depends on the action of thromboplastin and calcium.

Anticoagulants

Clot formation may be prevented by a number of substances as well as by vitamin K deficiency. Dicemerol, related to coumarin, which comes from clover, inhibits prothrombin synthesis in the liver. It may be used clinically when there is danger of thrombosis by reducing clotting tendency.

TABLE 16.1: Blood constituents

Compounds	Normal values	Possible pathology
Hemoglobin	14–16 g/100 mL whole blood	High in polycythemia. Low in anemias.
Non-protein nitrogen (NPN)	25–35 mg/100 mL whole blood	High in nephritis and Addison's disease.
Uric acid	3–5 mg/100 mL whole blood	High in gout.
Total plasma proteins	6.5–8.2 g/100 mL plasma	Low in nephrotic syndrome and malnutrition.
Cholesterol	150–250 mg/100 mL plasma or serum	High in nephrotic syndrome and hypothyroidism. Low in pernicious anemia and liver disease.
Glucose	80–110 mg/100 mL whole blood	High in diabetes. Low in Addison's disease.
CO_2 combining power	53–80 mL, CO_2/100 mL plasma	Low in acidosis, uncontrolled diabetes and nephritis.
Inorganic phosphates	3–4 mg/100 mL plasma or serum	High in renal rickets and nephritis. Low in infantile rickets.
Chloride	570–620 mg (as NaCl)/100 mL plasma or serum	High in nephritis. Low in fever or pneumonia.

Heparin

Heparin, a sulfated polysaccharide, which inhibits the formation of thrombin from prothrombin, is the most satisfactory anticoagulant, since it produces no change in the composition of the blood. However, oxalate and citrate have been most widely used, as they are cheaper. Use of more of these salts may bring appreciable changes in the distribution of water between the cells and plasma.

Potassium Oxalate

Potassium oxalate has been most commonly used, since it is more soluble. It acts by precipitating calcium ions as calcium oxalate.

Sodium Citrate

Citrate does not precipitate calcium, but converts it to non-ionized form. Citrated plasma is not as satisfactory as serum for calcium estimation.

Ethylenediaminetetraacetic acid (EDTA) and its salts act by chelating calcium ions.

Sodium Fluoride

Sodium fluoride also acts as an anticoagulant, but large amounts are required. For blood glucose estimation a mixture of sodium fluoride and potassium oxalate is used as fluoride acts as a preservative by inhibiting glycolytic enzymes.

FUNCTIONS OF BLOOD

1. Carrying the products of digestion from the small intestine to various organs and tissues.
2. Accepting oxygen in the lungs and releasing it in the tissues.
3. Carrying CO_2 from the tissues for elimination by the lungs.
4. Removal of waste products from tissues for excretion by the kidneys.
5. Maintenance of water balance and temperature control.
6. Synthesis of antibodies for the protection against bacterial infection.
7. Distribution of hormones, vitamins and enzymes to their sites of action.

Oxygen Transport

During respiration, gases CO_2 and O_2 are interchanged between the body and the environment. This process can occur due to the hemoglobin present in red blood cell (RBC). The function of the RBC is to carry the inhaled oxygen from lungs to tissues, where it is utilized for their growth, development and sustenance.

Hemoglobin is a globular protein. It consists of four polypeptide chains arranged in a tetrahedral configuration. Hemoglobin contains a non-protein constituent called heme. Heme is an iron porphyrin and is responsible for the red color of blood. Each of the polypeptide chains of hemoglobin is associated with one heme unit.

Hemoglobin combines with oxygen in the lungs (where oxygen is present in higher concentrations). Such a combination results in the formation of oxyhemoglobin. Myoglobin stores oxygen in the muscle tissues. In contrast to hemoglobin, it consists of only a single polypeptide chain and is associated with one heme unit.

Formation of CO_2 and its Distribution in Blood

Carbon dioxide is formed in large amounts in the body as the end product of normal metabolism. In tissues about 200 mL of CO_2 is formed per minute at rest and 4 liters at maximal exercise. CO_2 enters the bloodstream and from there reaches the lungs. The chief acid present in the blood is CO_2.

Carbon dioxide dissolves in water to form H_2CO_3, which on dissociation yields H^+ and HCO_3^-.

$$H_2O + CO_2 \rightleftharpoons H_2CO_3 \rightleftharpoons H^+ + HCO_3^-$$

The only alkali present as such in blood is bicarbonate (HCO_3). It dissociates in water as follows:

$$NaHCO_3 + H_2O \longrightarrow H_2CO_3 + NaOH$$

PLASMA PROTEINS

Plasma proteins constitute almost 70% of the plasma and are usually divided into three groups: albumin, globulins and fibrinogen. Approximately 55% of the plasma protein is albumin, 38.5% globulins and 6.5% is fibrinogen.

Albumin

Albumin, like other plasma proteins, cannot pass through the walls of the blood vessels (because they are colloids and colloids cannot pass through membranes). Since albumin is principal plasma protein and the smallest plasma protein both in size and weight (it consists of a single chain of 610 amino acids), it accounts for most of the colloid osmotic pressure of the blood.

This colloidal osmotic pressure is caused by the small amounts of plasma that pass through the capillary membranes and tend to accumulate at the venous end of the capillaries.

If the plasma proteins (primarily albumin) are present in decreased amounts (as during a low-protein diet or in nephritis), the osmotic pressure of the plasma decreases. This decreased osmotic pressure of the blood causes a greater net pressure outward at the arterial end of the capillary and a lower net inward venous pressure at the venous end of the capillary. When this occurs, water (fluid) accumulates in the tissues. Such a condition is known as edema.

Kwashiorkor

A severe protein deficiency disease, characterized by edema of the abdomen and extremities. In children, a swollen belly is characteristic. Kwashiorkor is caused by a drop in plasma protein particularly albumin. Under these conditions, water moves from the bloodstream into the tissues causing swelling.

Edema can also occur because of heart disease, whereby there is an increase in venous hydrostatic pressure. Many terminal illnesses cause edema. This becomes a serious problem and tapping and draining may be necessary. Concentrated albumin infusions (25 g in 100 mL diluent) are helpful in the treatment of shock, to increase the blood volume and to remove fluid from the tissues.

The amount of albumin present in the blood is lowered in liver disease because albumin is formed in the liver.

Another function of albumin in the blood is to act as a carrier for fatty acids, trace elements and many drugs.

Globulins

The globulins present in the plasma can be separated into different groups by a process known as electrophoresis, whereby charged protein particles migrate at varying rates to electrodes of opposite charge, with albumin migrating the fastest. The distribution of the plasma proteins during electrophoresis is as below.

The globulins are subdivided into α, β and γ. They form complexes (loose combination) with such substances as carbohydrates (mucoprotein and glycoprotein), lipids (lipoprotein) and metal ions (transferrin for Fe and ceruloplasmin for Cu). These complexes can be transported to all parts of the body.

The γ-globulin fraction (immunoglobulins) include the antibodies with which the body fights infectious diseases. γ-globulin has been found to contain as many as 20 different antibodies for immunity against such diseases as measles, infective hepatitis, poliomyelitis, mumps and influenza.

Some people lack the ability to make γ-globulin. These people are quite susceptible to infections because they have no antibodies to counteract such diseases. The lack of γ-globulin is called agammaglobulinemia and can be combated by the administration of γ-globulin.

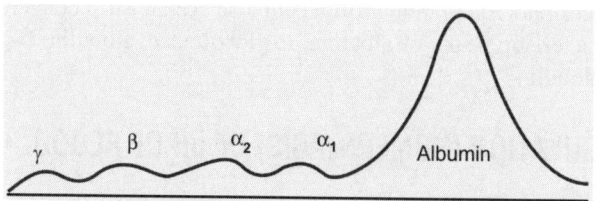

Fig. 16.1: Distribution of plasma proteins during electrophoresis

Albumin/Globulin Ratio

In severe liver disease, there is lowered concentration of plasma albumin, but globulin fraction may not decrease (as it is not synthesized by the liver). The albumin/globulin (A/G) ratio 1.2–1.7 may be reversed in liver disease.

SEPARATION OF PLASMA PROTEINS

The separation of plasma proteins can be done by following methods:
1. Salting out.
2. Electrophoresis.
3. Ultracentrifugation.
4. Immunoelectrophoresis.

Electrophoresis

One of the most powerful tools for separating mixtures of proteins is electrophoresis, which is used routinely in clinical laboratories. It is the movement of a charged particle in an electric field towards oppositely charged electrodes.

Principle

Proteins having different amounts of charge at a particular pH, when placed in an electric field, move at different rates. The rate of movement is determined by the charge/size ratio. It is directly proportional to the charge and inversely proportional to the size of the protein molecule.

In the clinical laboratory, the electrophoresis of plasma proteins (Fig. 16.1) is usually carried out at pH = 8.6. The plasma proteins have a negative charge and will migrate to the positive electrode (cathode) when placed in the electric field.

Electrophoretic scanning from cellulose acetate strip converts bands to characteristic peaks of albumin, α-globulin, α_2-globulin, β-globulin and γ-globulin.

REGULATION (HOMEOSTASIS) OF pH OF BLOOD

If pH is lower than 7.38, it is called acidosis. Life is threatened when pH is lowered below 7.25. Acidosis leads to CNS depression and coma, death occurs when pH is below 7.0. When pH is more than 7.42, it is alkalosis. It is very dangerous if pH is increased above 7.55. Alkalosis induces intramuscular hyperexcitability and tetany. Death occurs when pH is above 7.6.

The normal pH range of the blood is 7.38–7.42. When the pH falls below this range, the condition is called acidosis. Alkalosis occurs when the pH rises above its normal value. Acidosis is more common than alkalosis because many of the metabolic products produced during digestion are acidic.

Maintenance of Acid-base Balance (pH)

Nurses and other healthcare professionals are responsible for preventing, detecting and intervening in acid-base imbalance.

Three physical systems act independently to maintain a normal serum pH.

1. Blood buffers: Chemical buffering of excess acid or base by buffer systems in blood plasma and in cells.
2. Respiratory mechanism by the lungs: Excretion of acid by lungs.
3. Renal mechanism: Excretion of acid or regeneration of base by the kidneys.

$$\text{For normal pH} = \frac{20 \text{ parts base}}{\text{One part acid}} = \frac{HCO_2^-}{CO_2 + H_2CO_3} = 20$$

An increase in the denominator (acid) lowers pH; a decrease in the acid raises the pH.

Blood Buffers

The blood maintains its pH between 7.38 and 7.42 because of buffers. These buffers are present both in the plasma and in the RBCs. Those in the plasma are primarily sodium buffers; those in blood cells are mainly potassium buffers. Buffers are substances, usually a mixture of a weak acid and a salt of a weak acid that resist change in pH. The blood buffers consist of:
- Bicarbonate buffers
- Phosphate buffers
- Protein buffers (including hemoglobin and oxyhemoglobin).

Bicarbonate buffers: The bicarbonate buffer system in the red blood cells consists of carbonic acid (H_2CO_3) and potassium bicarbonate ($KHCO_3$). The bicarbonate buffer system in the blood plasma consists of carbonic acid and sodium bicarbonate ($NaHCO_3$). If a strong acid (such as HCl) is added to a sample of blood, it will react with the salt part of the buffer and undergo the following reactions:

$$HCl + KHCO_3 \longrightarrow H_2CO_3 + KCl \text{ (in blood cells)}$$
$$HCl + NaHCO_3 \longrightarrow H_2CO_3 + NaCl \text{ (in blood plasma)}$$

The carbonic acid (H_2CO_3) produced is part of the original buffer. Note that the strong acid HCl has been replaced by a very weak acid H_2CO_3. The other products, KCl and NaCl are neutral salts and will not affect the pH of the system. If a strong base, like KOH or NaOH is added to a sample of blood, the following reactions will occur with the bicarbonate buffer systems:

$$KOH + H_2CO_3 \longrightarrow KHCO_3 + H_2O \text{ (in blood cells)}$$
$$NaOH + H_2CO_3 \longrightarrow NaHCO_3 + H_2O \text{ (in blood plasma)}$$

The salts $KHCO_3$ and $NaHCO_3$ are part of the original buffer systems and the water produced is neutral, so the pH again is not affected. In both cases (reaction with a strong acid or a strong base) more of the buffer is produced plus a neutral compound. The bicarbonate buffers control the pH of blood and the phosphate buffers have an important role inside the cell and the urine.

Phosphate buffers: It consist of mixtures of K_2HPO_4 (basic phosphate) and KH_2PO_4 (acidic phosphate) (also Na_2HPO_4 and NaH_2PO_4) which function similarly as the bicarbonate buffers in neutralizing excess acid and base.

$$HCl + K_2HPO_4 \longrightarrow KH_2PO_4 + KCl$$
$$KOH + KH_2PO_4 \longrightarrow K_2HPO_4 + H_2O$$

Hemoglobin buffers: It accounts for more than half of the buffering action in the blood. These are hemoglobin buffers and oxyhemoglobin buffers:

$\left.\begin{array}{l}\text{HHb}\\ \text{KHb}\end{array}\right\}$ Hemoglobin buffers $\qquad$ $\left.\begin{array}{l}\text{HHbO}_2\\ \text{KHbO}_2\end{array}\right\}$ Oxyhemoglobin buffers

These buffers, as well as other proteins that act as buffers in the blood stream, pick up excess acid or base to help keep the pH of the blood at 7.38–7.42.

Respiratory Mechanism

The process of respiration, i.e. the intake of oxygen and removal of CO_2, requires the transport of these substances by blood. Since CO_2 reacts to form HCO_3^- and oxygen forms oxyhemoglobin, which is more acidic than hemoglobin, the respiratory process is involved in the delicate acid-base balance of the body. Maintenance of a constant pH of 7.38–7.42 is required for health.

$$CO_2 + H_2O \longrightarrow H_2 + CO_3$$
$$H_2CO_3 \longrightarrow H^+ + HCO_3^-$$

The respiratory center in the medulla of the brain is particularly sensitive to any change in the pH of the blood and immediately causes an increase in the rate and depth of breathing until excess CO_2 (and hence excess H^+) is removed. Changes brought about by respiration are rapid.

Renal Mechanism

Renal mechanism is by far the most effective mechanism, but it is slow, requiring hours to show result. The kidneys excrete more HCO_3^- and HPO_4^-, when the blood pH is too high and more H^+ (which it gains in exchange for Na^+) and $H_2PO_4^-$ when pH is too low.

The kidney can also increase its production of NH_3 (ammonia), which will trap H^+ to form NH_4, thus lowering the acidity of the blood. Since the cell membrane is not permeable to the charged NH_4, it is 'trapped' and excreted in the urine as ammonium salts. Ammonia is produced in the renal epithelial cells largely by the deamidation of glutamine taken up from the arterial blood.

$$\text{Glutamine} + H_2O \longrightarrow \text{Glutamic acid} + NH_3$$

Urine is slightly acidic because of the phosphates and sulfates, formed principally from catabolism of the food and extracted mainly as acid ions, $H_2PO_4^-$ and HSO_4^-. Also organic acids formed in metabolism are excreted by the kidney, if they do not undergo further metabolism.

TABLE 16.2: Typical changes in plasma pH, pCO_2 and HCO_3^- concentration for various acid-base disorders

Acid-base disorders	pH	$[HCO_3^-]$	pCO_2
Metabolic acidosis	↓	↓	↓
Metabolic alkalosis	↑	↑	↑
Respiratory acidosis	↓	↑	↑
Respiratory alkalosis	↑	↓	↓

Measurement of Acid-base Balance

The definite way of assessing the state of acid-base balance of the body is to determine the pH of the blood. But clinically this is not always possible. As an alternative method, determination of the CO_2 content of the plasma is considered suitable for clinical purposes. Typical changes in plasma pH, pCO_2 and HCO_3^- concentrations for various acid-base disorders are given in Table 16.2.

Disturbances in Homeostasis [H⁺] (Acidosis and Alkalosis—Acid-base Imbalance)

Changes in the CO_2 level in blood and corresponding changes in HCO_3^- and pH may be caused by respiratory acidosis, respiratory alkalosis, metabolic acidosis and metabolic alkalosis. If the pH is abnormally high or low, the alkalosis or acidosis is said to be uncompensated. Disturbances in the acid-base balance are known as acidosis and alkalosis and these occur mostly due to abnormalities in respiratory system or due to disturbances in metabolism. The principal effect of acidosis is depression of CNS through decreased synaptic transmission characterized by generalized weakness in CNS function. Severe acidosis can cause disorientation, coma and death. Alkalosis causes overexcitability of the deranged and peripheral nervous systems, characterized by numbness and light headedness. It can cause nervousness, muscle spasms or tetany, convulsions, loss of consciousness and death. Accordingly acidosis and alkalosis are classified as:

1. a. Respiratory acidosis.
   b. Respiratory alkalosis.
2. a. Metabolic acidosis.
   b. Metabolic alkalosis.

Acid-base disorders can be differentiated based on whether they have metabolic or respiratory etiologies.

Respiratory acidosis: It is caused by depression of the respiratory centers by drugs, e.g. barbiturate poisoning, narcotics ingestion. In pulmonary disorders (pneumonia) due to mechanical obstruction of air passage and during breathing of air with high CO_2 content, there will be a decrease in blood HCO_3^- content and increased levels of $CO_2/(H_2CO_3)$. The condition is compensated by the action of the kidneys.

The principal effect of respiratory acidosis is depression of central nervous system (CNS) through decreased synaptic transmission characterized by generalized weakness and deranged CNS function. Severe acidosis causes disorientation, coma and death.

Respiratory alkalosis: It is relatively uncommon. It is caused by hypoventilation as in high fever, hysteria, high altitudes and salicylate poisoning or due to dry hot weather. It can also occur during anesthetic procedures with manual control of breathing causing expulsion of CO_2 and in certain diseases of CNS affecting the respiratory system.

Respiratory alkalosis causes overexcitability of the central and peripheral nervous systems, characterized by numbness and lightheadedness. It can cause nervousness, muscle spasms or tetany, convulsions, loss of consciousness and death.

Metabolic acidosis: Results from increased generation or accumulation of acids or loss of base (i.e. bicarbonate). Simple, acute metabolic acidosis results in low blood pH or acidemia. Symptoms include headache, lethargy, nausea, vomiting and diarrhea. If left untreated, leads to coma and death.

In this condition, there is a deficit of plasma bicarbonate, without much change in the carbonic acid content. Metabolic acidosis can occur in the following conditions:
1. Uncontrolled diabetes, complicated with ketosis.
2. Vomiting with loss of fluid not containing acid.
3. Poisoning by an acid salt.
4. Starvation, high fever.
5. Violent exercise.
6. Lactic acidosis due to shock or hemorrhage.
7. Ingestion of acidifying salts like acetyl salicylic acid, phosphoric acid, HCl, NH_4Cl.
8. Renal insufficiency: Retention of acids normally produced, e.g. terminal stages of nephritis, destructive renal lesions, such as polycystic kidneys, pyelonephritis, renal TB.

The CO_2/HCO_3^- buffer system in blood reflects the changes in all buffer systems during disturbances. When pH falls, the ratio $HCO_3^-/CO_2 + H_2CO_3$ also decreases. Excess of CO_2 is blown off through lungs that brings back the original ratio.

$$pH = \frac{HCO_2}{CO_2 + H_2CO_3} = 20$$

Thus, acidosis is compensated by a respiratory response.

Metabolic alkalosis: Results from the administration or accumulation of acid (e.g. during gastric suctioning or loss of extracellular fluid containing more chloride than bicarbonate). Simple acute respiratory alkalosis results in a high blood pH or alkalemia. Symptoms include slow and shallow respiration, hyperactive reflexes often related to depletion of electrolytes.

In metabolic alkalosis, the bicarbonate content of the plasma is increased without undue changes in the carbonic acid content. Metabolic alkalosis occurs in the following conditions:

1. Ingestion of large doses of alkalies in the treatment of peptic ulcer.
2. Excessive vomiting with loss of large amount of gastric juice as in cases of intestinal obstruction.
3. Removal of large amounts of gastric secretion as in gastric suction.
   There is also loss of chloride. Compensation is attempted by a depression of respiration so that more CO_2 is retained.

Symptoms of metabolic acidosis: Symptoms include headache lethargy, nausea, vomiting and diarrhea. If left untreated, leads to coma and death.

Symptoms of metabolic alkalosis: Slow and shallow respiration, hyperactive reflexes (tetany) often related to depletion of electrolytes, atrial tachycardia and dysrhythmias.

QUESTIONS

1. What is the normal pH of blood? How is it regulated?
2. Describe the mechanism of regulation of acid-base balance in the body.
3. Write a short note on blood buffers.
4. What is the normal pH of blood? Name the buffer system and explain how they regulate the pH of the blood.
5. Write short notes on:
   A. Acidosis.
   B. Alkalosis.

MULTIPLE CHOICE QUESTIONS

6. **Normal pH of arterial blood is:**
   A. 4.35–4.45
   B. 6.35–6.45
   C. 6.95–7.25
   D. 7.35–7.45
7. **Mechanisms for the regulation of acid-base balance include:**
   A. Renal mechanism
   B. Respiratory mechanism
   C. Blood buffers
   D. All of the above
8. **The chief physiological buffer in the blood is:**
   A. Bicarbonate buffer
   B. Hemoglobin buffer
   C. Proteinate buffer
   D. Phosphate buffer
9. **The major acid produced in the body during oxidation of food in the cells is:**
   A. Hydrochloric acid
   B. Acetic acid
   C. Carbonic acid
   D. Phosphoric acid
10. **Renal mechanism for regulation of acid-base balance include:**
    A. Phosphate mechanism
    B. Bicarbonate mechanism
    C. Ammonia mechanism
    D. All of the above
11. **If the pH of the blood is 7.4, the ratio of $NaHCO_3/H_2CO_3$ will be:**
    A. 5:1
    B. 10:1
    C. 20:1
    D. 25:1
12. **In a solution containing phosphate buffer the pH will be 7.4, if the ratio of monohydrogen phosphate to dihydrogen phosphate is:**
    A. 4:1
    B. 5:1
    C. 10:1
    D. 20:1
13. **Metabolic acidosis can occur in all the following *except:***
    A. Diabetes mellitus
    B. Addison's disease
    C. Diarrhea
    D. Vomiting
14. **During compensation of respiratory alkalosis, all the following changes occur *except:***
    A. Decreased secretion of hydrogen ions by renal tubules
    B. Increased excretion of sodium in urine
    C. Increased excretion of bicarbonate in urine
    D. Increased excretion of ammonia in urine
15. **Metabolic alkalosis can occur in:**
    A. Renal failure
    B. Recurrent vomiting
    C. Severe diarrhea
    D. Excess use of carbonic anhydride inhibitors

16. All the following features are present in blood chemistry in uncompensated metabolic alkalosis *except:*
   A. Increased pH
   B. Increased bicarbonate
   C. Normal chloride
   D. Normal pCO_2

ANSWERS

6. (D)   7. (D)   8. (A)   9. (C)   10. (D)
11. (C)   12. (A)   13. (D)   14. (B)   15. (B)
16. (C)

17
CHAPTER

Urinalysis

COLLECTION OF URINE

Many urine estimations are carried out on timed specimens (24 hour). The accuracy of the result depends largely on that of urine collection. Therefore, more care should be taken to ensure that the collection of urine for 24 hours is done properly. For example, when a 24-hours collection is required between 10 AM on Monday and 10 AM on Tuesday, the following procedure should be adopted.

On Monday 10 AM, empty bladder completely and discard the specimen. Then collect all the urine passed in the bottle containing the preservative till 10 AM on Tuesday. The bladder is emptied at 10 AM on Tuesday and this is also added to the above pooled urine.

Preservative for Urine

A preservative must be added to the urine to prevent bacterial growth and destruction of the substance being estimated.

Hydrochloric acid: Acidification of the specimen is very satisfactory. 10 cc of concentrated HCl is adequate for 24-hours specimen. This is suitable for the determination of urea, ammonia, total nitrogen, calcium and phosphorus.

Toluene: It is a commonly used preservative. It is convenient for sodium, potassium, uric acid and protein analysis. This only prevents further surface contamination with bacteria.

Thymol: It is also used as a preservative (a few crystals or 5 mL of 10% solution). This is a satisfactory preservative for a wide range of substances. However, it cannot be used for the estimation of 17-oxosteroids using Zimmermann reaction.

COMPOSITION OF URINE

Color

Normal urine is clear and straw colored. The color is due to the pigment urochrome. The color is lighter when large amount of water is consumed, and darker in fevers and after excessive perspiration. In jaundice, the urine is yellow due to excretion of bile pigments. In alkaptonuria and methemoglobinemia, urine is dark brown in color.

Odor

Freshly voided urine has a mild aromatic odor. It develops ammoniacal odor on standing, due to the formation of ammonia by bacterial decomposition of urea. Urine in ketosis emits the smell of acetone.

Volume

The daily urinary output varies widely and is dependent on the fluid intake and environmental conditions. The volume excreted varies between 1,000–2,000 mL. Polyuria or increase in the volume of urine to more than 2,000 mL is seen in diabetes mellitus. A fall in the urinary output is termed as oliguria when excretion is less than 500 mL, which is found in renal failure, some diseases of the heart and lungs, fevers and diarrhea. Anuria, a complete cessation of urine output is seen in the terminal stages of renal failure (less than 50 mL).

Appearance

Normal urine is ordinarily clear and transparent when freshly voided. It may become cloudy on standing because of the precipitation of phosphates. Urine may be turbid when RBCs or pus cells are present.

Specific Gravity

Specific gravity varies from 1.010 to 1.030 depending upon water and food intake. It is determined in clinical practice by means of a urinometer. It consists of a weighted cylinder, which floats in urine and a stem calibrated in degrees of specific gravity usually from 1.000 to 1.060. The depth to which the urinometer sinks depends on the density of the urine. The instrument is usually calibrated for use at 15°C.

PROCEDURE

1. Fill the cylinder with urine without producing bubbles.
2. Float the urinometer so that it does not touch the sides.
3. Make the reading from the bottom meniscus.

Temperature Correction

The urinometer is usually calibrated for use at 15°C and specific gravity should be corrected to room temperature by adding, 0.001 for every 3°C above the temperature at which the urinometer is calibrated (15°C).

Room temperature = 30°C
Specific gravity read = 1.009
Temperature correction = $1.009 + 5 \times 0.001$
 = 1.014

Total Solids

Under normal conditions, the total solids present in about 1,500 mL of urine varies from 60 to 70 g. The output of urinary solids is influenced by the intake of fluid diet.

The total solids per liter of urine is obtained by multiplying the last two digits of the specific gravity by a factor of 2.6, which is called the Long's coefficient. If the specific gravity is 1.020, the total solids would be 52 g/L.

Reaction

Normally urine is acidic (pH = 6) in reaction due to monobasic salts of phosphoric acid plus small amounts of organic acids. The acidity of urine is influenced by diet, fluid intake and also by various drugs. Meat diet will increase acidity whereas fruit decreases. Fasting and starvation in which the body proteins are metabolized also tend to increase titrable acidity. Urine on standing turns alkaline due to the formation of ammonia by the bacterial decomposition of urea.

CONSTITUENTS OF NORMAL URINE

Normal urine is composed of water, inorganic salts and organic compounds.

Major Inorganic Ions

Anions = Cl^-, PO_4^{---}, SO_4^{--}
Cations = Na^+, K^+, Ca^{++}, Mg^{++}, $[NH_4]^+$

Organic Constituents

Non-protein Nitrogen

Non-protein nitrogen (NPN) is nitrogen in the blood that is not a constituent of protein, e.g. nitrogen associated with urea, uric acid, creatine, creatinine and polypeptides. NPN substances in urine are urea, creatine, creatinine, uric acid, amino acids, allantoin and hippuric acid.

Urea

About 25–30 g of urea is excreted daily in urine. As urea is the end product of protein metabolism, urea excretion in urine is an index of protein intake in diet. Urea in urine is increased in exaggerated protein metabolism, fevers and increased adrenocortical activity. It is decreased in the last stages of severe hepatic diseases and in acidosis.

Urea can be detected by sodium hypobromide test, where it undergoes decomposition to nitrogen on being exposed to the reagent and a brisk effervescence ensues.

Sodium hypobromide test: Add about 5 drops of sodium hypobromide solution to a test tube containing about 5 mL of the sample urine and note the brisk effervescence of the liberated nitrogen gas.

Urease test: The enzyme urease converts the urea into ammonia and carbonic acid both of which react with each other to form ammonium carbonate under experimental conditions. This results in an alkaline solution that can be detected by the addition of phenolphthalein indicator when a pink color is produced.

Procedure: Label two test tubes as 'test' and 'control' containing 5 mL of urine in each. Add 2 mL of urease suspension to the test tube marked as 'test' and 2 mL of inactivated urease suspensions to the test tube marked 'control'.

Incubate both the test tubes at room temperature for 15 minutes and then add 2 drops of phenolphthalein indicator solution to each test tube. Pink color will be produced in the test tube having active enzyme.

Uric Acid

Uric acid is derived as an end product of the breakdown of cellular nucleoproteins. The daily excretion is 0.6–1 g. An increase in the excretion of uric acid is observed in leukemia, in severe liver disease and in various stages of gout. Deposits of urates and uric acid in the joints and tissues are also characteristics of gout, so that this disease appears to be a form of arthritis.

Under certain conditions uric acid or urates crystallize in the kidneys and are called kidney stones or calculi. An increase in the nucleoproteins in the diet also causes an increased excretion of uric acid in the urine.

Schiff's test: Uric acid reduces ammoniacal silver nitrate solution to metabolic silver and can be detected by the conversion of colorless silver nitrate to silver, seen as a black precipitation. Wet a piece of filter paper with a few drops of ammoniacal $AgNO_3$ solution and add a couple of drops of the sample urine to it. Note the formation of black carbon.

Uric acid

Creatinine

Creatinine is the anhydride of creatine and it is in this form that creatine is excreted in normal health. It is a waste product formed from creatine phosphate, which is the stored form of energy in muscle. Skeletal muscle contains a reservoir of high-energy phosphoryl group in the form of creatine phosphate or phosphocreatine, which transfers its high energy phospho group to ADP to form ATP, catalyzed by creatine kinase.

Creatine phosphate maintains a high concentration of ATP in skeletal muscle during period of muscular exertion.

Under physiological pH and temperature, phosphocreatine spontaneously loses phosphoric acid, leaving behind creatine. Creatine loses water to form creatinine, which is excreted in urine.

Normal blood plasma contains 0.2–0.6 mg of creatine per 100 mL. In 24 hours urine, 1.5–2 g of creatinine is excreted by males and 0.8–1.5 g by females. 98% of the total creatine in the body is in the muscles of which 80% is in the phosphorylated form.

$$\underset{\substack{\text{Creatine phosphate}\\\text{(phosphocreatine)}}}{\overset{\displaystyle\text{HP}-\overset{\displaystyle\overset{\text{O}}{\|}}{\underset{\displaystyle\text{OH}}{\text{P}}}-\overset{\displaystyle\text{N}-\text{CH}_3}{\underset{}{\text{N}}}-\overset{\displaystyle\text{COOH}}{\underset{\displaystyle\text{CH}_2}{\text{C}=\text{NH}}}}{}} \xrightarrow[\text{ADP}\quad\text{ATP}]{\text{Creatine kinase}} \underset{\text{Creatinine}}{\overset{\displaystyle\text{HN}=\text{C}\underset{\displaystyle\underset{\displaystyle\text{CH}_3}{\text{N}}-\text{CH}_2}{\overset{\displaystyle\text{NH}_2\;\;\text{COOH}}{}}}{}}$$

$$\underset{\text{Creatine}}{\text{HN}=\text{C}\underset{\underset{\text{CH}_3}{\text{N}}-\overset{\text{COOH}}{\text{CH}_2}}{\overset{\text{NH}_2}{}}} \xrightarrow{-\text{H}_2\text{O}} \underset{\text{Creatinine}}{\text{HN}=\text{C}\underset{\underset{\text{CH}_3}{\text{N}}-\text{CH}_2}{\overset{\text{NH}-\text{CO}}{}}}$$

Creatine synthesis: Three amino acids, glycine, arginine and methionine participate in the synthesis, which takes place in two steps.

1. The first step involves transamination, by which the amidine group of arginine is transferred to glycine to form guanidinoacetate. This reaction is reversible and takes place in the kidneys. Arginine after losing the amidine group forms ornithine.
2. The second step involves transmethylation when the methyl group from activated methionine is transferred to guanidinoacetate to form creatine. This reaction takes place in the liver.

```
            Arginine  ←―――→ Glycine
            (amidine)
            Ornithine ←―――→ Guanidinoacetate
                                    +CH₃
      Phosphocreatine ←――――――― Creatine
          H₃PO₄  ↖              ↗ -H₂O
                  ↘ Creatinine ↙
```

Creatine coefficient is the urinary creatinine and creatine nitrogen expressed in mg/kg body weight. The value is elevated in muscular dystrophy. Normal range is 20–25 mg/kg for males and 15–21 mg/kg for females.

The estimation of creatinine is also helpful in finding out the nephrotic syndrome. The proteins and creatinine are estimated in the urine and expressed as a ratio. A ratio less than 0.2 rules out any renal pathology and a ratio more than 3.5 indicates nephrotic syndrome.

Jaffe's test: Creatinine is detected by its reaction with alkaline picrate solution to give an orange-colored creatinine picrate.

Procedure: Add 2 mL of saturated solution of picric acid and a few drops of 10% NaOH solution to about 2 mL of the sample urine. Perform a control test with water in place of urine. Observe the distinct orange color in the sample test tube and the yellow color in the control test tube.

ANALYSIS OF NORMAL URINE

Physical Examination

Note the color, appearance and odor. Test the acidity with blue or red litmus paper. Determine the specific gravity using urinometer. Apply the correction for temperature variation.

Chemical Examination

Calculate the total solids present and perform the following tests with the sample.

Test for Chlorides

Place 5 mL of albumin free urine in a test tube and add 3 drops of concentrated HNO_3 to prevent precipitation of protein. Add 5 drops of $AgNO_3$. White precipitate of AgCl indicates presence of chlorides.

Test for Phosphates

To 3 mL of urine add 1 mL of concentrated HNO_3 and 5 mL of ammonium molybdate and warm. A canary-yellow precipitate indicates the presence of phosphate.

Test for Inorganic Sulfates

To 3 mL of urine add 1 mL of concentrated HCl followed by 10% $BaCl_2$ solution. A white precipitate of $BaSO_4$ indicates inorganic sulfate. Filter and set aside the filtrate for the next experiment.

Test for Ethereal Sulfate

Take the above filtrate and boil. A white precipitate is formed again indicating the presence of ethereal sulfate.

Test for Ammonia

Boil urine with equal volume of 10% NaOH. Smell of ammonia gas indicates the presence of ammonium ion in the urine sample.

ANALYSIS OF PATHOLOGICAL URINE

In the case of abnormal urine, glucose, ketone bodies, proteins, blood, bile salts and bile pigments are tested in the clinical biochemical laboratory.

Test for Reducing Sugar: Benedict's Test

Reducing carbohydrates like glucose reduces $CuSO_4$ in alkaline media to insoluble Cu_2O. Color of the solution depends upon the particle size of Cu_2O formed.

Procedure: Take 5 mL of Benedict's qualitative reagent. Boil for a minute and add 8 drops (0.5 mL) of urine, boil for 2 minutes, cool and note the color change (Table 17.1).

TABLE 17.1: Benedict's test for reducing sugar

Colors	Indication
Green	0.5%
Yellow	1.0%
Orange	1.5%
Brick red	2.0% and above

Test for Proteins (Albumin)

Heat and Acetic Acid Test

Proteins are coagulated by boiling, CO_2 driven out of the solution, pH of the urine is increased, which may precipitate phosphates. Thus when a sample of urine is heated precipitate may be due to protein or phosphate. Addition of a few drops of acetic acid will dissolve phosphate, if present.

Procedure: Fill up two third of a test tube with urine. Boil the upper portion of the test tube. Add a drop of 2% acetic acid. A white cloud in the heated portion shows the presence of albumin.

Heller's Nitric Acid Test (Cold Test)

Cold test is a sensitive test is based on the fact that protein is converted into a meta protein, which is insoluble in concentrated mineral acids.

Procedure: Take 3 mL of concentrated HNO_3 in a test tube and pour 2 mL of urine along the sides. A white ring at the junction of the two layers shows the presence of proteins.

Sulfosalicylic Acid Test

Place 1 mL urine in a test tube, add 3% sulfosalicylic acid and allow to stand for 10 minutes. Presence of cloudiness is due to albumin.

Benzidine Test for Blood in Urine

Prepare a saturated benzidine solution in glacial acetic acid; mix well equal parts of benzidine solution and H_2O_2. Take 2 mL of urine and add 2 mL of this mixture. A green or deep blue color indicates presence of blood in urine.

Any catalyst or enzyme, which splits up H_2O_2 and liberates nascent oxygen will give this test. The pus cells (WBCs in urine) contain an enzyme called peroxidase, which can split H_2O_2 and liberate nascent oxygen. To test hemoglobin in presence of pus cells, the urine must be boiled to destroy the pus cells enzyme before performing this test.

Bile Salts and Bile Pigments

Normally bile salts and bile pigments do not enter in the general circulation, and therefore, they are absent in normal urine. But if there is intrahepatic or extrahepatic obstruction to the flow of bile, bile regurgitates into the general circulation and appears in urine as in obstructive jaundice. Bile pigments give urine a greenish yellow or brown color.

Hay's Test for Bile Salts

When powder of sulfur is sprinkled on the urine containing bile salt, the sulfur powder sinks due to lowering of surface tension by bile salts. A positive test indicates the liver damage or obstruction of bile duct.

Gmelin's Test for Bile Pigments

When concentrated HNO_3 is added to urine, there is a play of color. Green indicates presence of bile pigments. Nitric acid oxidizes bilirubin to form a series of colored compounds, biliverdin (green), bilicyanin (blue), choletelin (yellow), etc.

To 2 mL of concentrated HNO_3 in a test tube add 3 mL of sample urine slowly along the sides. Play of colors at the junction of the two layers indicates the presence of bile pigments.

Fouchet's Test for Bile Pigments

Add 5 mL of 10% $BaCl_2$ solution to about 10 mL of urine. Mix and filter. Pour a few drops of Fouchet's reagent ($FeCl_3$, the oxidizing agent) on the precipitate in the air-dried filter paper. In the presence of bile pigments, bilirubin turns green and blue due to oxidation [urobilinogen (UBG) and stercobilinogen (SBG)].

Ehrlich's Aldehyde Test for Urobilinogen

Take 10 mL of urine in a test tube. Add 2.5 mL of $BaCl_2$ solution and filter. Take 3 mL of filtrate add Ehrlich's aldehyde reagent (paradimethylaminobenzaldehyde) shake well and allow to stand for 3 minutes. Pink color indicates a positive test. UBG is absent in obstructive jaundice.

Acetone Bodies

The acetone bodies in urine include acetoacetic and β-hydroxybutyric acids in addition to acetone.

Rothera's Test for Acetone and Acetoacetic Acid

Take 3 mL of urine in a test tube and fully saturate with saturated ammonium sulfate. This is to precipitate and remove proteins, which may interfere with the test. Add 1 or 2 crystals of sodium nitroprusside. Mix well and add liquor ammonia. A permanganate colored ring indicates the presence of acetone and acetoacetic acid.

Gerhardt's Test for Acetoacetic Acid

To 5 mL of urine add 10% $FeCl_3$ solution drop by drop till a maximum precipitate of ferric phosphate is obtained. This is to eliminate the phosphate, which may otherwise obscure the color in the test. Filter and to the filtrate add excess of $FeCl_3$. A bordeaux wine red color indicates the presence of acetoacetic acid in urine.

QUESTIONS

1. What are the normal constituents of a given sample of urine? Describe the tests conducted to detect proteins and blood in a given sample of abnormal urine.
2. How do you test the following in urine?
   A. Blood.
   B. Protein.
   C. Sugar.
   D. Ketone bodies.
   E. Bile salts.
   F. Bile pigments.
3. Name the pathological constituents of urine. How are they detected in the laboratory?
4. Name the nitrogen constituents of urine. How are they identified (NPN substances)?

MULTIPLE CHOICE QUESTIONS

5. Urine turbidity may be caused by any of the following *except:*
   A. Phosphates
   B. Proteins
   C. RBCs
   D. WBCs
6. Urine pH tends:
   A. To remain below 4.5
   B. Remains above 8.0
   C. Same as that of blood
   D. Reflects the acid-base status of the body
7. Urine specific gravity 1.050 indicates:
   A. Presence of glucose or proteins in urine
   B. Excellent renal function
   C. Inappropriate excretion of ADH
   D. The need for dilution test
8. Ketonuria can occur and Rothera's test may be positive in all following situations *except:*
   A. A very high-fat diet
   B. In starvation
   C. Following ether anesthesia
   D. Diabetes mellitus
9. Urinary excretion of protein in 24-hours urine in normal individual is:
   A. 1–5 mg
   B. 5–20 mg
   C. 20–40 mg
   D. 50–100 mg

10. **Normal renal plasma flow in healthy adults ranges about:**
    A. 12.5 mL/min
    B. 200 mL/min
    C. 450 mL/min
    D. 574 mL/min

11. **In adults, the upper limit of normal serum creatinine concentration is:**
    A. 0.75 mg/dL
    B. 71.2 mg/dL
    C. 1.6 mg/dL
    D. 201 mg/dL

ANSWERS

5. (B)   6. (D)   7. (D)   8. (C)   9. (D)
10. (D) 11. (C)

18 CHAPTER
Renal Function Tests

FUNCTIONS OF A KIDNEY

The kidney not only excretes the non-volatile metabolic waste materials of the body, but also maintains the homeostasis of the body fluids. The kidney function is made up of the following five processes:
1. Filtration of protein-free plasma by glomeruli.
2. Selective reabsorption by the tubule.
3. Secretion by the tubule.
4. Maintenance of acid-base balance.
5. Formation of urine.

Urine is formed as a result of these four processes. A large volume of blood, approximately 1 L/min flows through the kidneys. The filtrate contains all other constituents of plasma except the proteins. It contains many substances necessary for normal metabolism such as water, glucose, amino acids and chlorides as well as substances to be rejected such as urea, creatinine and uric acid. Substances, which are necessary for the body are reabsorbed by the tubule along with nearly 99% of the water of the filtrate. Certain other substances are added to produce the final urine, which is passed out into the bladder at the rate of about 1 mL/min.

RENAL FUNCTION TESTS

The kidneys are the major excretory organs and they also maintain the acid-base, fluid and electrolyte balance. Therefore it is very important to detect any abnormal function of kidney as early as possible.

Renal functions tests are grouped into three:

1. Routine clinical tests which include:
   a. Complete urinalysis.
   b. Measurement of NPN in blood.
   c. Measurement of serum electrolytes.
2. Tests done for detailed assessment are:
   a. Clearance tests.
   b. Urinary and plasma osmolality.
   c. Concentration and dilution tests.
3. Tests done for specific diagnosis or research purposes.

Tests of Glomerular Function

The glomerular filtration rate (GFR) depends on the net pressure being exerted across the glomerular membrane, the physical nature of the membrane and the surface area of the membrane. GFR gives an index of the number of functioning glomeruli. This can be evaluated by:
1. Urea clearance test.
2. Inulin clearance test.
3. Creatinine clearance test.

Clearance: The clearance of any substance is defined as the volume of plasma/blood, which contains the amount of that substance excreted in 1 minute by the kidneys.

Blood Urea and Urea Clearance Test

The normal blood urea level ranges from 20 to 40 mg/100 mL. Urea clearance is the volume of plasma cleared of urea per minute.

$$\text{Urea clearance} = \frac{U \times V}{B}$$

Where U = Concentration of urea in urine (in mg/100 mL)
 V = Volume of urine (in mL/min)
 B = Concentration of urea in blood (in mg/100 mL)

Maximum urea clearance: Normal maximum urea clearance is 75 mL/min. When the volume of urine excreted per minute is 2 mL or more, urea clearance is maximum.

Standard urea clearance: When the urinary volume is less than 2 mL/min the urea clearance is reduced. Such clearance is termed as standard clearance and the average normal value is 54 mL/min.

Procedure for urea clearance test: The patient is asked to take a light breakfast with two glasses of water. The first sample of urine passed after the water intake is discarded. Time is noted. Two urine samples are collected at 1 hour interval along with two blood samples. Urea clearance is calculated using the formula UV/B. In severe renal failure the clearance falls below 20% of the average normal.

Creatinine Clearance Test

Creatinine clearance test is more than 100 mL/min in healthy adults. Creatinine clearance measurements correlate fairly closely with inulin clearance measurements except in patients in whom GFR is severely impaired. Because a portion of creatinine is secreted by tubules, the clearance value is slightly raised.

Procedure: Collected 24-hours urine. At the start of the collection period, usually at 8 AM, the patient is instructed to empty the bladder and to discard the specimen. After this, all the urine samples are collected and placed in toluene (preservative) till 8 AM the following day. The volume of pooled urine is noted.

A specimen of blood is collected during the period of urine collection. Creatinine clearance is calculated by using the formula $\frac{UV}{B}$.

The creatinine clearance is impaired in acute and chronic renal failure.

Inulin Clearance Test

Inulin clearance test is done to find GFR. Inulin is filtrated by the glomeruli, but neither secreted nor absorbed by the tubules. The amount of inulin excreted in each minute is the amount filtered by the glomeruli. The concentration of inulin in the glomerular filtrate is equal to that in the plasma. Thus the clearance value of inulin is the same as glomerular filtration rate.

During the period of urine collection, a constant plasma inulin level is maintained by intravenous drip. The normal inulin clearance value is about 125 mL/min.

Urine Concentration Test

Urine concentration test is designed to test the concentration power of the kidneys. The capacity of the kidneys to concentrate urine is a sensitive test to detect early loss of kidney function. The test is simple as it does not require any laboratory facilities.

At 6 PM give the patient, a meal with good protein content, but not morethan 200 mL of fluid to drink. Allow no more fluid after this meal. Discard any urine passed during the night. On the following morning collect three samples of urine as follows:

8 AM : Urine sample I
9 AM : Urine sample II
10 AM : Urine sample III

Measure the specific gravity of all the samples. The specific gravity of atleast one specimen should exceed 1.022. A maximum specific gravity of less than 1.022 indicates impaired renal function.

When the kidney loses its capacity to do osmotic work, the urinary solids must be excreted in more dilute solution. The advantage of this test is that it is useful for the detection of renal defect when the blood urea is normal.

Dilution Test

In addition to the loss in power of the kidneys to produce concentrated urine, there is also an impairment in its ability to excrete dilute urine.

In this test, no water is taken after midnight, the bladder is emptied at 7 AM and the patient is given 1,200 mL of water to drink in 30 minutes. Urine samples are collected hourly for next 4 hours, i.e. at 8, 9, 10 and 11 AM. The volume and specific gravity of each specimen are noted.

Specific gravity of atleast one sample should fall to 1.003 or below. Almost all the water drunk (1,200 mL) should be excreted within those 4 hours. When renal impairment is severe, volume may be less than 100 mL with the specific gravity of 1.010 or more.

Phenolsulfonphthalein Test or Phenol Red Excretion Test for Kidney Function

The phenolsulfonphthalein (PSP) test indicates a general loss of kidney function. The dye is non-toxic and is exclusively excreted by the kidney. After intravenous injection of the dye, the 15 minutes sample collected should contain 25% or more of the injected dye, which is estimated colorimetrically.

Measurement of Renal Blood/Plasma Flow

Renal blood flow can be determined by using para-aminohippuric acid, which at low blood concentration is removed entirely by the tubular excretion in a single circulation through the kidney. It is a measure of the plasma flow, which is normally 574 mL/min/1.73 m^2 body surface area.

QUESTION

1. Short notes on:
   A. Urea clearance test.
   B. Inulin clearance test.
   C. Creatinine clearance test.
   D. Urine concentration test.

MULTIPLE CHOICE QUESTIONS

2. All of the following substances have been used to estimate GFR *except:*
   A. Inulin   B. Creatinine
   C. Phenol red   D. Mannitol
3. Relationship between GFR and serum creatine concentration is:
   A. Non-existent   B. Inverse
   C. Direct   D. Indirect
4. Normal maximum urea clearance in adult averages about:
   A. 60   B. 65
   C. 70   D. 75
5. In patients with renal failure all the following are typically elevated in serum *except:*
   A. Urea nitrogen   B. Phosphate
   C. Uric acid   D. Albumin
6. Excretion of BSP primarily reflects:
   A. Liver function test   B. Glomerular filtration rate
   C. Maximal tubular excretory capacity   D. Kupffer cell activity
7. Kidney functions, which are important in maintaining acid-base balance include:
   A. Bicarbonate mechanism B. Ammonia mechanism
   C. Phosphate mechanism   D. None of the above

8. **Renal tubular functions can be assessed by:**
   A. Creatinine clearance test
   B. Inulin clearance test
   C. Urea clearance test
   D. Concentration and dilution tests
9. **Excretion of phenolsulfonphthalein (PSP) reflects:**
   A. Glomerular filtration rate
   B. Liver function
   C. Tubular excretory capacity
   D. None of the above
10. **Clearance is measured to assess quantitatively the rate of excretion of a given substance by the:**
    A. Liver
    B. Spleen
    C. Intestine
    D. Kidneys
11. **Creatinine clearance is decreased in:**
    A. Liver diseases
    B. Renal diseases
    C. Brain diseases
    D. Bone diseases

ANSWERS

2. (D)	3. (B)	4. (D)	5. (D)	6. (C)	
7. (D)	8. (D)	9. (C)	10. (D)	11. (B)	

CHAPTER 19

Abnormalities of Bilirubin Metabolism: Jaundice

JAUNDICE

Normal serum bilirubin concentration is almost 1 mg/100 mL. This is made up of 0.8 mg of bilirubin and 0.2 mg of bilirubin diglucuronide.

When the total bilirubin level exceeds 1 mg, the condition is called hyperbilirubinemia. Hyperbilirubinemia may be due to:
1. Production of more bilirubin than the normal liver can excrete.
2. The failure of damaged liver to excrete bilirubin produced in normal amounts.
3. Block in the excretion of bile.

In these cases, bilirubin accumulates in the blood and beyond 2.0 mg% it diffuses into the tissues, which then become yellow. This condition is called icterus or jaundice.

In hemolytic and hepatic jaundice, the liver looses the capacity to remove urobilinogen from the blood. Therefore, the urobilinogen in circulation in the liver is all excreted by the kidneys and the excess of urobilinogen appears in the urine (detected by Fouchet's test and Gmelin's test).

Bilirubin: Pigment Metabolism

Bilirubin is excreted in urine in the following diseases:
1. Obstructive jaundice.
2. Hepatic cirrhosis, infective hepatitis.
3. Hemolytic jaundice, following malaria, hemolytic anemia and non-compatible blood transfusions.

Three Different Types of Jaundice

Jaundice is of three different types, depending upon the ways in which it is caused.

Hemolytic (Prehepatic) Jaundice

Hemolytic jaundice is due to excessive destruction of RBCs. Since the cause is increased production of bilirubin and not an abnormality in the hepatic conjugation or excretion. It is characterized by the presence of only unconjugated bilirubin.

Hepatic Jaundice

Hepatic jaundice is due to the damage to parenchymal liver cells. Damage may be due to liver poisons, e.g. chloroform, carbon tetrachloride, phosphorus, toxins, hepatitis virus, etc.

Obstructive (Regurgitation or Posthepatic Jaundice)

Obstructive type is caused by an obstruction (blockage) of the bile duct, e.g. by gallstone, carcinoma of the bile duct or head or pancreas. Consequently the conjugated bilirubin returns to the blood and hence serum contains excessive amount of conjugated bilirubin.

van den Bergh Test for Serum Bilirubin

Bilirubin forms a reddish compound with the diazo reagent (diazotized sulfanilic acid) and can be estimated colorimetrically.

The bilirubin of bile is combined chemically (conjugated) with glucuronic acid to form the mono- and di-glucuronide salts of the bilirubin. Free bilirubin is very soluble. Conjugated bilirubin develops red color directly on addition of diazo reagent within 1 minute. Hence, it is known as 1 minute bilirubin or direct reacting bilirubin.

Normal blood plasma contains 0.2–0.8 mg% of the indirect type (unconjugated). The van den Bergh reaction in 1 minute will be negative. In jaundice, serum bilirubin level exceeds 2 mg%.

In hemolytic jaundice, indirect test is positive because of the accumulation of unconjugated bilirubin (insoluble).

In obstructive jaundice, direct test is positive because of accumulation of conjugated bilirubin (soluble).

In hepatic jaundice, the test is biphasic positive because of the increased levels of both conjugated and unconjugated bilirubin.

Differential Diagnosis of Jaundice

In differential diagnosis of jaundice, measurement of bilirubin in the serum is of great value. This is done by van den Bergh test. The test is based on the coupling of diazotized sulfanilic acid and bilirubin to produce a reddish purple azo compound, while conjugated bilirubin (bilirubin mono- and di-glucuronide water soluble) gives color with the reagent directly.

Abnormalities observed in bilirubin and its metabolism in the different types of jaundice are mentioned in Table 19.1.

TABLE 19.1: Abnormalities observed in bilirubin level in different types of jaundice

Bilirubin types	Hemolytic jaundice	Hepatic jaundice	Obstructive jaundice
Serum bilirubin	Increased	Increased	Increased
Total direct	Less than 20% of total	–	–
Indirect	Markedly increased	Variable	A slight increase
Urine bilinogen	Increased	Usually increased	May be present
Urine bile salts	Absent/increased	Increased	Markedly increased
Fecal urobilinogen	Markedly increased	Usually increased	Absent/low

Unconjugated bilirubin gives color only after adding methanol. Unconjugated bilirubin is insoluble in water, but soluble in methanol, thus conjugated bilirubin is called 'direct reacting' (1 minute bilirubin) bilirubin and free or unconjugated bilirubin is called 'indirect reacting' bilirubin.

For estimation of total bilirubin, serum is treated with van den Bergh reagent and methanol, and the color is read in a colorimeter. For estimation of conjugated bilirubin, serum is treated with the reagent and color is read. Difference between total bilirubin and conjugated bilirubin gives the free or unconjugated bilirubin.

Total bilirubin – Conjugated bilirubin = Free or unconjugated bilirubin. *van den Bergh reaction* with serum from hemolytic jaundice is an indirect one as the condition is characterized by a high level of unconjugated bilirubin. Reaction with normal serum is also an indirect one as the concentration of unconjugated bilirubin is much more than the conjugated bilirubin. Reaction with obstructive jaundice serum is 'direct' as the serum is characterized by a high level of conjugated bilirubin. Reaction with hepatic jaundice serum is also 'direct'.

Difference between Hemolytic Jaundice and Obstructive Jaundice with Respect to Excretion of Urobilirubin and Bilinogen

In hemolytic jaundice, the increased production of bilirubin in the tissues leads to increased production of urobilinogen, which appears in the urine in large amounts. Thus, Ehrlich test for urine bilirubin is distinctly positive. Since bilirubin is water insoluble, it is not excreted as urine in this condition. Thus, a combination of increased urobilinogen and no bilirubin in urine is suggestive of hemolytic jaundice.

In complete obstruction (obstructive jaundice) of the bile duct, no urobilinogen is found in the urine, since bilirubin does not reach the intestine. Since in this condition there is a high level of conjugated bilirubin (water soluble form) in blood, it is excreted in urine. Thus, Fouchet's test (for bilirubin) is distinctively positive. Thus, a combination of no urobilinogen and the presence of bilirubin in urine is suggestive of obstructive jaundice.

QUESTION

1. Short notes on:
    A. Jaundice.
    B. van den Bergh test.

MULTIPLE CHOICE QUESTIONS

2. **Test based on abnormalities of bile pigment metabolism is:**
    A. Creatinine clearance test
    B. Hippuric acid synthesis test
    C. van den Bergh test
    D. Rothera's test
3. **Obstruction of the common bile duct leads to:**
    A. Prehepatic jaundice
    B. Posthepatic jaundice
    C. Hepatic jaundice
    D. Physiological jaundice

4. **In case of jaundice, if there is no trace of bile pigments in urine, the most probable diagnosis is:**
   A. Infective jaundice
   B. Hemolytic jaundice
   C. Serum hepatitis
   D. Obstructive jaundice
5. **Jaundice is clinically detected in sclerae when serum bilirubin concentration reaches above:**
   A. 1–2 mg/100 mL
   B. 0.5–1 mg/100 mL
   C. 2–3 mg/100 mL
   D. 3–4 mg/100 mL
6. **In hemolytic jaundice, the urinary bilinogen is:**
   A. Normal
   B. Small amount is present
   C. Increased more than normal
   D. Absent

ANSWERS

2. (C)   3. (B)   4. (B)   5. (C)   6. (C)

20 Liver Function Tests

Liver performs numerous metabolic, secretory, excretory, storage and detoxifying functions. Several biochemical tests are available to test the functional efficiency of liver. The pathological processes that may be present singly or in combination are:
1. Liver cell damage caused by viral infections.
2. Cholestasis caused by impaired secretion of bile by the liver cells.
3. Reduced functional mass due to chronic liver damage.

LIVER FUNCTION TESTS

Chemical tests for the diagnosis and follow-up of liver diseases are:
1. Bilirubin metabolism and excretion.
2. Assessment of hepatic transport function—bromsulfalein (BSP) excretion test.
3. Plasma protein abnormalities (albumin/globulin ratio):
   a. Protein synthesized in the parenchymal cells.
   b. Abnormalities of immunoglobulin synthesis.
4. Estimation of plasma enzymes:
   a. Albumin phosphatase.
   b. Serum glutamic oxaloacetic transaminase (SGOT) or aspartate transaminase (AST).
   c. Serum glutamic pyruvic transaminase (SGPT) or alanine aminotransferase (ALT).
   d. Gamma-glutamyltransferase (γ-GT).

Test for Hepatic Transport Function

Bromsulfalein Excretion Test

A measured amount of an anionic dye is injected intravenously. The liver rapidly removes the dye and excretes in the bile. If the liver function is impaired, the excretion is delayed and larger portion of the dye remains in the serum. It is a very sensitive test and is most useful in liver cell damage without jaundice, in cirrhosis and chronic hepatitis.

Plasma Proteins (Albumin/Globulin Ratio)

The liver has dominant role in plasma protein synthesis, being the source of plasma albumin and fibrinogen along with other proteins associated with blood coagulation. The liver contributes important components of α- and β-globulin fractions and is also involved in the synthesis of γ-globulins. The serum albumin level is lowered in cirrhosis, in viral hepatitis, in nutritional liver disease and in neoplastic disease of liver. There is generally an equal simultaneous rise in globulin level with the γ-globulin accounting for much of the increase in total globulin of serum. While the serum γ-globulin content rarely exceeds 1.6 g/100 mL in healthy subjects, in liver diseases concentrations as high as 2–5 times the normal are seen. The normal serum albumin/globulin ratio is 2:1. In advanced liver disease, albumin is decreased and the globulin is increased so that albumin/globulin ratio is reversed.

Protein Electrophoresis

Electrophoresis gives abnormal patterns in liver diseases. In cirrhosis, serum albumin is reduced and the γ-globulin is increased. In cholestasis, there is an increase in the concentrations of α- and β-globulin factors.

Coagulation Factors (Prothrombin Time)

Prothrombin time is the time required for clotting to take place in citrated plasma to which optimum amounts of thromboplastin and calcium have been added. Prothrombin is formed by liver cells, vitamin K being required. When bile salts are not present in the intestine the absorption of vitamin K from intestine is impaired. The normal prothrombin time is 16–18 seconds. It is prolonged in jaundice and liver diseases.

Tests for Detecting Changes in Serum Proteins

In the thymol test, adding thymol in barbital buffer to serum, produces marked turbidity.
1. In the presence of liver disease (parenchymatous), flocculation appears on longer standing. Similarly in the presence of liver disease, diluted serum forms a flocculent precipitate when treated with a suspension of cephalin and cholesterol in water.
2. Using Biuret reagent: Total proteins may be determined and repeating this after suitable fractionation of serum, concentration of different type of proteins in the serum is obtained.
3. Serum enzymes: A number of enzymes in serum exihibit changes in activity during parenchymal liver disease and the following studies are routinely employed.
    a. Alkaline phosphatase:
    Alkaline phosphatase activity of the serum often assists in the differentiation of liver disease of parenchymal origin from that due to obstruction and other lesions of the biliary tract. Biliary obstruction is characterized by a persistent increase in alkaline phosphtase activity to two or more times the normal values (in the range of 1.5–4 units/100 mL in adults and 5–12 units/100 mL in children) with moderate changes occurring during hepatocellular disease.
    b. Amino transferases:
    Amino transferases or transaminases are used in the diagnosis of a variety of disorders, e.g.
    SGOT (old name) or AST (new name). This enzyme occurs in high concentration in heart muscles. Increased levels of AST in the bloodstream indicates, cirrhosis of the liver or myocardial infarction (which results from the reduction in blood flow to the heart muscle caused by a clot in the coronary artery).
    SGPT (old name) or ALT (new name) levels are increased during infective hepatitis (refer 'Transamination' of amino acids in Chapter 13).
    Elevated AST or SGOT is observed soon after exposure to hepatitis virus, even before the appearance of clinical symptoms with striking elevations to the extent of 20 or more times the normal at the onset of active illness. A similar rise may be observed on exposure to various chemicals and drugs, but in contrast, only

moderate increase occur in case of biliary obstruction, cholestatic syndrome or cirrhosis. ALT or SGPT is much more abundant in liver than in other tissues. However the rise of ALT in liver disease is often delayed and may not become evident until AST has begun to fall. Hence the specificity attributed to ALT often fails to workout in practice. Nevertheless, ALT activity remains high throughout the subsequent course of illness and returns to normal values much later than AST (as the former is cleared more slowly from the blood) and helps in monitoring the illness more effectively.

4. Gamma-glutamyltransferase (γ-*GT*): It is a letter index for the diagnosis of alcohol-induced liver disease.

MULTIPLE CHOICE QUESTIONS

1. **The following are the important liver function tests *except:***
   A. Urea clearance test
   B. Galactose clearance test
   C. Prothrombin time
   D. Bromsulfalein test

2. **In alcoholics, the marker enzyme estimated in serum is:**
   A. SGOT
   B. SGPT
   C. CPK
   D. γ-GT

ANSWERS

1. (A)   2. (D)

Part 2
Nutrition

21. Food, Nutrition and Health
22. Carbohydrates: Sugar, Starch and Fiber
23. Nutritional Aspects of Fats
24. Proteins
25. Mineral Metabolism
26. Water Metabolism
27. Cookery Rules and Preservation of Nutrients
28. Food Preservation: Principles and Methods
29. Foodborne Diseases
30. Food Laws and Food Standards
31. Hospital Diets
32. Budgeting for Balanced Diet
33. Assessment of Nutritional Status
34. Role of Nurse in Nutritional Programs
35. Nutrition in Pregnancy
36. Nutrition in Infancy
37. Menu for Preschool, School-age Children and Adolescents
38. Geriatric Nutrition
39. Naturopathic Medicine
40. Diet Therapy

21 Food, Nutrition and Health
CHAPTER

HISTORY

Nutrition as a new field of study is about 100 years old. Even though Hippocrates had recognized diet on a component of health as early as 300 BC, only during the past 100 years, people began to realize the importance of carbohydrates, lipids and proteins for normal growth and development. The next nutrition breakthrough was the discovery of vitamins—vitamin A in 1913, vitamin C in 1919, vitamin D in 1925, vitamin K in 1935, vitamin E in 1936, vitamin B_1 (thiamine) in 1936, vitamin B_2 (riboflavin) in 1935, vitamin B_6 (pyridoxine) in 1936, vitamin B_9 (folic acid) in 1948 and so on.

Nutrition was officially recognized as an independent field of study only in 1928 with the formation of American Institute of Nurtrition. It took about half a century more for nutrition to achieve its current status as one of the most talked about scientific disciplines.

Nutrition encompasses not only the study of vitamins, minerals and other foods, but also diverse subjects as alcohol, caffeine and pesticides. Besides, nutrition research tries to find out the impact of food on body by examining the progress in allied fields, such as physics, chemistry, biochemistry and immunology.

CONCEPTS

Nutrition

Nutrition is defined as the science of food and its relationship to health. It is food at work in the body. It includes everything that happens to food. It is the study of nutrients and processes by which they are used by the body. It is concerned with the part played by nutrients in the body growth, development and maintenance.

Dietetics

Dietetics are the practical application of the principles of nutrition, which includes planning of meals for the healthy as well as the sick. Good nutrition means maintenance of nutritional status that enables us to grow well and enjoy good health.

Food

Food is vital for human existence just as air and water. Food may be defined as anything eaten or drunk, which meets the needs of tissue building, regulation and protection of the body and its energy needs. It is the raw material from which bodies are made. Intake of right kinds and amounts of foods can ensure good nutrition and health, which may be evident in one's appearance, well-being and efficiency.

Food is basic to life. The food, we eat is digested and assimilated in the body and used for its growth and development. Food also provides the necessary energy for doing work. The selection of best food for promoting good health is by trial and error. Use of milk of different mammals as food for infants has been practiced from very early times. Man has shown great foresight and ingenuity in cultivating a variety of food grains, fruits, vegetables, oil seeds and nuts, and rearing of animals and birds for food. The food that is ingested by the body is digested, absorbed and metabolized.

Diet

Diet refers to whatever people eat, drink each day. It includes the normal diet people consume and the diet people consume in groups (hotel diet), but will also be modified for the sick as part of their therapy (diet therapy).

NUTRIENTS

Useful chemical substances derived from the food by the body are called nutrients. Human beings require more than 45 different nutrients for their well-being. Nutrients include:
- Carbohydrates
- Lipids
- Proteins
- Water
- Minerals
- Vitamins.

Classification

1. Major nutrients (macronutrients): Carbohydrates, lipids, proteins and water.
2. Minor nutrients (micronutrients): Vitamins and minerals.

Major Nutrients

Are utilized for energy converted to structural components of cells or are stored as fat, depending on their level of supply, e.g. carbohydrates form 65%–80%, proteins 7%–15% and lipids 10%–13% of food. The proper utilization of these nutrients requires, appropriate concentrations of micronutrients.

Minor Nutrients

Unlike carbohydrates, lipids and proteins, vitamins and minerals do not supply energy or calories, instead they regulate the metabolism. There are eight B complex vitamins each with its special functions.

Scientific research have shown that to some extent, we are really what we eat. With this, many consumers have become more confused than ever about how to incorporate the research findings into their food habits. With the amount of nutrition information and the number of alternative foods ever on the increase, choosing a healthy diet is becoming more and more challenging; queries may arise, such as:

Should I take vitamin substitute or antioxidants? Do diet pills work? Can a sports drink enhance my performance? Can vitamin C supplement prevent cancer and heart diseases? Fruits, vegetables and tea are loaded with antioxidants, but can their beneficial effect be captured in a pill?

NUTRITION AND HEALTH

The basic study of nutrition is of primary importance as:
1. It is fundamental for own health.
2. It is essential for the health and well-being of patients and clients from the time of eating till it is utilized for various functions. The scope of such study involves:
    a. Nutrition helps growth and development.
    b. Prevents malnutrition.
    c. Resists infection.
    d. Prevents diseases.

Growth and Development

Good nutrition is essential for attainment of normal growth and development both physical and intellectual. Learning and behavior are affected by malnutrition. Nutrition controls human beings from womb-to-tomb. Malnutrition during pregnancy affects the growth of the fetus.

NUTRITIONAL PROBLEMS IN INDIA

A survey in South India has revealed that about 1% children aged 1–5 years showed signs of kwashiorkor, 2% marasmus and 3%–5% vitamins A deficiency. Community studies have shown that many mothers give only breast milk to children up to 2 years. Thus, no additional food is added to the child's diet. Papaya, which is rich in vitamin A is considered as a food, which produce more heat that will cause miscarriage, hence is avoided by pregnant women. It is a belief that, if a pregnant woman eats more, the baby will be big and delivery difficult, so expectant mothers are not fed adequately both in quality and quantity (Table 21.1).

TABLE 21.1: Nutritional problems in India

Problem	Features
Low birth weight	Less than 2.5 kg
Stillbirth	Birth of dead baby
Kwashiorkor	Protein deficiency between 1 and 4 year
Anemia	20% adolescent girls and 90% pregnant women
Stunted growth	Height and weight not ideal
Night blindness	Vitamin A deficiency after 50 year
Cataract	Vitamin A and vitamin C deficiency
Goiter	Iodine deficiency in females
Underweight	50% adults
Overweight	15% Mumbai school children are obese
Diabetes	Female less, about 10% of the total population and about 1/5 above age 50 suffer
Hypertension	Male and female suffer more in urban areas
Cardiac problems	More in males
Cancer	More in females

The Hunger and malnutrition surgery report 2011 covered 7,300 households in 112 districts across 9 states and more than 1 lakh children and 74,000 mothers. Following are some of the key findings of the surgery:

1. 42% children under 5 are underweight; 59% are stunted.
2. 66% of mothers did not attend school. Rates of child underweight and stunting are higher among mothers with low levels of education.
3. By 2 years, 42% children are underweight and 58% stunted in the 100 focus districts.
4. Prevalence of child underweight has decreased from 53% in 2004 to 42% in 2011.
5. Birth weight:
   a. Under 2.5 kg at birth and continue to stay underweight 50%.
   b. Over 2.5 kg at birth, but underweight now 34%.
   c. Under 2.5 kg at birth and stunted now 62%.
   d. Over 2.5 kg at birth, but stunted now 50%.
6. Prevalence of malnutrition is significantly higher among children from low-income families particularly Muslims, Scheduled Castes and Scheduled Tribes although rates of malnutrition are significant among middle and high-income families.

We cannot hope for a healthy future for India with such a large number of malnourished children. The government cannot solely depend on Integrated Child Development Services (ICDS) to solve the issue. The government is launching a strengthened and restructured ICDS, to start a multisectoral program for 200 high burden districts and initiate a nationwide communication campaign against malnutrition.

INDIA'S HIGH CHILD MORTALITY RATE—NATIONAL SHAME

The 'Child Mortality Estimate Report 2012' released by the United Nations Children's Emergency Fund (UNICEF) shows India in a poor light. It led the whole world by recording deaths of 16.55 lakh children under the age of 5 in 2011. Among the five countries that accounted for more than 50% of such deaths, India's figure was more than the combined figures in Nigeria, the Democratic Republic of Congo and Pakistan. Though China has the world's largest population, it is far behind India in child mortality. For a country that claims to have crossed the threshold of development, these figures should serve as an eye-opener.

Causes of Malnutrition in India

Malnutrition implies imperfect assimilation or inadequate nutrition or both. It is more common among children, pregnant ladies and nursing mothers. Its effects are kwashiorkor, marasmus, xerophthalmia, beriberi, pellagra, goiter, rickets, etc. Malnutrition also predisposes to diseases, such as tuberculosis, diarrhea and parasitic infections. Causes of malnutrition in India:
1. Population growth: Food production is not keeping pace with population growth.
2. Agriculture: Food production is adversely affected by unpredictable rainfall, unprecedented drought and floods. Fragmentation of land holdings and socioeconomic conditions are also responsible.
3. Parasitic and infective diseases are responsible for decreased intestinal absorption.
4. Religions and cultural food facts: These prevent people from using the locally available nutritious foods. Cooking methods also depend on tradition.
5. Illiteracy and ignorance about balanced diet: Poverty does not allow a large chunk of the population to go to school and get education including balanced diet.

National Nutritional Policy

India's nutritional policy was formulated in the year 1993 by an act of the parliament with the following goals:
1. Reduction of incidence of low birth weight.
2. Elimination of nutritional blindness.
3. Reduction of anemia to 20% in pregnant women.
4. Universal iodination of common salt to lower-iodine deficiency disorders to less than 1%.
5. Establish special care to geriatric (old age) nutrition.
6. Increase annual food grain production to 250 metric tons.
7. Steps to create household food security through poverty alleviation.
8. Decrease incidence of moderate and severe malnutrition in children.
9. Promotion of appropriate diets and healthy lifestyle.

These goals are to be achieved by applying certain short-term interventions as well as long-term interventions.

Short-term Interventions or Direct Interventions

1. Expanding the nutrition intervention net (ICDS).
2. Empowering mothers with nutrition and health education.
3. Teaching the adolescent girl to avoid anemia.
4. Ensuring better nutritional coverage for expectant women.
5. Controlling micronutrient deficiencies and fortifying essential foods with nutrients.

Long-term Interventions or Development Policy Instruments

1. Food security.
2. Improvement of dietary pattern.
3. Increasing purchase power of the population.
4. Streamlining and expanding Public Distribution System (PDS).
5. Strengthening health and family welfare programs.
6. Nutrition and public education.
7. Education and literacy.
8. Nutrition and surveillance.
9. Information and communication.
10. Ensure community participation.

A nutritional plan of action was formulated in 1995 to implement the short-and long-term policy instruments with sectorial commitment by the following nutrition related ministries:

1. Agriculture.
2. Food production.
3. Civil supplies.
4. Public distribution.
5. Education and literacy.
6. Health and family welfare.
7. Preventive care.
8. Information and broadcasting.
9. Awareness.
10. Forestry and environment protection.
11. Labor.
12. Rural, urban and tribal development.
13. Transport communications.
14. Formation of high-level committees/councils for identifying factors affecting food and nutrition.

FACTORS INFLUENCING FOOD HABITS AND SELECTION OF FOODSTUFFS

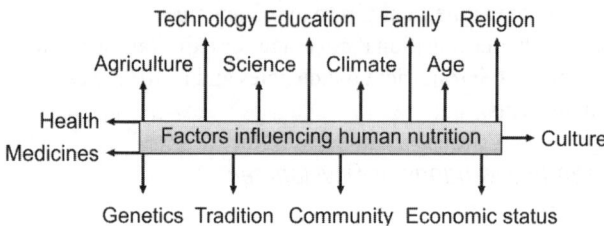

Fig. 21.1: Factors influencing nutrition

1. Superstitions.
2. Social and cultural factors.
3. Religious factors.
4. Income.
5. Geography/availability.
6. Advertising and media.

Superstitions and Cultural Factors

Food habits are handed over from generation-to-generation in the society particularly in the developing countries (Fig. 21.1). Though these factors have very little or no scientific basis, people rigidly adhere to them. In many parts of India, pregnant women are not allowed to consume papaya as it is believed that papaya produces a lot of heat in the body, which in turn induces abortion. Pineapple also is not given for the same reason. Pregnant ladies are given milk with a few strands of saffron in it as it would supposedly result in a baby with a very fair complexion. Consumption of a lot of garlic is for secretion of milk. In parts of Bengal, people believe that consumption of tongue of goat by children will make them more talkative.

Religious Belief

Hindus do not eat beef, since cow is an animal sacred to them. Among Hindus some communities do not eat fruits, onions and garlic. Many Hindus are vegetarians. Jains do not eat curds and do not eat after sunset. The central tenet of Buddhism is vegetarianism. To eat meat is to destroy the seeds of compassion. All plant foods are considered appropriate to eat except the 'five pungent foods' garlic, onions, leeks, scallions and chives. These foods are considered unclean and are believed to generate lust when eaten cooked and to induce rage when eaten raw. Islamic food laws prohibit the consumption of 'unclean' foods, such as swine and animals killed in a manner that prevents their blood from being fully drained from their bodies. Jews do not eat pork and shellfish. It is a custom in most communities in India, that women and girls eat only after men and boys finish their eating. Thus, the health of the female is affected as they eat poorly with the leftover food.

Child Rearing Practices

Another factor that blocks the normal food patterns in India is child rearing practices. The late introduction of weaning foods, prolonged breastfeeding and the adoption of commercially produced baby foods play an important part in the nutrition of children and have adverse effects in their growth and development.

The traditional cooking practices also act as a barrier to achieve a balanced diet, e.g. using polished rice, draining away the rice water and prolonged boiling of vegetables add to the great loss of nutrients in the diet of Indians, which lead to nutritional deficiencies.

Geography/Availability

In the olden days, human beings would eat whatever was available to satisfy hunger. The food man got was the type he could cultivate in his locality. Rice is the main food crop grown in tropical areas.

The nutrition value of natural foods do not vary from country-to-country. But there is a great variation in the composition of prepared foods, such as bread, biscuits, cakes, etc. due to variation in recipes and basic ingredients used in different regions.

EXCHANGE LISTS

In 1950, the American Diabetes Association developed a system of food lists to help diabetic patients to select foods in their diet. Since, India is a large country, there are three agencies who have brought out similar exchange lists. These agencies are the dietetic departments of major regional hospitals.

Each list includes a group of foods, which supply about the same calories in the portions indicated. Each food choice within a list is called 'exchange'.

It represents an amount of food that has almost the same macronutrition value as other foods in the same group. The exchange lists are very useful in diet planning in hospitals and personal diet management in homes.

To determine what nutrients we need each day and how much to keep us in good health, a lot of research has been done. The results of these studies have been used to workout the nutritional requirements of Indian people. After adding a factor safety, the recommended dietary allowances (RDAs) for Indians have been set up. RDA has been defined as the amount of nutrient that would meet the nutritional requirements of 97%–98% of people in a group.

An advisory committee of Indian Council of Medical Research (ICMR) is responsible for the setting up, review and revision of these RDAs.

INCOME

Financial resources determine the type of food consume. Depending on the availability one selects the food. People in lower income groups in India consume, a combination of cereals and cheaply available green leafy vegetables, roots and tubers. People of higher income groups, can choose food from all groups irrespective of season.

FUNCTIONS OF FOOD

1. Provide energy.
2. Bodybuilding.
3. Regulating the activities of the body including:
   a. Beating of the heart.
   b. Maintenance of body temperature.
   c. Muscle contraction.
   d. Clotting of blood.
   e. Control of water balance.
   f. Elimination of the waste products of the body.
4. Provide resistance to diseases.
5. Social function: Feasts are served on specific stages of life—birth, naming ceremonies, birthdays, marriages, etc. Prasad is distributed in temples. Pedhas are distributed to announce success in exams or birth of a baby. Laddus are associated with Deepawali and marriages, cakes with Christmas and weddings. Refreshments served at get together and meetings create a relaxed atmosphere.

6. Psychological functions of food: Breastfeeding provides closeness and security to the child. Food also satisfy some emotional needs like security, attention and friendship and acceptance. Food can be used as a weapon to fight against diseases. An insecure child sometimes refuses food, so that mother will be concerned about the child and how to meet its demand.

Role of Food and its Medicinal Value

Most deficiency diseases have been eliminated in the West by abundance of food supplies. Yet diseases related to malnutrition in the form of dietary excess and imbalance are quite common in the Western countries. Four of the ten leading causes of death—heart diseases, cancer, stroke and diabetes have been linked to diet.

Poor dietary habits and a sedentary lifestyle together account for 3 lakh deaths in the United States (US) every year. Dietary factors account for a third or more of all cases of both cancer and heart diseases. A high-fat diet raises risk of some types of cancer, heart diseases and obesity, which in turn contribute to a number of other problems including diabetes and high-blood pressure. Studies carried out have shown that the quality of diets consumed by people in the United Kingdom (UK) and United States of America (USA) during the period 1911–1960 have been steadily increasing and consequently the growth rate of children also was increasing during the same period. After 1960, the growth rate of children did not show any significant improvement showing that the diet had been adequate for providing maximum growth in children. On the other hand, the rate of growth of children in the developing countries continues to be poor. The children are malnutritioned, emaciated and stunted.

Resistance to Infection

Malnutrition predisposes the body to infections like tuberculosis. It also influences the course and outcome of many diseases. Infections in turn aggregate malnutrition.

Nutritional Status

Nutritional status is the state of body as the results of the foods consumed and their use by the body. Nutritional status can be good, fair or poor.

The characteristics of good nutritional status are alert, good natured personality, a well-developed body, with normal weight for height, well-developed and firm muscles, healthy skin, reddish pink color of eyelids and membranes of mouth, good layer of subcutaneous fat, clear eyes, smooth and glossy hair, good general health. Appetite, digestion and elimination are normal. Well-nourished persons are more likely to be mentally and physically alert and have a positive outlook on life. They are able to resist infections more than undernourished persons. They have extended years of normal functioning and ever increasing life expectancy.

Malnutrition

Malnutrition means an undesirable kind of nutrition leading to ill health. It results in a lack, excess or imbalance of nutrients in diet. It includes undernutrition and overnutrition. Undernutrition is a state of an insufficient supply of essential nutrients. Overnutrition refers to an excessive intake of one or more nutrients, which creates a stress in bodily functions.

Causes

1. Social factors:
   a. People themselves.
      - Income
      - Ignorance
      - Illiteracy.
   b. Increased birth rate results in over population.
   c. Cultural factors, food fads, attitudes, faulty food habits.
      - Religious beliefs
      - Traditional child rearing practices
      - Traditional cooking and eating habits.
2. Agriculture:
   a. Lack of rain.
   b. Poor soil.
   c. Insects and pests.
   d. Inadequate storage facilities for food grains.

Malnutrition can be primarily due to insufficient supply of one or more essential nutrients or it can be secondary, which means it results from an error in metabolism and drugs used in treatment.

Malnutrition is directly responsible for certain specific nutritional deficiency diseases like kwashiorkor, marasmus, vitamin A deficiency, anemia, goiter, etc. Good nutrition is therefore essential for prevention of diseases and promotion of good health.

Mortality and Morbidity

The indirect effect of malnutrition on the community are long lasting. A high general death rate, high infant-mortality rate (IMR) high sickness rate and lower life expectancy. Over nutrition is responsible for obesity, diabetes, hypertension, cardiovascular diseases, renal diseases and diseases of the liver and gallbladder.

Thus, food plays a prominent role in providing physical, mental and social well-being, which is the World Health Organization (WHO) definition of health.

CLASSIFICATION OF FOOD

Based on its Origin

1. Foods of animal origin.
2. Foods of vegetable origin.

Based on Chemical Composition

1. Proteins.
2. Fats.
3. Carbohydrates.
4. Minerals.
5. Vitamins.

Based on its Function

1. Bodybuilding foods—amino acids, proteins.
2. Energy giving foods—carbohydrates (wheat, rice).
3. Protective foods—vitamins and minerals (vegetables).

Based on Nutrition Value

Five Food Group System

1. Cereals and millets.
2. Pulses and legumes.
3. Milk, milk products and meat.

4. Fruits and vegetables.
5. Fats and sugars.

Based on their functions, foods are grouped into energy-yielding foods, bodybuilding foods and protective foods. Carbohydrates, fats and proteins release energy on metabolism in body.

Cereals like rice, wheat, ragi and maize, roots and tubers like potato, sweet potato and tapioca are good sources of carbohydrate. Fats are more concentrated source of energy. Proteins are considered as bodybuilding food even though they can supply energy as well. Protein, calcium, phosphorus, iron and water are bodybuilding nutrients.

Protein foods like milk, meat, fish, eggs, pulses, grams and nuts are essential to build our tissues and to form blood.

Our body functions are regulated by water, minerals and vitamins. They are called the protective foods. Water is necessary for various body processes.

Vitamins are essential for regulating the body processes, such as growth, muscular coordination of various organs and functions of several organs like eyes, ears, nose and skin.

Minerals like calcium helps in controlling blood clotting, muscular contraction and for efficiency of heart muscles. Iron is essential for blood formation. Iodine is necessary for regulating body functions through the thyroid gland.

FOOD GUIDE PYRAMID: A GUIDE TO DAILY FOOD CHOICE

One of the most helpful, easy to use diet planning tools is the food guide pyramid (Fig. 21.2), which separates foods into specific groups and then specifies the number of servings form each group to each day. The placement of this five food groups on the pyramid emphasizes their role in the diet. The grains that form the base should serve as the foundation of a healthy diet because breads, cereals, rice and wheat are high in carbohydrates and low in fat. The grains are followed by fruits and vegetables, which supply the vitamins, minerals and fiber. The next level suggests eating smaller amounts of dairy products as well as meat, poultry, fish, beans, eggs and nuts. While foods from these group provides proteins, calcium, iron, zinc and other nutrients, they often contain large amount of fat and should be chosen carefully.

Not considered one of the food groups, the tip of the pyramid consists of fats, oils and sweets. They supply lot of fat and/or calories and few nutrients. These items should be added to diet sparingly.

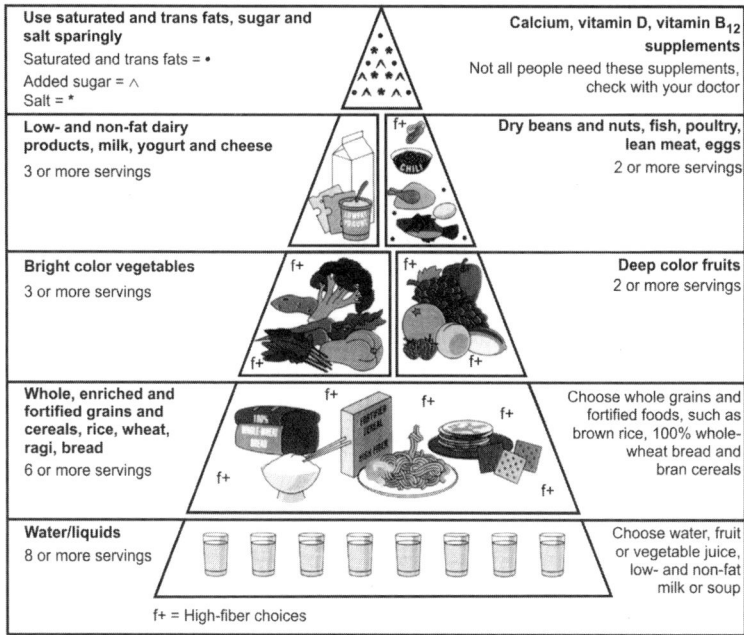

Fig. 21.2: Food guide pyramid for older adults

Calorie

The qualitative food requirements are estimated in term of energy in calories.

Physiologic calorie or kilocalorie (kcal) is the unit of energy, which is the amount of heat necessary to raise the temperature of 1 kg of water by 1°C, from 14.5°C to 15.5°C. This is 1,000 times the physical calorie unit. The international unit of energy is Joule (J) (1 kcal = 42 kJ).

Calorie Value of Food

Carbohydrates: 4 kcal/g
Fat: 9 kcal/g
Proteins: 4 kcal/g

RESPIRATORY QUOTIENT

The respiratory quotient (RQ) is the ratio of the volume of CO_2 eliminated to the volume of O_2 utilized.

$$RQ = \frac{\text{Volume of } CO_2 \text{ eliminated}}{\text{Volume of } O_2 \text{ utilized}}$$

Carbohydrates

The RQ is 1 because in carbohydrate diet, the volume of CO_2 produced is the same as the volume of O_2 consumed.

$$C_6H_{12}O_6 + 6O_2 \longrightarrow 6CO_2 + 6H_2O$$

$$RQ = \frac{CO_2 \text{ produced}}{O_2 \text{ consumed}} = \frac{6}{6} = 1$$

Fats: RQ for fat is about 0.7.

Protein: RQ for protein is about 0.8.

Mixed Diets

In mixed diets, containing varying proportions of proteins, fats and carbohydrates, the RQ is about 0.85.

Clinical Conditions

Respiratory quotient (RQ) increases in acidosis and fever. RQ decreases in alkalosis, uncontrolled diabetes mellitus and starvation.

Significance of RQ

Respiratory quotient (RQ) denotes the type of food burning in the body.

FACTORS AFFECTING ENERGY EXPENDITURE

1. The basal metabolic rate (BMR).
2. Specific dynamic action (SDA) or the thermogenic effect of food.
3. Physical activity.
4. Environmental temperature.

BASAL METABOLIC RATE

The basal metabolic rate (BMR) is the energy expenditure necessary to maintain basic physiologic conditions such as:
1. The activity of the heart.
2. Respiration.
3. Conduction of nerve impulses.
4. Ion transport across membranes.
5. Reabsorption in the kidney.
6. Metabolic activity, such as synthesis of macromolecules under standard conditions.

About 60% or more of the energy the average person spends goes to support the ongoing metabolic work of the body cells, the basic metabolism. This is the work that goes on all the time, without conscious awareness. The beating of the heart, the inhaling and exhaling of air, the maintenance of the body temperature and sending the nerve and hormonal messages to direct these activities are the basal procedures that maintain life. Basal metabolic needs are surprisingly large. A person whose total energy expenditure amounts to 2,000 cal/day spends as much as 1,200–1,400 calories to support usual metabolism.

Definition

The BMR is defined as the energy expenditure of a subject at complete physical and mental rest, awake (and not during sleep) having normal body temperature and in the postabsorption state (12 hours after the last meal) and 8–12 hours after any significant physical activity.

Measurement

Basal metabolism can be measured by:
1. Calorimeter directly by measuring the heat dissipated under basic conditions.
2. Indirectly by measuring oxygen consumption.

Factors Affecting BMR

Basal metabolic rate differs among different individuals. It depends on:
1. Variable factors.
2. Invariable factors.

Variable Factors Affecting BMR

1. **Nutritional state:** BMR is low in starvation and undernourishment as compared to well-fed state. Starvation leads to an adaptive decrease in BMR, which results from a decrease in lean body mass.
2. **Body size or surface area:** The BMR is directly proportional to the surface area of the subject. Larger the surface area, greater will be the heat loss and equally higher will be the heat production and BMR.
3. **Body composition:** The BMR is proportionate to lean body mass (LBM). LBM is the body weight minus non-essential (storage triacylglycerol) weight. Adipose tissue is not as metabolically active as lean body mass. BMR is often expressed as per kilogram of LMB or fat free mass. Therefore, higher the percentage of adipose tissue in the body lower the BMR per kilogram body weight.
4. **Endocrinal or hormonal state:** In hyperthyroidism, the BMR is increased and in hypothyroidism it may be decreased by up to 40%, leading to weight loss.
5. **Environmental temperature or climate:** In colder climate the BMR is higher and in tropical climate the BMR is proportionately low. Stress, anxiety and disease states, especially infections, fever, burns and cancer also increases the BMR.
6. **Drugs:** Smoking (nicotine), coffee (caffeine) and tea (theophylline) increase the BMR whereas β-blockers tend to decrease energy expenditure.

Invariable Factors Affecting BMR

1. **Gender or sex:** The BMR of males is slightly higher than that of females particularly due to:
   a. Women's lower percentage of muscle mass (LBM) and higher percentage of adipose tissue (that has lower rate of metabolism) when compared to men of the same body weight.
   b. The difference in sex hormone profile of the two genders.
2. **Age:** Decrease in BMR with increasing age is probably related to loss of muscle mass (LBM) and replacement of muscle with adipose tissue that has lower rate of metabolism.

Normal Value

BMR values are expressed as 'kcal or kJ/m^2' of body surface per hour. In adults, BMR for healthy males is 40 kcal (168 kJ) per hour and healthy females is 37 kcal (155 kJ) per hour.

This means that the total caloric expenditure in 24 hours to complete basal state is 1,800 kcal (7,500 kJ) for adult males and 1,400 kcal (5,859 kJ) for females assuming that the total body surface across are 1.8 m^2 and 1.6 m^2 respectively.

Clinical Applications

1. BMR estimation is used to diagnose thyroid disorders.
2. BMR is used in calculating food and drugs.

THERMOGENIC EFFECT [SPECIFIC DYNAMIC ACTION (SDA)] OF FOOD

Another component of energy expenditure in man is the diet induced thermogenesis also known as postprandial thermogenesis.

This is the energy expended in the digestion, absorption, storage and subsequent processing of food. This is called thermogenic effect of processing of food because these processes require energy and generate heat. The thermogenic effect of food is equivalent to almost 5%–10% of total energy expenditure.

This effect was originally attributed solely to the metabolic processing of protein and was termed specific dynamic action (SDA), but is now recognized as an effect produced by the consumption of all dietary fuels.

The consumption of protein produces the greatest increase in energy loss compared to fat or carbohydrates as shown below:

Protein: 20%–30% of intake.
Fat: 2.5%–4% of intake.
Carbohydrate: 5%–6% of intake.

PHYSICAL ACTIVITY

Physical activity is the largest variable affecting energy expenditure and represents 20%–40% of the energy expenditure.

The energy requirements of an adult in India was reviewed by the 'expert group' of the FAO/WHO in terms of reference man and reference woman. The reference man is in the age group of 20–39 years. With a weight of 55 kg without any disease and with a capacity to perform 8 hours of moderate activity. When not engaged in work, a reference man spends 8 hours in bed and 4–6 hours in moving around or in a sitting position and 2 hours either walking or doing household activities.

TABLE 21.2: Energy allowances for various groups

Category	Reference body weight	Activity	Energy allowances (kcal)
Man	55 kg	Light Moderate Heavy	2,400 2,800 3,900
Woman	45 kg	Light Moderate Heavy	1,900 2,200
	Pregnancy	2nd and 3rd trimester	+300
	Lactation	First 6 month 6–12 month	+550 +400

In the case of a reference woman, the difference is only in her body weight (45 kg). Instead of the physical activity of the occupation, the woman does household duties. Other conditions are the same in case of a reference man.

The energy expenditure for men and woman is calculated considering their internal and external activities. The FAO/WHO expert group (1983) made the following recommendations (Table 21.2).

Additional energy is needed for the growth of the fetus, placenta and tissues during pregnancy. The BMR is also increased due to increased internal activities. Daily 150 kcal during the first semester and 300 kcal during the rest of the pregnancy is recommended. The energy cost during the term of pregnancy is 62,500 kcal. Additional energy requirements during lactation is for the secretion of milk. For a normal output of 850 mL/day, during the first 6 months, 550 kcal/day is recommended.

The activities, which demand maximum energy are in the following order: Walking very fast, severe exercise, running, swimming, sawing wood, laborer work, carpentry, metal and industrial work, walking slowly, laundry work and ironing.

Classification of Activities Based on Occupation

Sedentary

Male: Teacher, tailor, priest, executive, shoe maker, retired personnel, landlords, peon.
Female: Teacher, nurse, housewife, executive.

Moderate

Male: Fisherman, weaver, driver, porter, fitter, turner, carpenter, agricultural laborer.
Female: Servant maid, basket maker, beedi maker.

Heavy

Male: Stonecutter, blacksmith, mine worker, wood cutter.
Female: Stonecutter, etc.

Environmental Temperature

Environmental temperature affects the metabolic rate. Low temperature increases energy expenditure by inducing shivering and non-shivering thermogenesis.

Shivering provides a regulated means of producing heat by measuring muscle activity in response to cold stress.

Another mechanism, non-shivering thermogenesis can also produce heat in response to cold stress. The site of non-shivering thermogenesis is the brown adipose tissue.

High temperature also has an effect on energy expenditure by increasing heat loss through sweating.

Calculating the Energy Requirements for Indians

Important factors for the calculation of the daily energy requirement are sex, height, weight and activity.

BODY MASS INDEX/QUETELET'S INDEX

The basal mass index (BMI) is used as a reference standard for assessing the prevalence of obesity in the community.

$$BMI = \frac{\text{Weight in kilograms}}{\text{Height in meters}}$$

Ideal body mass index for Indian woman = 19–24.
Ideal body mass index for Indian man = 20–26.
Once the BMI exceeds the normal limit, the person can be termed as overweight or obese.

A person is conswwidered overweight with BMI of 25 or more and obese with a BMI of 30 and above.

22

Carbohydrates: Sugar, Starch and Fiber

CHAPTER

CARBOHYDRATES

They are widely distributed in plants in which they are formed from carbon dioxide of the atmosphere by photosynthesis.

Sources of Carbohydrates

Following are main sources of carbohydrates:
1. Starch: These are present in cereals, roots and tubers, e.g. rice, wheat, ragi, pulses, potatoes, tapioca, yam and colocasia.
2. Sugars:
   a. Monosaccharides (simple sugars), e.g. glucose, fructose and galactose.
   b. Disaccharides (double sugars), e.g. sucrose, lactose and maltose.
   c. Polysaccharides (complex carbohydrates), e.g. cellulose.

Functions of Carbohydrates

1. They supply energy for body functions, for doing work and for the cells. They burn in the body at the rate of 4 kcal/g.
2. They are essential for the absorption of fats.
3. They have a sparing action on proteins.
4. They provide carbon skeleton for the synthesis of some non-essential amino acids.
5. Some carbohydrates are present in tissue constituents.
6. They add flavor to the diet.

Special Tissue Function

Carbohydrates serve many special functions in body tissues and organs.

Liver: Glycogen reserves in the liver and muscles provide a constant exchange with the body's overall energy balance systems. These reserves especially in the liver, protect cells from depressed metabolic functions and resulting injury.

Protein and fat: Carbohydrates helps to regulate both protein and fat metabolism.

Requirements

No daily allowances has been fixed for carbohydrates. The body has specific need for carbohydrates as a source of energy for brain and other tissue cells.

The carbohydrates calorie should be at least 40% in a well-balanced diet. The range of carbohydrates requirement is given below:

Adults	: 50%–70%
Expecting and lactating mothers	: 40%–50%
Infants	: 40%–50%
Preschool children	: 40%–60%
Other children and adolescents	: 60%–70%

A minimum of 100 g carbohydrates are needed in the diet to ensure efficient oxidation of fat. Most diets supply more. If the proteins supply about 10% of the calories, fats 20%, then carbohydrates must supply the remaining 70% calories. Being the cheapest source of food energy, it supplies up to 80% of the calories in the low cost Indian food.

Reserve Fuel Supply

Glycogen reserves supply the backup fuel. The total amount of carbohydrate in the body, including both glycogen and blood glucose is relatively small. Without constant supply, the total amount of available glucose provides enough energy for only half a day of moderate activity. Therefore to maintain a normal blood glucose level and prevent breakdown of fat and protein in tissues, individuals must eat carbohydrate rich food regularly to meet their energy requirements.

Dietary Fiber: Uses

Dietary fiber is the high fibrous lining found in vegetables, fruits and cereals. It is hard to digest and has no nutritional value.

Fiber has two forms, insoluble and soluble.

Insoluble Fibers

Insoluble fibers in wheat bran hold water in the colon, thus increasing bulk, which stimulates the muscles of the digestion tracts so that they retain their health and tone.

The toned muscles can move easily more waste products through the colon for excretion. This prevents constipation.

Soluble Fibers

1. The type in beans and oats reduce the risk of heart and artery disease—atherosclerosis, by lowering the level of cholesterol in the blood.
2. It helps prevent constipation by forming large bulk of feces and helps in gastrointestinal (GI) motility (roughage action).
3. Dietary fiber improves glucose tolerance by the body. It diminishes the rate of glucose absorption from intestine.
4. Soluble fiber found in the legumes and fruits like gums and pectins can lower blood cholesterol probably by binding to bile acids and dietary cholesterol, thus preventing their absorption.
5. By increasing bulk and needing more chewing, cellulose may reduce the food intake. Thus, it can help obese persons to reduce total energy intake and loose weight.
6. Satiety value: Fiber add bulk to the food stuff and gives a sensation of fullness of stomach. Thus satiety is achieved without consumption of excess calories.
7. It also slows down carbohydrate absorption thereby reducing blood glucose and insulin need for diabetics.
8. Large soft stools dilute potential carcinogens. Rapid transit of stools may reduce the content of carcinogens in colon mucosa and thus reduce the risk of colon cancer.

Adverse Effects of Dietary Fibers

1. Intestinal absorption of some minerals and trace elements is decreased.
2. Intestinal bacteria ferment some fibers causing flatulence and abdominal discomfort.
3. An excessive intake of fiber results in intestinal obstruction, if it is not accompanied by water.
4. If fiber intake is suddenly increased, complaints like cramming, diarrhea, excessive intestinal gas are common. To minimize these

effects, fiber content of diet should be gradually increased over a period of several weeks.
5. Dietary fiber is best taken from natural foods and not from fiber supplements. Food source provide a variety of fibers, vitamins and minerals in combination, whereas fiber supplements do not supplement any nutrients.

Sugar Substitutes

Artificial sweetners are used by people who wish to reduce their calorie intake. Two commonly available sugar substitutes are saccharin and aspartame.

1. *Saccharin:* O-sulfobenzimide is 300–500 times as sweet as sucrose and pass through the body unchanged. It has been used in beverages and desserts. It has no adverse effects. The only drawback is it leaves a bitter after taste.
2. *Aspartame:* is a dipeptide of two amino acids, aspartic acid and phenylalanine. Its trade names are NutraSweet and Equal. As the dipeptides are unstable to heat, this sweetner cannot be used in cooked and baked foods. People who suffer from phenylketonuria (PKU) should avoid aspartame.

Carbohydrate Excess: Clinical Problems

1. Obesity: It is very easy and common to eat sweets/mithais, candy and soft drinks in excess of one's needs. Most of these contain excess of carbohydrates. When the energy intake exceeds expenditure, the excess is deposited as fat leading to obesity and over weight. Obesity is a predisposing factor for a number of health problems.
2. Dental caries: If sugar remains in contact with teeth, it can lead to tooth decay. If it is not checked, it may lead to dental caries. Chewing sweets makes it remain longer periods, unless children are taught to rinse their mouth thoroughly after eating candy and also food.

23 Nutritional Aspects of Fats

FATS

Dietary fats are divided into two types (Table 23.1):
- Visible fats: Butter, ghee, oil
- Invisible fats: Egg, fish, meat, cereals, oil seeds.

TABLE 23.1: Important sources of fats

Sources	Fat %
Rich sources	
Pure oils and fats	100
Ghee and vanaspathi	100
Butter	80–81
Good sources	
Nuts and oil seeds	40–60
Milk powder	26
Eggs	14
Meat and fish	10–15
Fair sources	
Cow milk	4
Buffalo milk	7
Whole pulses	3.5
Whole cereals and millets	2.3

Fat Requirements of Individuals

1. Infants: Birth to 1 year—25%–30% of total calories from fat.
2. Children and adolescents (1–8 year)—15%–20% of total calories from fat.
3. Adults expectant and nursing mothers—10%–20% of total calories from fat.

Atleast 50% of the fat should consist of oils rich in essential fatty acids (EFA).

Fat is required for:
1. Energy needs.
2. Essential fatty acid needs about 10% of the total energy need is met by the invisible fat in the diet.

A minimum of 5% of the total energy is needed as visible fat. This works out 12 g of fat per day. A higher level intake of 20 g/day is desirable to provide energy and palatability for normal adults. To meet the EFA needs, the diet should contain at least 20 g of vegetable oil, which is an excellent source of linoleic acid (EFA).

An upper limit of 20 g/day of fat intake is desirable to prevent heart ailments. Recommended fat intake is 20%–30% of daily calorie requirement, which should contain about 30% polyunsaturated fatty acids (PUFA). Visible fat should be restricted to 10% of the calorie intake.

FUNCTIONS OF LIPIDS

The lipids present in the diet, animal and human body are:
1. Triglycerides (neutral fats).
2. Phospholipids.
3. Cholesterol (present only in animal fats).

Functions of Triglycerides (Neutral Fat)

1. It is a concentrated source of energy yielding 9 kcal/g, i.e. more than twice the energy supplied by carbohydrates and proteins per unit weight.
2. 95% of lipids in food is triglycerides.
3. Fats reduce the bulk of the diet as they produce twice as much calories as carbohydrates per unit weight. Further starchy food absorbs a lot of water during cooking and reduces the bulk of the diet.

4. Fat is essential for absorption of fat-soluble vitamins, i.e. vitamins A, D, E and K especially carotenoids (provitamins).
5. Some animal fats, e.g. mutton and fish liver oils are good sources of vitamin A. Most vegetable fat are good sources of vitamin E. Red palm oil is a good source of carotene. Certain vegetable fats are rich sources of essential fatty acid, e.g. linoleic acid.
6. Fats are deposited in the adipose tissue and serve as a reserve source of energy during starvation and illness. Further, adipose tissue functions as an insulating material against cold and physical injury.
7. Fats provide aroma and flavor to food. Fats improve the palatability and gives a feeling of fullness to the stomach.

Functions of Phospholipids

1. They are present in plasma in combination with proteins and lipoproteins, which are involved in the transport of fat and cholesterol.
2. They are important constituents of all membranes.
3. They are concerned with selective cation transport across the erythrocytic membrane.
4. They form a part of certain enzymes, e.g. cytochrome oxidase, succinic oxidase.
5. They are present in the mitochondria in large amounts and are essential for the organization and function of the mitochondrial electron transport system.
6. They are essential components of thromboplastin, a factor in blood coagulation.
7. They are present in large amounts in nerve tissues and essential for their function.

Functions of Cholesterol

1. As a precursor of bile acids.
2. Precursor for some steroids.
3. As a precursor for the formation of dehydrocholesterol in the skin for conversion to vitamin D by UV rays present in sunlight.
4. It is present in all membranes and is essential for maintaining the cell membranes in good condition.
5. Present in large amounts in the nerve tissues and is essential for their function.

ESSENTIAL FATTY ACIDS

Deficiency of essential fatty acids (EFA) leads to the cessation of growth and development of the skin and hemorrhage. Scales also develop on the dorsal and plantar surfaces of feet and around the ears. Hair is lost from the face and the back, blood may appear in the urine.

Phrynoderma: EFA Deficiency

Phrynoderma is also known as 'toad skin'. This condition is characterized by the presence of horny papular eruptions on the posterior and lateral aspects of the limbs, on the back and buttocks. Phrynoderma is rapidly cured by the administration of linseed or sunflower seed oil, rich in EFA along with vitamin B complex.

Other Effects of EFA Deficiency

1. Integrity of cell membranes and cell functions.
2. Certain enzyme systems.
3. Reproduction and lactation.
4. Transfer of cholesterol.
5. Water balance.

EFA Contents of Vegetable Sources

Sunflower, niger seed, cotton seed, linseed, corn, walnut, sesame and soybean oils are rich sources of EFA (40%–78%). These oils must form atleast 50% of fat in diet.

FATS AND HEART AILMENT

Fat is essential for health, but too much of it is harmful. The well to do section of Indians have a high intake of saturated fats from milk, sweets, egg and meat. They lead a very sedentary lifestyle. Their energy intake is in excess of actual needs, which leads to obesity and dangerous plasma lipid profiles. If unchecked this causes atherosclerosis, high blood pressure and many cardiac diseases. Reducing total fats, saturated fats and maintaining a low cholesterol diet are necessary for disease prevention and health promotion.

To Lower Blood Cholesterol Levels

1. Eat no more than 30% calories as fat.
2. Eat no more than 8%–10% of calories as saturated fat.
3. Eat no more than 10% calories as polyunsaturated fats.
4. Monounsaturated fats must make up to 10%–15% calories.
5. Limit daily cholesterol intake to less than 200 mg.

CHAPTER 24

Proteins

Proteins are classified into complete proteins, partially incomplete proteins and incomplete proteins based on the presence of essential amino acids in them. The presence of amino acids helps a protein to perform all functions of proteins in our body. A complete protein food contains all essential amino acids in correct proportions. It helps the protein to promote growth, maintenance and repair. Examples of complete protein foods are fish, egg and milk.

Partially incomplete proteins lack some essential amino acids and so they help to maintain our body and only moderate growth occurs. Wheat proteins and vegetable proteins are good examples.

Incomplete proteins neither help maintenance nor growth. Gelatin, zein grains and fruits are examples.

When a mixture of protein from different sources is consumed, mutual supplementation takes place. For example, rice or wheat protein is low in lysine whereas pulse is rich in lysine and low in methionine. Rice is rich in methionine and a mutual supplementation results when rice and pulse are consumed together.

PROTEIN QUALITY

Protein quality depends on the kinds and amounts of essential amino acids present in the food proteins. Qualitative data regarding the suitability to meet the protein requirements of the body have been obtained by the experiments on animals and human beings.

Biological Value

Biological value (BV) measures the quality of dietary proteins utilized by the animal for meeting its protein needs for maintenance and growth.

Groups of albino rats (28 days old) were fed successively on the following diet for a period of 10 days.
1. Protein free diet.
2. Diet containing 10% of protein to be tested.

Urine and feces were collected by keeping the rats in metabolism cages. Records of food intake were maintained. The diet, urine and feces are analyzed for nitrogen (N).

$$\text{Biological value} = \frac{\text{Nitrogen digested} - \text{Nitrogen lost in metabolism} \times 100}{\text{N retained by the body (dietary N} - \text{fecal N)}}$$

The quality of protein is directly related to BV. The BV increases with the increase in the percentage of nitrogen absorbed, being retained. The BV of milk is 84, brown rice is 73 and whole wheat is 65.

Net Protein Utilization

Net protein utilization (NPU) is the digestability of protein multiplied by its BV.

Protein Efficiency Ratio

Protein efficiency ratio (PER) is not based on intake and output of food protein residues. Therefore, it is less accurate than BV and NPU. But the technique is easy and also easy to use. In this method, a known amount of test protein in an adequate diet is fed to young rats for 4 weeks under standard conditions and the weight gain is determined. The PER is obtained by dividing the weight gain by grams of protein fed.

$$\text{Protein efficiency ratio} = \frac{\text{Weight gain in grams}}{\text{Protein fed in grams}}$$

The PER of milk is 3 and polished rice is 2.2.

Chemical Score

Chemical score is the ratio between the content of the most limiting amino acid in the test protein to the content of the same amino acid in egg protein expressed as a percentage. Since egg protein contains all essential amino acids in adequate amounts and possesses the highest nutrition value among dietary proteins, it is given the chemical score of 100.

The most limiting amino acid in milk is the α-amino acids. Chemical score of milk protein is:

$$\frac{3.4}{5.5} \times 100 = 61.81$$

The chemical score of gelatin and zein is 0.

RECOMMENDED DIETARY ALLOWANCE

The requirement of the body for protein as recommended by nitrogen balance studies is 0.5–0.6 g/kg of the body weight in adults when the source of protein supplies amino acids in the proportion needed by the body. In practice, the supply may not be in the required proportions. Therefore, the recommended dietary allowance of protein is raised to 1.0 g/kg body weight for adults. The daily recommended protein intake for normal men, women and children and at the time of pregnancy and lactation is given in Table 24.1.

During infancy, pregnancy and lactation, there is an increased demand of protein for growth. Persons suffering from burns or wasting diseases such as tuberculosis and rheumatic fever also need additional protein for regulation of wasted tissues. Similarly, more protein in the diet is required in case of blood losses due to excessive menstruation, hemorrhages and blood donation.

TABLE 24.1: Daily recommended protein intake

Particulars of the individual	Proteins in gram per day
Man (60 kg)	60
Woman (50 kg)	50
Woman, pregnant (later half of pregnancy)	65
Woman, nursing mother 0–6 month of lactation	75
Infant	
0–6 month	21 g/kg body weight
7–12 month	1.6 g/kg body weight
Children	
1–3 year	21
4–6 year	29
7–9 year	40
Girls	
13–15 year	67
16–18 year	60
Boys	
13–15 year	67
16–18 year	75

DIETARY SOURCES OF PROTEINS

Protein contents of some common foodstuffs are given in Table 24.2.

Plant Sources
The plant sources are cereal grains, pulses, nuts, legumes.

Animal Sources
The animal sources are meat, fish, poultry, eggs, milk and milk products.

TABLE 24.2: Protein content of some foodstuffs

Foodstuff	Protein content in g/100 g
Plant foods	
Bengal gram dal	20.8
Black gram dal	24.0
Cow pea	24.1
Green gram	24.5
Horse gram	22.0
Kesari dal	28.2
Soybean	43.2
Ground nut	25.0
Cashew nut	21.2
Almond	20.8
Pistachio	19.8
Walnut	15.8
Animal foods	
Milk	3.2
Meat	18.0
Egg	13.0
Fish	15.0
Paneer (cheese)	18.3

FUNCTIONS OF PROTEINS

Primary Tissue Building

Protein is the fundamental structural material of every cell in the body. The primary functions are to repair the worn out, wasted or damaged tissue and build up new tissue. Thus, protein meets the growth needs and maintains tissue health during adult years. In addition to bodybuilding functions, protein has other body functions related to energy, water balance, metabolism and body's defence mechanism.

Energy System

Carbohydrates are the primary fuel source for the body assisted by fat as stored fuel. In times of need (e.g. starvation), protein may also furnish additional fuel to sustain heat and energy. Fuel supplied by protein is 4 kcal/g (like carbohydrates).

Water Balance

Plasma proteins, especially albumin, help to control water balance throughout the body by exerting osmotic pressure to maintain internal circulation of body fluids and capillary blood flow.

Metabolism

Protein aids metabolic functions through enzymes, hormones and transport agents. Digestive and cell hormones are hormones that control metabolic functions. Enzymes that are necessary for the digestion of carbohydrates (amylase), fats (lipase) and proteins (protease) are all proteins. Proteins also act as vehicles, in which nutrients are carried throughout the body. Lipoproteins are necessary to transport fats in the water soluble blood supply. Other examples are hemoglobin and transferrin, the iron transport proteins in blood. Hormones such as insulin and glucagon are also proteins that have a major role in the metabolism of glucose.

Body's Defence System

Protein is used to build special white blood cells (lymphocytes) and antibodies as part of body's immune system to help defend against infection and diseases.

Energy Supply

A small part of body's need for energy (about 6%–12%) is supplied by products of protein metabolism.

PROTEIN DEFICIENCY

Kwashiorkor, marasmus and marasmic kwashiorkor are known as protein energy or caloric malnutrition (PEM or PCM).

Kwashiorkor

In Greek, 'kwashiorkor' means displaced child, when the next baby is born. This is widely prevalent in weaned infants and preschool children due to lack of proteins, calories, vitamins and minerals. It usually occurs in age group 1–4 years. Following symptoms are observed—muscle wasting, moon face, edemas, mental change, grey hairs, neurosis, fatty liver, psychomotor changes, Bitot's spots, angular stomatitis, mottled enamel, poor appetite and weight loss.

Marasmus

In Greek, 'marasmus' means withering. It usually occurs at earlier age than kwashiorkor widely prevalent in age group of 0–12 months, i.e. before 1 year. It is caused by both protein and caloric deficiencies. Marasmic child shows old man's appearance with just skin and bones. Other signs and symptoms are growth failure more severe than kwashiorkor, edema is absent, acid stool, dehydration, lack of subcutaneous fat and apathy.

Marasmic Kwashiorkor

In this condition, both kwashiorkor and marasmic symptoms are noticed. 50 calories and protein allowances are needed more than the daily requirements.

Treatment

High-quality protien and adequate amounts of calories are required.

Protein	=	3.5 g/day.
Calories	=	150–200 kcal/kg body weight.
Vitamin A	=	50,000 international units.
Iron	=	Iron salt and folic acid tablets are prescribed.
Electrolytes	=	KCl 3–4 g/day. $MgCl_2$ 5 g/day.

Protein Food

The protein foods are albumin water, dal water, soy milk, breast milk, puddings, egg flip, scrambled egg, dal payasam, nutrition porridge, fruit juice with milk, skimmed milk.

PROTEIN-CALORIE MALNUTRITION IN CHILDREN

Deficiency of protein foods during growth period produces kwashiorkor and marasmus (Table 24.3). Protein-calorie malnutrition is one of the largest nutritional problems of India.

TABLE 24.3: Salient features of kwashiorkor and marasmus

Kwashiorkor	Marasmus
1. Moderate to severe failure of growth	1. Severe muscle wasting
2. Lack of proper involvement of muscle and lack of muscle tone	2. Lack of subcutaneous fat
3. Presence of edema, potbelly in children	3. High incidence of diarrhea
4. Dry and flaky skin	4. Severe growth failure
5. Hair turns reddish	5. Decreased blood protein
6. Anorexial diarrhea	6. Skin changes
7. Low hemoglobin level	7. General severity leads to mental retardation
8. Decreased production of amylase, trypsin and lipases	8. Period of recovery is much longer
9. Patient recovers within a short period of time	

Treatment and Prevention

1. In developing countries, breastfeeding should be encouraged to ensure adequate supply of nutrients and antigens.
2. Foodstuffs that contain sufficient amounts of amino acids should be provided.
3. Improvement of sanitation and program of immunization.
4. Fluids with electrolytes of sodium and potassium to maintain electrolytic balance.

EFFECT OF EXCESS

When diet rich in protein are eaten, the excess protein is oxidized and nitrogen is excreted as urea. The excess protein is used mainly as a source of energy. Prolonged feeding of high-protein diets will be a strain on the kidneys and may produce hypertrophy of the kidneys. The diet consumed by Eskimos provide practical evidence that human beings can maintain good health over long periods of high-protein diets. Human beings may live on meat alone for a year when sufficient fat was supplied as a source of calorie.

Protein Excess: Clinical Problems

Though protein is a vital need of the body, intake of excess creates stress on the body function. The liver has to deaminize the excess amino acids and synthesize urea. The loss of calcium in urine is increased with high-protein intake. High protein from animal foods carries undesirable saturated fats also along with it.

As protein foods are expensive, their increased intake might lead to lesser intake of nutrient-rich foods and thus, reduce the quality of the diet. Adequate protein is good, but excess is not desirable.

NUTRITION

Health and weight depend on nutrition. Consume these foods for better nutrition and health:
1. Red, orange and green colored fruits and vegetables (guava, amla, papaya, mango, tomato, carrot, pumpkin).
2. Whole grain cereals (whole or broken wheat brown rice).
3. Coarse grains (bajra, ragi, jowar).
4. Sprouted grams.
5. Soybean.
6. Dark green leafy vegetables.
7. Mushroom.
8. Marine fish.
9. Iodized salt:
    a. These provide additional health benefits besides microminerals, macrominerals and fiber.
    b. Prevent nutritional deficiencies.
    c. Reduce risk of degenerative diseases like diabetes, hypertensions, cardiovascular disease, cancer, etc.
    d. Promote growth, development and immunity.
    e. Improve productivity.

25 Mineral Metabolism

CHAPTER

Minerals are inorganic elements required for a variety of functions. The minerals required by the human body are grouped into macrominerals and microminerals (trace elements) (Table 25.1). The macrominerals are required in amounts in excess of 100 mg/day. The microminerals are required in amounts less than 100 mg/day.

MACROMINERALS

CALCIUM

Calcium is the most abundant mineral present in the body.

TABLE 25.1: Minerals required in human nutrition

Macrominerals	Microminerals or trace elements
Calcium	Iron
Phosphorus	Copper
Sodium	Iodine
Potassium	Manganese
Chlorine	Zinc
Magnesium	Molybdenum
Sulfur	Cobalt
	Fluorine
	Selenium
	Chromium

Dietary Sources

Milk and milk products, meat, fish, cereals, pulses and green leafy vegetables.

Recommended Dietary Allowance Per Day

- Infants: 300–500 mg/day
- Children: 800–1,200 mg/day
- Adults: 800 mg/day
- Women during pregnancy, lactation and teenagers: 1,200 mg/day.

Absorption

Mainly occurs in duodenum by energy-dependent process. Absorption is increased by:
1. Vitamin D through its active form calciferol, i.e. 1,25-dihydroxycholecalciferol induces the synthesis of calcium-binding protein in the intestinal epithelial cells and promotes calcium absorption.
2. Gastric acidity, sugars like lactose promote calcium uptake by intestinal cells.

Absorption is decreased by oxalates, phytates, fatty acids—these form insoluble salts with calcium.

Distribution

1. Total content in the body = 1–1.5 kg.
2. 99% is present in the bone and teeth as hydroxyapatite.
3. 1% is present in blood and tissues.
4. Normal serum level 9–11 mg/100 mL.

Functions

Intracellular calcium is involved in:
1. Muscle contraction.
2. Release of hormones, neurotransmitter and neuromodulators.
3. Activation of a number of enzymes.
4. Glycogen metabolism.
5. Cell division.

Extracellular calcium provide calcium ion for the:
1. Maintenance of intracellular calcium.
2. Bone mineralization.
3. Blood coagulation.
4. Membrane excitability.
5. Plasma membrane potential.

Ca:P Product

The product of calcium (Ca) and phosphate (P) is around 50 in children and 40 in adults. In rickets, it is less than 30. The product of Ca:P is important for calcification of bones.

Clinical Significance

Hypercalcemia

Serum calcium level is more than 12 mg%. It is seen in hyperpara-thyroidism, hypervitaminosis 'D' and malignancies.

Features: Most patients have no symptoms, but if untreated, they may develop kidney stone, polyuria, bone pain and pancreatitis.

Hypocalcemia

Hypocalcemia leads to osteoporosis and tetany.

Tetany: This is a more serious and life-threatening condition. This provokes a characteristic hyperexcitable state of the nerves and muscles.

Symptoms: It include numbness of extremities, nerve irritability and spasms of muscles.

Causes: The causes are as follows:
- Hypoparathyroidism
- Rickets
- Osteomalacia.

Total serum calcium level may be less than 7 mg%.

Osteoporosis: Increased demineralization of bones. Therefore, there is a loss of bone mass. Seen in elderly people and postmenopausal women. Results in increased incidence of fractures.

Treated with calcium, vitamin D supplementation and estrogen administration.

Rickets

Defective calcification of bones. Decreased level of vitamin D in the body. Decreased Ca and P due to dietary deficiency. Serum Ca and P levels are low. Ca:P product is less than 30.

Increased alkaline phosphatase activity is seen.

PHOSPHORUS

Phosphorus is a widely distributed important element in the human body. Adults contain about 400–700 g of phosphorus, about 80% of which is combined with calcium in bones and teeth. It is present in the form of organic and inorganic phosphates.

Functions

1. Constituent of bones and teeth: Inorganic phosphorus is a major constituent of hydroxyapatite in bone, thereby playing an important part in structural support of the body.
2. Acid-base regulation: Mixture of HPO_4^{2-} and $H_2PO_4^-$ constitutes the phosphate buffer for maintaining the pH of body fluids.
3. Energy storage and transfer reactions: High-energy compounds, e.g. ATP, ADP, creatine phosphate, which store and transport energy.
4. Essential constituent: Phosphate is an essential part of phospholipids of cell membrane, include acids (RNA and DNA), nucleotides (NAD, NADP, cAMP and cCMP).
5. Enzyme action: Phosphate present in nucleotides, some of which function as coenzymes are pyridoxal phosphate, thiamine pyrophosphate, NADP and flavin coenzymes.
6. Regulation of enzymes activity: Phosphorylation and dephosphorylation of enzymes modify the activity of many enzymes.

Dietary Sources

The foods rich in calcium are also rich in phosphorus namely milk, cheese, beans, eggs, cereals, fish and meat.

Recommended Dietary Allowance Per Day

For both men and women, recommended dietary allowance (RDA) per day is 800 mg/day. The amount during pregnancy and lactation is 1,200 mg/day.

Normal Values

Serum: 3–4 mg% in adults.
4–6 mg% in children.

Clinical Significance

Hypophosphatemia

Seen in rickets, hyperparathyroidism.

Hyperphosphatemia

Occurs in hypoparathyriodism, hypervitaminosis D and in renal failure.

SODIUM

Sodium is the major cation of the extracellular fluid. The total sodium in an average man is 1.8 g/kg weight of which approximately 75% is exchangeable and 25% is non-exchangeable, which is incorporated into tissues such as bone. Most of the exchangeable sodium is in the extracellular fluid. Normal serum sodium (Na^+) level is 135–145 mEq/L.

Functions

1. Sodium maintains the osmotic pressure and water balance.
2. It is a constituent of buffer and involved in the maintenance of acid-base balance.
3. It maintains the muscle and nerve irritability.
4. It is involved in cell membrane permeability.
5. To raise the osmotic pressure, thereby maintaining the volume of blood.
6. To regulate the electrolyte and pH balance of extracellular compartment.
7. To control electric potentials of excitable tissues such as nerve and muscle.
8. Helps in active transport of glucose, galactose and amino acids across the intestinal mucosa.

Clinical Conditions Related to Plasma Sodium Level Alteration

Hypernatremia

Hypernatremia is an increase in serum sodium concentration above the normal range of 135–145 mEq/L.

Causes: The causes of hypernatremia are as follows:
1. *Water depletion:* May arise from a decreased intake of or excessive loss with normal sodium content, e.g. diabetes insipidus.
2. *Water and sodium depletion:* If more water than sodium is lost, e.g. diabetes mellitus (osmotic diuresis) and excessive sweating and diarrhea in children.
3. *Excessive sodium intake or retention:* In the ECF due to excessive aldosterone secretion, e.g. Conn's syndrome and Cushing's syndrome.

Symptoms: If hypernatremia is due to water loss, then the symptoms are those of dehydration and if it is due to excess salt gain, it leads to hypertension and edema.

Hyponatremia

Hyponatremia is a significant fall in serum sodium concentration below the normal range of 135–145 mEq/L.

Causes: The causes of hyponatremia are as follows:
1. *Retention of water*: Retention of water dilutes the constituents of the extracellular space causing hyponatremia, e.g. in heart failure, liver disease, nephrotic syndrome, renal failure, syndrome of inappropriate ADH secretion (SIADH).
2. *Loss of sodium*: This occurs only when there is pathological sodium loss. Such losses may be from gastrointestinal tract, e.g. vomiting, diarrhea, fistula and in urine. Urinary loss may be due to aldosterone deficiency (Addison's disease).

Symptoms: Constant thirst, muscle cramps, nausea, vomiting, abdominal cramps.

Dietary Sources

Table salt (NaCl), fatty foods, milk, baking soda, baking powder, carrot and tomato.

Recommended Dietary Allowance Per Day

1. 1–5 g.
2. 5 g NaCl is recommended for adults without history of hypertension.
3. 1 g of NaCl per day with history of hypertension.

Na⁺-K⁺ Pump

Na^+,K^+-ATPase transports Na^+ from the intracellular compartments against electrochemical gradient. It also transports K^+ intracellularly. The pump requires energy, which is obtained from the hydrolysis of ATP. This in turn helps in maintaining high concentration of sodium in the extracellular fluid and potassium in the intracellular fluid.

POTASSIUM

Potassium is the main intracellular cation. About 98% of total potassium is in cells and 2% in ECF. Most of the body's potassium is found in muscles.

Dietary Sources

Fresh vegetables, fruits like oranges and bananas, whole grain, meat, milk, legumes and tender coconut water. Average diet provides 4 g K^+/day.

Recommended Dietary Allowance Per Day

The RDA per day for potassium is 2–5 g.

Serum Potassium

The concentration in serum is 4.5 mEq/L. Serum potassium concentration does not vary appreciably in response to water loss or retention. But even a small change in intracellular potassium concentration will cause a big change in serum potassium contents.

Metabolic Functions

1. Potassium maintains the intracellular osmotic pressure, water balance and acid-base balance.
2. It influences neuromuscular activity of cardiac and skeletal muscles.
3. Several glycolytic muscles need potassium for their formation.

4. Potassium is required for transmission of nerve impulses.
5. Nuclear activity and protein synthesis are dependent on potassium.

Clinical Significance

Hyperkalemia

Hyperkalemia is due to increased serum potassium and occurs in the following conditions:
1. Renal failure.
2. Advanced dehydration.
3. Addison's disease.
4. Shock.
5. Intravenous administration of excess amount of potassium.

Hypokalemia

Hypokalemia is due to low levels of serum potassium and occurs in case of:
1. Diarrhea and vomiting.
2. Metabolic alkalosis.
3. Familial periodic paralysis.
4. Overactivity of adrenal cortex (Cushing's syndrome).
5. Prolonged administration of diuretics because of excretion of potassium in urine.
6. During heart failure.

CHLORIDE

Chloride is the major anion in the extracellular space.

Dietary Sources

Common salt, whole grains, leafy vegetables, eggs, milk.

Recommended Dietary Allowance Per Day

The RDA per day for chloride is 2–5 g.

Normal Level

The normal serum level is 95–110 mEq/L.

Functions

1. As a part of sodium chloride, chloride is essential for water balance, regulating osmotic pressure and acid-base balance.
2. Chloride is essential for the formation of HCl by the gastric mucosa and for activation of enzyme amylase.
3. It is involved in chloride shift.

Clinical Significance

Hypochloremia

Seen in low-salt diet, persistent vomiting, renal tubular damage, excessive sweating, Addison's disease.

Hyperchloremia

Seen in Cushing's syndrome, decreased renal flow, excessive saline therapy and excess steroid therapy.

SULFUR

The body receives sulfur through proteins as sulfur-containing amino acids, e.g. methionine and cysteine.

Dietary Sources

Plant and animal proteins, legumes, eggs, cereals and cauliflower.

Functions

Sulfur is a constituent of:
1. Protein.
2. Glycosaminoglycans, e.g. heparin and chondroitin sulfate.
3. Bile acids, e.g. taurocholic acid.
4. Compounds like insulin and glutathione.

Excretion

Sulfur is excreted by the kidneys in urine in the form of inorganic, organic and ethereal sulfate.

MAGNESIUM

Magnesium is the second most abundant intracellular cation after potassium.

Function

1. Magnesium is a cofactor for more than 300 enzymes in the body.
2. In oxidative phosphorylation, glycolysis, cell replication, nucleotide metabolism, protein synthesis and many ATP-dependent reactions.
3. Magnesium along with sodium, potassium and calcium controls the neuromuscular irritability.
4. It is an important constituent of bone and teeth.

Dietary Sources

Abundant in the chlorophyll of green leafy vegetables, cereals and meat.

Recommended Dietary Allowance Per Day

The RDA of the adult man is 350 mg/day and for woman it is 300 mg/day.

MICROMINERALS

COPPER

Dietary Sources

Fish, liver, nuts, green vegetables, meat, egg. Milk is a poor source.

Dietary Requirement

The requirement of copper in diet per day is 2–3 mg.

Function

1. Copper-containing enzymes include cytochrome oxidase, lysyl oxidase, tyrosinase.
2. It converts ferrous iron into ferric iron, the transport form of iron.
3. It is necessary for the synthesis of hemoglobin.

ZINC

Dietary Sources
Meat, egg, fish, beans, nuts, oil seeds and vegetables.

Dietary Requirement
The requirement of zinc in diet per day is 15–30 mg.

Function

1. Zinc is a component of enzymes like:
   - Carbonic anhydrase
   - Alcohol dehydrogenase
   - Alkaline phosphatase
   - Superoxide dismutase
   - Carboxypeptidase
   - DNA polymerase.
2. It is used for the storage and secretion of insulin from the B cells of pancreas. Zinc with insulin prolongs half-life of insulin.
3. To maintain normal levels of vitamin A. It helps in the release of vitamin A from liver into blood and thus increases its plasma level and its utilization in rhodopsin synthesis.
4. It is important in taste sensation.
5. Zinc plays an important role in expression of genetic potential in synthesis, repair, structural integrity of nucleic acids.
6. Zinc stabilizes membrane structures and gives protection at the cellular level by preventing lipid peroxidation and reducing free radical formation.
7. It is required for normal growth and reproduction.
8. It is also included in native structure of insulin.
9. It is an important element in wound healing, as it is a necessary factor in the biosynthesis and integrity of connective tissue.
10. Zinc stabilizes structure of protein and nucleic acids.

Absorption and Excretion
Approximately 20%–30% of ingested dietary zinc is absorbed in small intestine. It is transported in blood plasma mostly by albumin and $\alpha 2$-macroglobulin. Zinc is excreted in urine, bile, pancreatic fluid and in milk in lactating mothers.

SELENIUM

Selenium is present in the body as selenium analogues of sulfur-containing amino acids, e.g. selenomethionine, selenocysteine.

Dietary Sources

Liver, kidneys, seafoods, cereals.

Recommended Dietary Allowance Per Day

The RDA per day for selenium is 50–200 mg.

Functions

1. Along with vitamin E, it prevents membrane lipid peroxidation.
2. It prevents hepatic necrosis, muscular dystrophy.
3. Selenium acts as a prosthetic group of enzyme glutathione peroxidase, which is present in cell cytosol and mitochondria and functions to reduce H_2O_2. This enzyme protects the cells against the damage caused by H_2O_2 and acts as an antioxidant.
4. To protect from carcinogenic chemicals.
5. It reduces the requirement of vitamin E.

Selenium Deficiency

Causes liver necrosis, pancreatic degeneration, cardiomyopathy, muscular dystrophy and infertility.

Excess (Toxicity)

Selenosis is due to excessive intake of selenium. It leads to weight loss, dermatitis, diarrhea and emotional disturbances.

IODINE

There is about 25–30 mg of iodine (I_2) in the body. Of this about 33% is present in the thyroid gland. Skin and skeleton contain small amounts. Nearly half of the I_2 in the body is in the muscles.

Dietary Sources

Seafood, drinking water, iodized table salt, onions and vegetables grown in soil-containing iodine.

Recommended Dietary Allowance Per Day

The RDA per day for iodine is 150 μg.

Functions

Required for the synthesis of thyroid hormones thyroxine (T4) and triiodothyronine (T3). T3 is more active than T4.

Deficiency Manifestation

Deficiency occurs in several parts of the world. In high altitude regions like Himalayan region, water plants and soil are deficient in iodine. A deficiency of iodine in children leads to cretinism and in adults, endemic goiter.

Goiter

Goiter is an enlarged thyroid with decreased thyroid hormone production. An iodine deficiency in adults stimulates the proliferation of thyroid epithelial cells, resulting in the enlargement of the thyroid gland. The thyroid gland collects iodine from the blood and uses it to make thyroid hormones. In iodine deficiency, the thyroid gland undergoes compensatory enlargement in order to extract iodine from blood more efficiently.

When mothers suffer from prolonged iodine deficiency, they give birth to babies, who are physically and mentally deformed.

Goitrogenic factors: Excessive intake of cabbage, cauliflower and radish leads to goiter. The compound responsible is 5-vinyl, 2-thio-oxazolidone, which binds to iodine.

Potassium iodide or iodate is used for the fortification of table salt to prevent goiter.

IRON

Total body iron in an adult body is 3–5 g. Iron-containing compounds in the body are:

- Hemoglobin
- Myoglobin
- Catalase and peroxidase
- Cytochrome b, c, aa3
- Ferritin and hemosiderin
- Transferrin.

Dietary Sources

Liver, meat, fish, egg yolk, green leafy vegetables, whole wheat, legumes, cashew nuts, molasses, dates. Milk is a poor source of iron.

Recommended Dietary Allowance Per Day

- Adult male: 10 mg/day
- Adult female: 18 mg/day (to compensate losses during the menstruation)
- Pregnancy and lactation: 40 mg/day (to replenish the stores)
- Children: 10–15 mg/day.

Iron is stored in the liver, spleen and bone marrow in the form of protein ferritin. Men have higher stores of ferritin than women.

Utilization of Iron

Iron needs of the body is met by:
1. Use of iron released from RBCs over and over again.
2. Absorption of iron from diet.
3. Use of stored ferritin.

Absorption of iron from food takes place mostly in the duodenum and the small intestine. Only 3%–10% of iron is absorbed by a well-nourished adult.

Iron found in the food is mainly in the ferric (Fe^{3+}) form, which is bound to proteins or organic acids. In the acid medium provided by the gastric HCl, the ferric form is released from the foods. Ascorbic acid and cysteine convert ferric iron (Fe^{3+}) to ferrous iron (Fe^{2+}). Iron in the ferrous form is soluble and readily absorbed.

Factors Influencing Iron Absorption

Factors, Which Promote Iron Absorption

Acidity, ascorbic acid and cysteine increase iron absorption.

Factors, Which Decreases Iron Absorption

Phytates, oxalate, phosphates, alkaline pH, malabsorption syndromes.

Transport in the Plasma

The iron released from the mucosal cells enter the portal blood, mostly in the ferrous state. In the plasma, Fe^{2+} is oxidized rapidly to the ferric state (Fe^{3+}) and is then incorporated into a specific iron-binding protein, transferrin. Ceruloplasmin exerts a catalytic activity (serum ferroxidase) in plasma to convert Fe^{2+} into Fe^{3+} form.

Storage of Iron

Iron is stored in the liver, spleen and bone marrow in the form of ferritin. In the mucosal cells of intestine, ferritin is the temporary storage form of iron.

Hemosiderin is another iron storage protein. Hemosiderin accumulates in the body (spleen, liver) when the supply of iron is in excess of body demands.

Excretion

Iron loss from the body is around 1 mg/day, which may occur through bile or through sloughing of GI epithelium.

Iron is not excreted in urine.

Deficiency of Iron

Anemia

Anemia is a condition where the hemoglobin level is lowered in the blood. When the hemoglobin falls below 12.5 g/100 mL of blood, it results in the diminished oxygen-carrying power of the blood. Iron deficiency anemia is otherwise known as hypochromic anemia. In this condition, the number of RBCs is not much reduced, but the quantity of hemoglobin is less.

Causes: Hemorrhage, malabsorption, hookworm infestation, inadequate dietary intake.

Manifestation: Generalized weakness, sluggish metabolic activities, loss of appetite, retarded growth.

Hemosiderosis

Occurs due to excess of iron in the body. Seen in patients with repeated blood transfusions, prolonged iron injunctions. Hemosiderin is deposited in the cells. Seen in Bantu tribal people of Africa who cook food in iron pots.

Hemochromatosis

Hemochromatosis is a rare disease where iron is directly deposited in tissues like liver, spleen, pancreas and skin. It is characterized by bronze pigmentation of the skin, cirrhosis of the liver and pancreatic fibrosis. This leads to bronze diabetes.

MANGANESE

About 20 mg of manganese is present in an adult. Bones, liver, pancreas, kidney and pituitary gland contain manganese.

Sources

Cereals, bean, dried beans, peas, green vegetables and nuts are good sources. Tea and coffee have high manganese content. But animal foods are relatively poor in it.

Manganese functions in many enzyme systems. It activates certain enzymes, which take part in the digestion and metabolism of carbohydrates, proteins and lipids. It plays an important part in the synthesis of cholesterol, fatty acids, RNA and ATP. Manganese deficiency in human beings is not known.

CHROMIUM

An adult body contains about 6 mg of chromium present in skin, hair, muscles, brain, adrenal glands and in body fats.

An important function of chromium is its role in glucose tolerance factor formation in the body. Chromium niacin factor helps the action of insulin on glucose. Chromium is also essential for activating enzymes involved in carbohydrate, protein and fat digestion and metabolism.

Sources

Organ meat like liver meat, whole grain cereals and brewer's yeast are good sources of chromium.

Requirements

For healthy adults it is 0.05–20 mg/day.

COBALT

Cobalt is necessary for the biological activity of vitamin B_{12}. It also takes part in enzymatic action and thyroid function.

Dietary Sources

Cereals beans, peas and organ meats like kidney and liver.

Recommended Dietary Allowance Per Day

Not established. Deficiency of cobalt is not common among human beings.

Deficiency Manifestation

A cobalt deficiency is accompanied by all the signs and symptoms of B_{12} deficiency. The most important is anemia.

FLUORINE

Dietary Sources

The body receives fluorine mainly from drinking water. Some sea fish and tea also contain small amounts of fluoride.

Recommended Dietary Allowance Per Day

The RDA per day for fluorine is 1.4–4 mg.

Absorption and Excretion

Inorganic fluoride is absorbed readily in the stomach and small intestine, and distributed entirely to bone and teeth. Almost 50% of the daily intake is excreted through urine.

Functions

Fluoride is required for the proper formation of bone and teeth. Fluoride become incorporated into hydroxyapatite, the crystalline mineral of bones and teeth to form fluoroapatite, which increases hardness of bone and teeth and provide protection against dental caries and attack by acids.

Deficiency Syndromes

Deficiency of fluoride leads to dental caries and osteoporosis.

Toxicity

1. Excessive amount of fluoride can result in dental fluorosis. This condition results in teeth with a patch, dull white, even chalk looking appearance. A brown mottled appearance can also occur.
2. It is known to inhibit several enzymes especially enolase of glycolysis.

MOLYBDENUM

Dietary Sources

Whole grain cereals, dried beans, peas and dark green vegetables and legumes.

Recommended Dietary Allowance Per Day

The RDA per day for molybdenum is 0.15–0.5 mg.

Functions

Molybdenum serves as a cofactor for metalloenzymes. It is incorporated into:
- Xanthine oxidase
- Aldehyde oxidase
- Sulfite oxidase.

Absorption and Excretion

Dietary molybdenum is readily absorbed by the intestine and is excreted in urine and bile.

Deficiency Manifestation

Deficiency causes xanthinuria with low plasma and urinary uric acid concentration.

SUMMARY

Principal functions and deficiency manifestations of various micronutrients and macronutrients are summarized in Table 25.2 and very important minerals below are listed:

- Ca   Helps form strong teeth and bones
- Cl_2 Helps to form stomach acids (HCl) for digestion
- Cu   Needed for healthy RBCs
- I_2 Needed for thyroid glands to control rate of energy used by cells
- Fe   Helps RBCs carry oxygen
- Mg   Needed for healthy nerve cells
- P   Helps build strong teeth and bones
- L   Help nerves to send signals and also helps keep fluids in cells
- Na   Help nerves to send signals
- Zn   Needed for tissue growth.

TABLE 25.2: Principal functions and deficiency manifestations of macrominerals and microminerals

Elements	Metabolic functions	Deficiency manifestation
Macrominerals		
Sodium	Principal extracellular cation, buffer constituent, water and acid-base balance, cell membrane permeability	Dehydration, acidosis, excess leads to edema and hypertension
Potassium	Principal intracellular cation, buffer constituent, water and acid-base balance, neuromuscular irritability	Muscle weakness, paralysis and mental confusion, acidosis
Chloride	Principal extracellular anion, electrolyte, osmotic and acid-base balance, gastric HCl formation	Deficiency secondary to vomiting and diarrhea
Calcium	Constituent of bone and teeth, blood clotting, regulation of nerve, muscle and hormone functions	Tetany, muscle cramps, convulsions, osteoporosis, rickets
Phosphorus	Constituent of bone and teeth, nucleic acids, NAD, FAD, ATP, etc.; required for energy metabolism	Growth retardation, skeletal deformities, muscle weakness, cardiac arrhythmia
Magnesium	Cofactor for phosphate transferring enzymes, constituent of bones and teeth, muscle contraction, nerve transmission	Muscle spasms, tetany, convulsions, osteoporosis, rickets
Sulfur	Constituent of proteins, bile acid, glycosaminoglycans, vitamins like thiamine, lipoic acid, involved in detoxification reactions	Unknown

Contd...

Contd...

Elements	Metabolic functions	Deficiency manifestation
Microminerals		
Chromium	Helps the action of insulin on glucose	Impaired glucose metabolism
Cobalt	Constituent of vitamin B_{12}	Macrocytic anemia
Copper	Constituent of oxidase enzymes, e.g. tyrosinase, cytochrome oxidase, ferroxidase and ceruloplasmin; iron absorption and mobilization	Microcytic hypochromic anemia, depigmentation of skin, hair; excessive deposition in liver in Wilson's disease
Fluoride	Constituent of bone and teeth, strengthens bone and teeth.	Dental caries
Iodine	Constituent of thyroid hormones (T3 and T4)	Cretinism in children and goiter in adults
Iron	Constituent of hem and non-hem compounds and transport, storage of O_2	Microcytic anemia
Manganese	Cofactor for number of enzymes, e.g. arginase, carboxylase, kinases, etc.	Not well defined
Molybdenum	Constituent of xanthine oxidase, sulfite oxidase and aldehyde oxidase	Xanthinuria
Selenium	Antioxidant, cofactor for glutathione peroxidase, protects cell against membrane lipid peroxidation	Cardiomyopathy
Zinc	Cofactor for enzymes in DNA, RNA and protein synthesis, constituent of insulin, carbonic anhydrase, carboxypeptidase, LDH, alcohol dehydrogenase, alkaline phosphatase, etc.	Growth failure, impaired wound healing, defects in taste and smell, loss of appetite

26 CHAPTER

Water Metabolism

WATER

Water is the commonest liquid with the most uncommon properties. Water content of the body changes with age. It is almost 75% in the newborn and decreases to less than 50% in older individuals. Water content is maximum in brain tissue and least in adipose tissue.

Water is distributed throughout the body, being closely associated with the distribution of electrolytes in the body. It is present in the body both inside and outside the cells. There are two water compartments in the body.
1. Intracellular water (water present inside the cell).
2. Extracellular water (water present outside the cell) is further subdivided into:
   a. Plasma.
   b. Interstitial fluid.
   c. Dense connective tissue, i.e. water content in the bones and cartilages.
   d. Transcellular fluids.

Importance (Functions) of Water

1. Water acts as a carrier of nutritive elements to tissues and removes waste materials from tissues.
2. It provides the media in which chemical reactions of the body take place.
3. The fluidity of blood is because of water.
4. It is the solvent for electrolytes and regulates the electrolytic balance of the body. It maintains the equilibrium of osmotic pressure exerted by the solutes dissolved in water.

5. It is a regulator of body temperature, because of its high specific heat, it can absorb or give off heat without any appreciable change in temperature. Also, because of its high latent heat, it provides the mechanism for the regulation of heat loss by sensible (sweating) and insensible (through the respiratory tract) perspiration.

Water Balance

Water balance is maintained by a body when water gained by the body is equal to the water lost from the body (Table 26.1).

ELECTROLYTES

Electrolytes are positively and negatively charged ions, which are in solution in all body fluids. Normal cellular functions and survival require electrolytes, which are maintained within narrow limits. The concentration of electrolytes are expressed as milliequivalent/liter (mEq/L).

Distribution of Electrolytes

Total concentration of cations and anions in each compartment [extracellular fluid (ECF) and intracellular fluid (ICF)] is equal to maintain electrical neutrality. The concentration of electrolytes in ECF and ICF is shown in Table 26.2.

Sodium is the principal cation of the ECF and comprises over 90% of the total cations, but is very low in ICF.

Potassium by contrast is the principal cation of the ICF and has a low concentration in ECF.

Similar differences exist with the anions. Chloride (Cl^-) and bicarbonate (HCO_3^-) predominate in the ECF, while phosphate is the principal anion within the cells.

TABLE 26.1: Average water balances in normal adult

Water intake (in mL/day)		Water output (in mL/day)	
Water intake as such	= 1,200	Water excreted in urine	= 1,500
Water intake in diet	= 1,200	Water excreted in stools	= 50
Water produced during metabolism	= 300	Water lost through skin and lungs	= 1,150
Total intake	= 2,700	Total output	= 2,700

TABLE 26.2: Electrolytes content of ECF and ICF

Ions	Extracellular fluid (mEq/L)	Intracellular fluid (mEq/L)
Cations		
Na^+	142	10
K^+	5	150
Ca^{++}	5	2
Mg^{++}	3	40
Total	155	202
Anions		
Cl^-	100	2
HCO_3^-	27	10
HPO_4^-	2	140
SO_4^-	1	5
Organic acids	6	5
Protein	16	40
Total	152	202

The four ions in the plasma, Na^+, K^+ Cl^- and HCO_3^- exert the greatest influence on water balance and acid-base balance.

The body water balance is closely associated with the balance of dissolved electrolytes, the most important of which are Na^+ and K^+. The osmotic pressure of ECF is determined by the concentration of Na^+ as it accounts for over 90% of the osmolality. Thus, Na^+ concentration determines the ECF volume because water flows from or into other compartment to restore osmotic homeostasis if disturbed. K^+ similarly determines intracellular osmolality to a large extent.

DISORDERS OF WATER AND ELECTROLYTE BALANCES

Dehydration

Dehydration is defined as a state in which loss of water exceeds the intake as a result, of which the body's waste contents get reduced and the body is in negative water balance. Dehydration may be of two types:
1. Due to pure water deficiency without loss of electrolytes called simple dehydration.
2. Due to combined deficiency of water and electrolyte sodium.

Overhydration or Water Intoxication

Overhydration is a state of water excess or water intoxication. A normal healthy individual can consume a large volume of water without producing any deleterious effect, as the normal individual has the capacity to excrete large volume of dilute urine, when excess of free water without electrolyte is given.

More often water intoxication results due to the retention of excess water in the body, which can occur due to:
1. Renal failure.
2. Excessive administration of fluids parenterally.
3. Hypersecretion of ADH [syndrome of inappropriate ADH (SIADH) secretion].

Symptoms of Overhydration

Nausea, vomiting, headache, muscular weakness, confusion and in severe cases, convulsions, coma and even death.

27 CHAPTER
Cookery Rules and Preservation of Nutrients

PURPOSE OF COOKING

Cooking is an art. It is linked with the dietary habits and cultural pattern of the people. Food preparation requires creativity in blending of flavor, texture as well as color. To achieve high quality of products with efficient use of time, money and material, one should have knowledge of the effect of heat in its various forms on the nutrients present in the food. All the methods of preparation are based on certain principles and the physical and chemical characteristic of various food groups.

AIMS AND OBJECTIVES OF COOKING FOOD

1. Cooking makes food attractive in appearance.
2. Cooking makes the food soft, making it easily chewable, masticated and easily digestible. Complex foods are split into simple substances during cooking. This helps the body to absorb and utilize the food more readily than raw food.
3. Cooking partly sterilizes the food. It kills the microorganism at 40°C and makes food safe for consumption. Above 40°C, the growth of bacteria decreases rapidly and in general it ceases above 45°C. Non-sporing bacteria are killed at temperature above 60°C for varying periods of time.

    For instance, to make milk safe, it is pasteurized at 62.8°C for 30 minutes. Boiling kills living cells with the exception of spores in a few second. Spore-bearing bacteria take 4–5 hours of boiling to be destroyed. To destroy them in a shorter time, higher temperatures are used.

4. Cooking brings about physical and chemical changes in food whereby color, texture and appearance are improved. This increases palatability, taste and digestibility of food.
5. Cooking enhances the availability of some nutrients, e.g. it destroys tryptophan inhibitors present in the protein foods. This makes trypsin freely available to the body. Similarly, starch is more easily available to the body after cooking.
6. Cooking also improves the storage quality of food. Boiling sterilizes the milk, which can then be stored for a longer time.
7. Cooking helps to make food more digestible. Complex foods are usually split into simpler substances during cooking. This helps the body to absorb and utilize food more readily than raw food.
8. Some vegetables like soybeans naturally contain some antinutritional factors such as hemagglutinins and trypsin inhibitors. These can be destroyed only by heating and cooling.
9. Cooking makes food more attractive in appearance and therefore more appetizing.
10. Cooking helps to prepare innumerable products from the same food materials and provide variety and avoid monotony.
11. Cooking enables mixing of different foods in order to provide good quality preparations with other nutrients.
12. Cooking helps to provide a balanced diet. The different ingredients combined together in one dish make it easier to provide a balanced meal.

METHODS OF COOKING

Heat can be transferred to food by conduction, convection, radiation or microwave energy.

Conduction

In conduction, heat flows from source to food. For efficient conduction from one hot surface to another, the area of contact has to be as large as possible. Hence, the bottom of pans should be flat and thick, e.g. steaming, poaching.

Convection

When a liquid or air is heated, the parts nearest to the heat becomes warm and less dense. Roasting is mainly by convection, e.g. baking.

Radiation

When heat radiations reach food, only the surface is heated by them. They do not penetrate the food. The rest of the food is cooked by conduction and to a less extent by convention, e.g. boiling or toasting of bread.

COOKING MEDIA

Food can be cooked in various media or no media at all. Air, water, steam and fat or their combinations are used as cooking media. Food can be cooked by a combination of media, e.g. upma and halwa involve the combination of fat and water.

Cooking in Air

Grilling, roasting and baking take place in air. Roasting and baking are essentially the same. The term roasting is used to cook meat and baking is used for breads, buns, cakes and biscuits. Food is cooked partially in dry heat and partially in moist heat.

Cooking in Water

Boiling or simmering involves cooking in water. The medium transferring heat is water.

While the correct preparation of ingredients and correct mixing are necessary, greater skill is needed in actual cooking. Some of the different methods of cooking include roasting, baking, frying, boiling, poaching, steaming, stewing, braising, broiling and grilling.

Roasting

Spit roasting: Is done only with good quality meat. The food is brought in contact with direct flame in front of a bright fire. The food is basted over with fat and is turned regularly to ensure even cooking and browning. Roast meats have an excellent flavor and are served in large hotels and special restaurants, e.g. barbecued meat.

Oven roasting: This is done in a closed oven with the aid of fat. First-class meat, poultry and vegetables are put into a fairly hot oven for 5–10 minutes and temperature is lowered to allow the joint to be cooked. Cooking in a moderate oven for a longer time produces a better cooked joint than cooking at a higher temperature for shorter period. Aluminium foil is now used in oven roasting. The joint is larded or raised with fat. This method of cooking is an improvement on oven roasting as the meat retains its moisture and flavor.

Pot roasting: This is for cooking small joint and birds when no oven is available. A thick heavy pan is essential and enough fat is melted to cover the bottom of the pan. The joint is browned when the fat is hot. The joint is then placed on a couple of skewers to prevent the joint from sticking to the pan. The pan is then covered tightly with the lid and cooked over a very low fire.

Baking

Bread, cakes, pastries, puddings, potatoes and vegetables are cooked by baking. The food is surrounded by hot air in a closed oven. The action of the dry heat is modified by steam arising when the food is being cooked.

Frying

Here the food is brought in contact with hot fat. Even though fried foods are a bit difficult to digest, if the frying is carefully carried out, the fried food is suitable for normal people. Frying provides variety, keeping quality is better and the food is really appetizing. Two types of frying are shallow fat frying and deep fat frying.

Shallow fat frying: This method is applied to precooked food unless the food takes very little time to cook (omelette, liver, etc). Only a little fat is used and the food is turned over to get both sides equally browned. Fat absorption is more in shallow frying than in deep fat frying.

Deep fat frying: A large quantity of fat is required to completely immerse the food. The large amount of fat will need extra time for heating. However, extra care is needed to prevent overheating of fat, which will spoil both the fat and food. Both sweets and savories can be cooked by this method. Food cooked by deep fat frying has a better look than that cooked by shallow frying, as food is evenly browned.

Boiling

Food is cooked by surrounding it by boiling or simmering liquid (stock or water). Only sufficient amount of liquid should be used just to cover the items to be cooked. Vegetables grown above the ground are cooked in boiled salted water and vegetables grown below the ground are cooked in cold salted water. Dry vegetables are cooked in cold water. Salt is added only after the vegetables become soft. Fish is put into hot liquid and allowed to simmer.

Poaching

Poaching is cooking slowly in a minimum amount of liquid, which is not allowed to boil, but kept below boiling point. Fish, eggs and fruits are poached. While poaching eggs, a little vinegar is added to the liquid for quick coagulation and to prevent disintegration.

Steaming

Steaming is a slow process of cooking and used for easily cooked food. The food to be cooked is surrounded by plenty of steam by placing in steam or boiling water.

Advantages: Steaming are as follows:
1. All nourishment and flavors are preserved in the food.
2. Food by this method is easily digested.
3. Food cannot be overcooked.

Stewing

Stewing is a very gentle method of cooking in a cold pan with only a small quantity of liquid. Meat and vegetables may be cooked and served together to make an appetizing dish saving fuel and labor. Even tough meat, unripe fruits and vegetables are made tender by this slow moist method. All nourishment and flavors are retained and hence food is very appetizing and healthy.

Grilling/Boiling

In boiling, food is cooked uncovered on a hot metal grill or a frying pan. The pan or grill is oiled slightly to prevent sticking.

Microwave Cooking

Microwave is electromagnetic radiation similar to that found in radio, radar or TV. Microwaves penetrate the food and are absorbed. The heating is very fast. Foods placed in the microwave oven are heated by microwaves from all the directions. This helps in easy cooking.

Pressure Cooking

Steam cooking are of three types—steam cooking, waterless cooking and pressure cooking. In steaming, food is cooked by steam from added water. In waterless cooking, the steam originates from food itself.

Pressure cooking is a device to reduce the cooking time by increasing the pressure so that the boiling point is quickly reached. The food is cooked as a result of steam condensation on food, e.g. rice, dal, puttu.

CHANGES IN COOKING

When food is subjected to heat, many changes take place. Some carbohydrates, lipids and proteins are destroyed. Some changes are beneficial. Heat treatment also improves food presentation.

Changes in carbohydrates: Starch molecules when heated with water, swell and break, which permit quicker enzymatic digestion, thereby increasing the digestibility of carbohydrates. When starch is subjected to dry heat, the starch breaks down to dextrins, e.g. roasting of bread/vermicelli.

Changes in lipids: Due to heat, fats undergo oxidative changes. Exposure of fats to high temperature gives a volatile odor and unpleasant taste. Rancidity, which gives food an unpleasant oily flavor is the result of exposure to oxygen (air) and water (moisture).

Changes in proteins: The main effect of heat on proteins is deamination. This results in destruction of microorganisms and some enzymes present in food. Cooking would destroy some toxins present in food, like the enzymes that affect the health seriously, e.g. legumes contains trypsin inhibitors, antivitamins, etc. which otherwise when consumed may inhibit hemoglobin. These are destroyed by heat.

Changes in vitamins and minerals: Some vitamins and minerals are lost by bleaching, oxidation of water-soluble nutrients and destruction by heat. Vitamin C is lost due to exposure to air. The media of cooking also destroy nutrients. Minerals are mainly destroyed by heating.

Changes in colors: Various colors of food are affected by heat, e.g. chlorophyll of greens, carotenoids of carrot, anthocyanin of beetroot, onion and red cabbage, and myoglobin of meat. Not only heat, but also acid/alkali brings about changes in colors of food. Therefore, cooking conditions should be combined in such a way that there is minimum loss of nutrients.

28
CHAPTER

Food Preservation: Principles and Methods

FOOD PRESERVATION

Food preservation is the science dealing with the process of prevention of decay or spoilage of food, thus allowing it to be stored in a fit condition for future use. The process used may be varied with the period of storage. It may be as simple as boiling milk to preserve it for 24 hours or pickling vegetables, fish or meat to last for a year.

Need for Food Preservation

There is always a shortage of food in developing countries like India due to demands of the growing population. Increasing production to meet the shortage results in wastage due to inadequate facilities available for storage and preservation. It is therefore, very important to improve and expand facilities for storage and preservation of food. Preservation increases availability of foods, thus improving the nutrition of the people. Availability of seasonal foods throughout the year also helps in stabilizing prices of food stuffs.

Causes of Food Spoilage

Food is spoiled due to the action of microorganisms such as mold, yeast and bacteria or by the action of enzymes present in foods or due to infestation with insects and worms. Enzymes are biological catalysts produced by living cells. They are proteins and hence denatured by heat. Enzymes include those present in the food as well as those from the microorganisms. Some microorganisms can exist either in the vegetative form or in the highly resistant spore form.

Bacteria are unicellular organisms. They occur in different sizes and shape and are classified as cocci, bacilli, vibrios and spirilla. Some of them need oxygen for growth (aerobic), while others will grow only when oxygen is absent (anaerobic). They are classified into three groups as per temperature requirement.

Thermophiles require temperature above 45°C. Mesophiles need temperature below 20°C–25°C. Psychrophiles need temperatures below 20°C. Foods likely to be spoiled by bacteria are vegetables, milk, milk products, eggs, meat and fish. Foods liable to be spoiled by yeast are fruit juices, syrups, molasses, honey, jams and jellies.

Principles of Food Preservation

1. Prevention or delay of microbial decomposition by:
   a. Keeping out microorganisms (asepsis).
   b. Removal of microorganisms, e.g. by filtration.
   c. Inhibiting the growth and activity of microbes by the use of lower temperature, drying, anaerobic conditions or chemicals.
2. Destroying the microorganisms by radiation or by heat.
3. Preventing or delay of self-decomposition of the food by:
   a. Destroying or inactivation of food enzymes, e.g. by blanching or boiling.
   b. Prevention or delay of purely chemical reactions, e.g. prevention of oxidation by antioxidants.
   c. Prevention of damage by insects and rodents.

Methods of Food Preservation

There are two methods used for food preservation.
1. *Bacteriostatic methods:* These methods inhibit the growth and multiplication of microorganisms in food, e.g. freezing, dehydration, pickling, salting and smoking.
2. *Bactericidal methods:* In this methods the microorganisms are killed, e.g. cooking, canning and irradiation.

Cold Storage and Freezing

Refrigeration is widely used both in homes and in commercial plants as a mean of maintaining the low temperature necessary for storage of perishable foods. Microorganisms are much less active at low temperature even though they may not be destroyed by severe cold.

Fresh milk and fish are kept just above the freezing point. A refrigerator thermometer is kept in the refrigerator at all times. Left over foods from a meal should not stay out of refrigeration longer than 2 hours. Certain fruits and vegetables also keep better when cold.

Boiling

Boiling food at 100°C kills all vegetative cells and spores of molds and yeast, but not bacterial spores. Cooking of rice, vegetables, meat, etc. is usually done in homes by boiling. Many foods are preserved at home by boiling, e.g. milk. Cooked food can be preserved from 12 to 24 hours at room temperature.

Canning

If the effectiveness of pasteurization and sterilization has to last for a long time, the material thus treated must be protected from fresh contamination by canning. Various foods, e.g. fruit juices, milk, baby foods, soups and fish are preserved by canning. The food is first sterilized at temperature above 100°C for a few seconds and then cooked and filled in presterilized containers in a sterile atmosphere. There is some loss of heat-labile vitamins during the process of canning.

Addition of Salt or Sugar

Certain chemicals are useful in preserving food, either by retarding or preventing the growth of microorganisms. These may be either added to the product or produced in it by fermentation. Dry salting is used for the preservation of tamarind, raw mango, amla, fish and meat. Pickling of mango, lemon, fish and meat is by addition of 15%–20% salt. Rasgulla and gulab jamun are preserved by sugar syrup. The principle is high osmotic pressure produced by salt or sugar.

Jams and Marmalades

Jams and marmalades are prepared by boiling the fruit pulp or shredded fruit peels with sugar (above 55% by weight) to a thick consistency, firm enough to hold the fruit tissues in position. Later on, they are packed hot into glass jars or tin cans and sealed. The same process is used for jellies except that fruit juices are used in place of fruit pulps. The high concentration of sugar (68%) binds the moisture, making it not available for microorganism, to grow and multiply. Anaerobic conditions are obtained by sealing. Application of heat, kills most of the molds and yeast. All these increase the shelf life of the products.

pH

Low pH inhibits the growth of many organisms. Vinegar used in pickling is acetic acid. Citric acid is added to many fruit squashes, jams and jellies to increase acidity and to prevent mold growth. Formation of curd from milk is an example of lactic acid produced from lactose. The lactic acid inhibits the growth of bacteria. By adding certain condiments along with salt, certain foods like mangoes, vegetables, meat and fish are preserved.

Chemical Preservation

Benzoic acid is used to preserve fruits, fruit juices, squash and jams because it is soluble in water and easily mixes up with food products. Potassium metabisulfite or sodium metabisulfite is used to preserve colorless food stuff such as fruits, juices and squash. These preservatives, on reaction with fruit acids liberate sulfur dioxide (SO_2), which is quite effective in killing the harmful microbes present in food. SO_2 is a bleaching agent and cannot be used as a preservative for colored food materials.

CHAPTER 29

Foodborne Diseases

TYPES OF FOODBORNE DISEASES

Foodborne diseases are of two types:
1. Food intoxication.
2. Infection.

Food Intoxication

Occurs when a chemical or toxin transmitted through food causes the body to malfunction. For example, vomiting, nausea, abdominal cramps, sweating and chills by eating food contaminated by *Staphylococcus aureus*. Enterotoxin of this bacteria causes severe gastrointestinal distress. The time between the consumption of the food and the appearance of symptoms can range from 1–6 hours. Recovery takes about a day or two and mortality is very low.

Pasteurization kills all staphylococci present in food/milk. Refrigeration of food immediately after cooking prevents the growth and formation of enterotoxins by *Staphylococcus*. Personnel suffering from staphylococcal infection such as colds and boils should not be allowed to handle foods.

Clostridium botulinum is a spore forming, anaerobic bacteria found in the soil. Foods such as fish, meat, beans, peas and corn are likely to be contaminated with its spores. If this contaminated food is not given sufficient heat treatment during canning, these spores survive and the *C. botulinum* will multiply in the can as it is anaerobic and produces botulism, a severe form of food poisoning. The toxin is killed by heating the food for 15 minutes.

Poisoning by Other Organisms

Molds, especially of the *Aspergillus* species cause aflatoxins in groundnuts and sometimes in cereals like wheat, rice and jower. These aflatoxins can cause death in poultry and cancer in rats, but no illness has been so far reported in human beings.

Poisonous Plants and Animals

Certain varieties of mushrooms are poisonous and could be fatal if consumed. Snakeroot poisoning could result from drinking milk from cows that have been fed on this poisonous food. Seafoods like crabs and prawns may cause food poisoning.

Foodborne Infections

Foodborne infections occur as a result of eating food that contains living organisms such as bacteria, viruses or parasites. Ingested in large amounts, these microorganisms can cause infection in the digestive tracts and other parts of the body, e.g. *Vibrio* bacteria often present in raw seafoods like oysters and prawns. Inside the body, the bacteria settle down fast and cause abrupt onset of chills, fever or prostration.

Lathyrism

Lathyrism is a disease seen in India and Spain where there is a high concentration of the pulse, kesari dal *(Lathyrus sativus)* in specific regions of the countries.

In India, lathyrism is seen in Madhya Pradesh, the border districts of Uttar Pradesh, Bihar and Orissa. In the districts of Reva and Satna in MP, 2.6% of the population is affected. Lathyrism is 10 times more common in men than in women. In women, the disease is not set in during reproductive years.

Kesari dal is cheap and is consumed by people in the low economic stratum. Among them, *Lathyrus sativus* constitute about 40% of the diet.

The toxic factor in *Lathyrus sativus* is the water-soluble β-N-oxalylamino-L-alanine (BOAA).

Clinical manifestations: The disease affects only the pyramidal tracts. The onset is sudden, usually after exertion or exposure to cold, with the contraction of calf muscles during sleep and pain in the lower back. A static paralysis of the lower limbs develops with rigidity, weakness, exaggerated knee and ankle jerks and ankle clonus.

Prevention: Lathyrism can be prevented. The contaminated dal is made safe for consumption by soaking the pulses in four times its volume of hot water for an hour. This removes not only 90% of the BOAA, but also the water-soluble vitamin B complex. The water is removed and the pulse is sundried and ground to make flour. Parboiling the dal, a process similar to that for rice, preserves its B complex vitamins.

CHAPTER 30
Food Laws and Food Standards

PREVENTION OF FOOD ADULTERATION ACT, 1954

The Prevention of Food Adulteration Act (PFA) 1954 came into effect from June 1, 1955. The purpose of the act is to ensure that food articles sold to the consumers are pure and wholesome, also to prevent deception or fraud and to ensure fair trade practices. The act was amended in 1964 and 1976 to plug the loopholes and to ensure deterrent punishment to the offenders.

As per the act, food can be considered adulterated, when any one of the following modes (or acts) are resorted to:

1. Admixture of inferior or cheaper substance.
2. Extraction of certain quality ingredients from the food.
3. Preparing or packing under insanitary conditions.
4. Sale of insect infested food.
5. Obtaining food materials from a diseased animal.
6. Incorporation of a poisonous component.
7. Entry of injurious constituents from the container used.
8. Use of coloring matter other than or in greater quantities than that approved for the food.
9. Sale of substandard products, which may or may not be injurious to health. These are all prohibited acts under the PFA Act.

Persons found guilty of selling such adulterated food, can be convicted. The severity of sentence would depend on the gravity of the offence. Tests for adulterations in daily use items is detailed in Table 30.1.

FRUIT PRODUCTS ORDER

The Government of India promulgated a Fruit Products Order (FPO) in 1946 and amended it in 1955. The order lays down the statutory minimum standards in respect of the quality of various facilities. Packing fruits and vegetables of a standard below the minimum prescribed standard is punishable under law. Periodical inspection by government inspectors are also conducted to ensure conformity of standard by processor.

MEAT PRODUCTS ORDER

Meat Products Order makes it illegal to transport meat unless it has been prepared and processed according to the provision of the order and carries the mark of inspection. It provides the means to:
1. Detect and destroy meat of diseased animals.
2. Ensure that the preparation and handling of meat products be conducted in a clean and sanitary manner.
3. Prevent the use of harmful substances in meat foods.
4. See that every cut of meat is inspected before sale to ensure its wholesomeness.

The order also lays down rules and conditions to be adopted per selecting disease-free animals, slaughterhouse practices and further treatment of the meat as to maintain the meat in a wholesome manner without disease-producing pathogens.

ENFORCEMENT

The FPO and PFA are enforced by the Department of Health. Under the law, slaughterhouses, markets, factories, warehouses and other establishments involved in food trade may be inspected to ascertain that the raw materials, as well as the processing, packaging and storage facilities are clean, and up to the minimum standard as per the law. The food inspectors from the department are authorized to sieze, destroy or relabel the adulterated, misbranded products and legal action initiated against the offenders as considered necessary. The court may impose rigorous imprisonment and/or fine.

MISBRANDING

A food is considered as misbranded, if it has a label, which gives false or misleading information about the product. Failure to specify weight, measure, names of additives (color, flavorings and preservatives), limitations in use of the product are all considered as misbranding of food, which is a punishable offence under law.

In addition, voluntary agencies such as Indian Standards Institute (ISI), Directorate of Marketing and Inspection have also laid down quality standards for food. These are voluntary.

ISI Standards

Indian Standards Institute consists of representatives of government, consumers and industry to formulate ISI standards for vegetable and fruit products, spices and condiments, processed foods and animal products. When these standards are accepted, the manufacturers are allowed to use the ISI label on each unit of their products.

Agmark Standard

Agmark standard was setup by the Directorate of Marketing and Inspection, Government of India, by the Agricultural Produce Act, 1937. The act defines quality of cereals, spices, oil seeds, oil, butter, ghee, legumes, eggs, etc. The commodities are graded into grades 1, 2, 3 and 4 or special, good, fair and ordinary. These standards also specify the types of packaging to be used for different products.

The ISI standards and the Agmark standards have benefited the manufacturer and the consumer.

TABLE 30.1: Some simple tests to detect adulteration in items of daily use

Food article	Possible adulterant	Tests
Artificial milk	Urea, starch, detergent	Add bromocresol blue (an indicator) to the suspected milk. If it gives dark blue color, it indicates the presence of urea in it. Add bromocresol purple to the milk and if it gives faint blue color, it indicates the presence of detergent. Add a few drops of iodine solution to the milk. If it turns blue, the presence of starch is confirmed.
Milk	Added water	Specific gravity of the milk can be checked by lactometer. A reasonably good quality milk has 1.030–1.034.
	Fat/cream removed	Non-sticking of milk to the dipped finger, is an indication of removal of fat.
Ghee and butter	Hydrogenated fat (vanaspati)	Dissolve 1 teaspoon of sugar in 11 mL of hydrochloric acid (HCl) and 10 cc of melted ghee/butter. Shake for 1 minute and allow it to remain for 10 minutes. If vanaspati is there, the aqueous layer becomes red.
Edible oils	Argemone oil	Add concentrated nitric acid (HNO_3) to the sample. A red to reddish brown color in the acid layer, indicates the presence of argemone oil.
	Castor oil	Dissolve some oil in petroleum ether in a test tube and cool it with ice. Presence of turbidity within 5 minute, indicate the presence of castor oil.
	Mineral oil	Take 2 mL of oil and add equal quantity of 2N alcoholic potash. Heat in boiling water bath for few minute and add 10 mL of water. If there is turbidity, it shows the presence of mineral oil.
Chilli powder	Colored sawdust, brick powder or talcum	Add the sample chilli powder on the surface of water, sawdust will float. Upon heating, the talcum or brick powder will leave large quantity of ash.

Contd...

Contd...

Food Laws and Food Standards

Food article	Possible adulterant	Tests
Turmeric powder	Harmful colors like metanil yellow	Add concentrated hydrochloric acid (HCl) to a solution of turmeric powder. A magenta red color develops upon dilution with water. The red color disappears if turmeric is pure, the red color will persist, if metanil yellow is present.
	Starch	Add few drops of iodine solution to the sample and if it turns blue, it indicates the presence of starch.
Powdered sugar (icing sugar)	Washing soda	Add few drops of HCl, if it gives foam, it indicates the presence of washing soda. The red litmus turns blue, if soda is present.
Cardamom	Oil is extracted	The extracted pods will be white whereas the genuine ones are green. They appear shrunk.
Cloves	Oil is extracted	The oil extracted cloves are dull in color and have less aroma besides being short in size.
Silver foils	Aluminium foil	The genuine silver foil burns completely leaving a glittering white spherical ball of mass.
Saffron	Scented colored hair of maize	The pieces of pure saffron do not break easily whereas maize hair breaks quite easily. Pure saffron gets dissolved easily in water whereas the adulterated material remains undissolved. Pure saffron will have one end bulging and thick, while the adulterated has uniform size.
Tea	Used tea, dried colored leaves	Spread the tea leaves mixed with water on a white paper. If adulterant is present, color of the paper will change.

Contd...

Contd...

Food article	Possible adulterant	Tests
Red gram dal	Kesari dal, which causes lathyrism, a disease causes disfunctioning of legs and hands	Kesari dal is bit orange in color and has different size compared with red dal.
Honey	Jaggery syrup	Mix one spoon of honey in boiling water. Pure honey would not dissolve in water whereas syrup will. Pure honey burns, while adulterated honey burns with a sound.
Sweets like jalebi, ice creams, sherbets, etc.	Metanil yellow (a banned local tar dye)	Extract with lukewarm water from the article, add a few drops of concentrated HCl. A magenta color shows up, if metanil yellow is present.
Asafoetida (hing)	Artificial aroma	Pure hing dissolves in water producing milky white emulsion.
	Colored resins or glue	If ignited, pure hing burns with a bright flame.

CHAPTER 31

Hospital Diets

TYPES OF HOSPITAL DIETS

Hospital diets suitable for feeding are:
1. Clear-fluid diets.
2. Full-fluid diets.
3. Soft diets.

Clear-fluid Diets

Clear fluids are prescribed for patients with marked intolerance. An acute illness may produce nausea, vomiting, anorexia, distention and diarrhea. Clear-fluid diets are meant to provide very few calories and makeup the water loss in the body. Clear-fluid diets include:
1. Tender coconut water.
2. Clear fruit juices.
3. Glucose water.
4. Albumin water.
5. Clear vegetable or meat soup.
6. Whey water.

The clear fluids are used for 1 or 2 days, till the patient is able to retain and digest a more liberal liquid diet.

Full-fluid Diet

Full-fluid diet bridges the gap between clear fluid and soft diet. These consist of inclusion of eggs, milk, cereals, porridges, conjees or gruels, vegetable, chicken or mutton soup, fruit milk shakes, etc. This diet will meet the minimum requirement of all protein calories, vitamins and minerals.

Soft Diet

Soft diet bridges the gap between acute illness and convalescence. It is used in acute infection following surgery and for patients unable to chew. The soft diet is:
1. Made of simple foods.
2. Easily digestible.
3. Contains no fiber.
4. Near to a normal diet.
5. Not highly spiced or seasoned.

It is nutritionally adequate when planned on the basis of normal diet.

PREPARATION OF SIMPLE BEVERAGES AND DIFFERENT TYPES OF FOOD

Fluid Diets

1. Beverages: Tea, coffee, barley water, fruit juice and raw tomato juice.
2. Milk preparations: Whey curd, butter milk, lactic acid milk.
3. Egg preparation: Egg flip, albumin water, soft-cooked egg, hard-cooked egg, scrambled or buttered egg and poached egg.
4. Soups: Dal soup, vegetables and bones.

Beverages

Tea

Have ready water, which has just started boiling. Do not use water, which has been boiling for sometime as it spoils the flavor. When it boils, pour a little into the teapot (1 teaspoon) to warm it. Empty out this water and put the tea into the pot (1 teaspoon of tea to each person) pour the boiling water over the tea and allow to stand for 3–5 minutes. Strain and pour. Dilute with hot water if desired, add a few drops of lime or lemon juice and sugar to taste.

Black Coffee

One heaped teaspoon of pure coffee powder and 300 mL of freshly boiled water. Heat the coffee jug thoroughly. Put the coffee in the jug. Pour boiling water and allow to stand near the fire for 10 minutes. Strain, reheat and serve as black coffee with sugar/jaggery, if desired.

Barley Water

Add 50 g of pearl barley and one pint of cold water. Blanch the barley by covering with cold water. Simmer the barley slowly, with one part of water till it is reduced to two thirds of a pint (about 1½ hours) and strain. A fresh supply should be made at least twice daily. Lime juice may be added to the water before boiling, if desired and sugar added to taste.

Fruit Juice

Fruit juice may be prepared from fresh fruit or by dilution of commercially prepared fruit squashes. Remove the juice from citrous fruit by means of a squeezer, strain, dilute with water and add sugar or glucose to taste.

Raw Tomato Juice

Select ripe, juicy tomatoes, pour boiling water over the tomatoes and let stand for 2 minutes to loosen the skin. Remove skin, mash the tomatoes and press through the strainer as much of the juice and soft part as possible. Add salt/pepper or sugar to taste.

Milk Preparations

Whey

Whey is prepared from curds. It contains fats, sugar, salts and vitamins, but no protein. Breakup the curds with a fork, then drain off whey by straining through gauze.

Egg Preparations

Albumin Water

Take the whites of two eggs, add one cup of water. Put into a wide necked bottle, cork it and shake thoroughly. Add a little lime juice and sugar. If preferred, orange juice may be substituted for lime juice.

Egg Flip or Eggnog

Beat an egg thoroughly (yolks not used in albumin water preparation may be used here) and add 250 mL of milk, stir well and strain before serving. This may be flavored with sugar, cinnamon or lime juice. If desired, it may be added to coffee, tea or cocoa.

Soft-cooked Egg

Place egg in cold water and bring it to boil. Let it boil for about half a minute, remove with spoon. Lower the egg gently with a spoon into a saucepan of boiling water deep enough to cover it. Put the lid on the pan and allow to stand for 4–5 minutes. Serve immediately after the egg is removed from hot water.

Hard-cooked Egg

Place egg in hot water and keep it at simmering temperature for 10–15 minutes according to the size of the egg and how hard it is required. If the egg is to be used cold, it should be cooled immediately after cooking by placing in cold water. The shell may then be removed easily.

Scrambled or Buttered Egg

Beat the egg well, adding salt and pepper and a tablespoon of milk. Melt just enough butter in a saucepan to cover the bottom of the pan. Put the egg and cook slowly over a very gentle heat, stirring lightly to prevent the egg from sticking to the pan. The egg should be soft and creamy, when cooked and should be served immediately.

Poached Egg

Use a small pan with water coming about two thirds up the pan. Add a level teaspoon of salt and a teaspoon of vinegar to each pint of water used. This helps to set the egg. Bring the water almost to boiling point, break the egg into cup, taking care to keep it whole and slide it gently into water. Tilt the pan and with a tablespoon gently gather the white round the york. Simmer until the white is nicely set (about 3 minutes) lift out the egg carefully, draining off the water and serve on hot buttered toast.

Soups

Dal Soup

Dal—½ cup, water—2 cups, onion—1, ghee or oil—1 teaspoon. Salt to taste.

   Grind the dal firmly, chop and fry the onion, mix all the ingredients and boil for 20–30 minutes.

Vegetable Soup

Half a cup small part butter (about 1 teaspoon) salt and pepper, cups of meat stock (meat stock water in which bones or meat had been simmered shortly for a long time).

Prepare and slice the vegetables. Place in a saucepan and melted butter for a few minutes. Add the boiling stock, salt and pepper to taste and boil gently until the vegetables are tender. Mix 45 g flour with a little cold stock, add boiling stock stirring continually, then return the flour mixture to the soup and boil until thickened. If desired, the vegetables may be rubbed through a strainer, before thickening the soup.

LIGHT DIETS

Steamed Fish

Clean the fish and cut it into pieces. Drain water carefully. Sprinkle a little pepper and salt on the fish, fold into two, lay on a buttered plate and cover with buttered paper and lid. Place the plate over a pan of boiling water and steam for 15–20 minutes or until the fish looks quite white and the flakes separate easily. Serve on a hot dish with juice poured over it. A small piece of lime or lemon may be served with the fish.

Light Cereal Preparations

Double boiled rice
Rice: 2 tablespoons.
Milk: 240 mL, water or milk (water mixed).

Wash the rice and add it to the milk. Simmer gently for 1–1½ hours, till it is reduced to a pulpy mass. Add sugar if desired, before serving. Cooking in a double boiler or milk cooker is more easily regulated than in an ordinary sauce pan.

Ragi Conjee

Ragi, after being ground, should be sifted two or three times through muslin. One tablespoon of ragi flour stored to be mixed, till smooth, with a little cold water. Then gradually add 30 mL boiling water with a pinch of salt and boil for 15 minutes. If preferred, half milk and half water may be used.

Arrowroot Conjee

Arrowroot: 1 tablespoon
Boiling water: 125 mL
Cold water: 2 tablespoons
Hot milk: 125 mL
Salt: ¼ tea spoon
Sugar to taste

Mix the arrowroot powder to a smooth paste with the cold water and add the boiling water gradually. Boil for 10 minutes, stirring constantly. Then add milk and salt, and boil for 10 minutes. Before serving add sugar, if desired.

Sago Porridge

Sago: 2 tablespoons
Milk: 150 mL
Water: 150 mL
Pinch of salt
Sugar to taste

Wash the sago, add milk and water. Bring it to the boiling point, gently stirring in between. After it starts boiling, simmer gently for 15–20 minutes. Add salt and sugar to taste. Serve hot.

If milk and sugar are added to the conjee it is called porridge.

32

CHAPTER

Budgeting for Balanced Diet

PLANS FOR FOOD BUDGET

In practice, one must make daily menus for a week and base the food purchase on them. This step is essential whether the plan is for a single person, a family or an institution. Food purchase is guided by nutrient needs and the food budget. Planning helps to make the best use of the available money to meet needs of the family.

The food choices within a group can be guided by one's food budget. The steps, which help to get the best returns for food expenditure include:
1. Buying the staple food, dals and pulses in bulk, when the prices are competitive just after the harvest.
2. Buying milk and milk products from government daily outlets.
3. Buying fruits and vegetables from main markets at competitive rates.
4. Buying seasonal vegetables and fruits.
5. Buying sugar, jaggery in bulk from wholesale dealers.
6. Buying oils from wholesale depots in bulk.
7. Make butter and ghee at home.
8. Buying spices in bulk and prepare the spices mix at home.

There are several government programs, which subsidize foods for the various socioeconomic strata. These include rationed food grains, food given to children in grade schools to ensure attendance, school level programs and supplementary feeding of expectant and nursing mothers. These programs help to meet the nutritional needs. To some extent, these reduce the food budget of the family.

SELECTION, STORAGE AND PREPARATION OF FOOD

1. Plan the daily diet for family so that it contains food from each of the five food groups. The diet should be varied to make it more appetizing.

2. Buy foods, which are in season because they will be cheaper and plenty. Buy atleast one, which can be served as raw.
3. Select fruits and vegetables, which look fresh. Buy just enough for one day.
4. Discard any damaged or decayed portion and store in a well-ventilated container or keep safe in a cool place from the sun. Keep potatoes and onions open in a dry place.
5. Clean and wash vegetables and fruits, before cutting to preserve nutrients. Do not soak cut vegetables in water.
6. Well-scrubbed vegetables and fruits do need to be peeled or scraped before cooking or eating. Vegetables such as potatoes cooked with their skins retain more nutrients.
7. Clean and cut vegetables just before cooking or serving raw in order to preserve nutrients.
8. Many kinds of leaves and tops of vegetables, e.g. beetroot, radish, cauliflower, knolkhol, turnip, drumstick and carrot are rich in protein nutrients and should be used in curries or other dishes.
9. Preserve nutrients in food during cooking by:
   a. Cooking with minimum amount of water, not throwing away excess water after cooking rice or vegetables and using any amount of water left, for making a soup or drink by adding savory or sweet seasonings.
   b. If cereals or dals are soaked before cooking, use the same water for cooking because it contains dissolved nutrients.
   c. Covering root vegetables so as to cook them in their own steam and also to reduce cooking time.
   d. Cooking leafy green vegetables quickly in a little boiled water.
   e. Not using soda to preserve the color of vegetables or to soften them, because it destroys nutrients.
   f. Avoiding over cooking or reheating vegetables or keeping them warm on the fire as these practices destroy the nutrients.

FOOD GROUPS AND GUIDELINES FOR FOOD SELECTION

Foods are classified into different groups based on their nutritive value. These groups are:
1. Cereals and millets.
2. Pulses (legumes).
3. Nuts and oil seeds.
4. Vegetables.

5. Fruits.
6. Milk and milk products.
7. Eggs.
8. Meat, fish and other animal foods.
9. Fats and oils.
10. Sugar and other carbohydrate foods.
11. Spices and condiments.

Nutritional importance of the above food groups are briefly explained.

Cereals and Millets

Cereals contain 6%–12% of proteins and vitamins like thiamine, niacin, pantothenic acid and vitamin B_6. They also contain minerals like phosphorus and iron. Cereals are poor in calcium except ragi, which is a rich source of calcium (poor man's milk). Cereals are deficient in vitamin A, D, B_{12} and C.

Cereals and millets form the staple food of majority of the population in developing countries because milk, fruits and fish are very expensive and beyond the reach of many. Puffed cereals are consumed widely as a snack.

If the cereals consumed is milled rice, it should be at least partly substituted by undermilled or parboiled rice, whole wheat or ragi.

Pulses (Legumes)

Pulses are rich in proteins (20%–24%). They are also good sources of vitamin B and minerals, but deficient in vitamin A, D, B_{12} and C. They are palatable and tasty. Puffed pulses are consumed by majority of low-income group families as snack.

Pulses contain antidigestive factor trypsin inhibitor, which gets destroyed during cooking. Germination of pulses increases their vitamin content. Combination of cereals and pulses provide enough protein of high biological value.

Nuts and Oil Seeds

Nuts and oil seeds are also rich sources of proteins (20%–40%). Some are rich in calcium, e.g. sesame seeds. Richest in protein is soybean. They are also good sources of fats, B complex vitamins, vitamin E and minerals like phosphorus and iron.

The common nuts used in tropical countries are coconuts, cashew nuts, groundnuts and walnuts. They are ideal foods for supplying high calories in a palatable form and are used in milk substitutes for infants.

Vegetables

Vegetables include green leafy vegetables, roots and tubers and other vegetables.

Green leafy vegetables are rich in β-carotene (provitamin A), riboflavin, folic acid, vitamin C and calcium. Because of their cellulose content (cellulose is not digested in man) they form the bulk of fecal matter and avoid constipation.

Roots and tubers like potatoes, sweet potato, tapioca and carrots are good sources of carbohydrates and poor sources proteins. They can act as partial substitutes for cereals. Excess consumption may cause protein-calorie malnutrition.

Other vegetables include snakegourd, cucumber, ash gourd and drumstick. Some of them are rich in vitamin C. Yellow pumpkin is a rich source of β-carotene.

Fruits

Many fruits like amla (Indian gooseberry) guava and citrous fruits are rich in vitamin C. Apple, grapes and banana are poor sources of vitamin C. Banana is rich in potassium and is the cheapest and most extensively used fruit in India. Mango and papaya are good sources of β-carotene.

Milk and Milk Products

Milk is rich in protein, carbohydrates, fat, vitamin and minerals like calcium. It is deficient only in iron, vitamin C and D. Milk proteins are first class proteins containing all the essential amino acids and therefore have high biological value. Milk is used as a complete food for infants and as supplement in the diets of children and adults.

Full Fat Milk Powder

Contains about 25%–26% fat. It is reconstituted by adding warm water (7 times its weight). It is a substitute for fresh milk.

Skimmed Milk Powder

Skimmed milk powder is prepared from fat-free milk. It contains 35% proteins, but no fat or vitamin A. It is used as a supplement to the diet for children.

Dahi, lassi, butter, ghee, khoya and chana are some of the other milk products used.

Eggs

Eggs of hen or duck contain protein of high biological value (13%). It is a rich source of vitamin A, B complex vitamins and a fair source of vitamin D, but does not contain vitamin C. Egg yolk contains saturated fatty acids, which increase cholesterol level.

Egg is used as a supplement to the diet of infants. A large number of vegetarians eat eggs and non-vegetarians usually take eggs during breakfast.

Eggs are digested completely and therefore form ideal nutritive food for acutely ill and convalescent patients and in the diseases of the colon.

Meat, Fish and Other Animal Foods

Meat is rich in protein, which contains all essential amino acids and high biological value. It does not contain vitamin A, D or C, but is a fair source of vitamin B. High-meat diet is indicated in protein malnutrition, anemias and nephrosis. Liver is rich in protein (18%–20%) vitamin A and B complex especially B_{12}.

Fish contains 18%–20% of protein of high biological value. It is fair source of vitamin B. Fat fishes are rich in vitamin A and D. Large fishes are rich in phosphorus and small fishes in calcium (as they are eaten with their bones).

Fats and Oils

Butter, ghee and vanaspati are good sources of vitamin A. Common vegetable oils do not contain vitamin A. Many fats and oils are good sources of vitamin E. They are used for taste, as sources of energy and for providing the required quantity of essential fatty acids.

Sugar and Other Carbohydrate Foods

Cane sugar, jaggery, glucose, honey and custard powder are used as a source of energy. Honey and jaggery also contain small quantities of vitamins.

Condiments and Spices

The essential oils present in them improve flavor and enhances the taste of food. They stimulate appetite. They irritate the intestine and help excretion of bowels in constipated persons.

FUNCTIONAL CLASSIFICATION OF FOODS

Functionally foods are divided into:
1. Energy-yielding foods.
2. Bodybuilding foods.
3. Protective foods.

Energy-yielding Foods

Foods rich in carbohydrates and fats and also pure fats, and carbohydrates. Cereals also provide in addition to energy, the greater part of the proteins, certain minerals and vitamins in the diets of the low-income groups in the developing countries.

Bodybuilding Foods

Foods rich in protein are called bodybuilding foods. For example:
1. Milk, eggs, meat, fish. They contain protein of high biological value.
2. Pulses, oil seeds and nuts containing proteins of medium nutritive value.

Protective Foods

Foods rich in proteins, vitamins and minerals are called protective foods. They are of two types:
1. Foods rich in proteins, vitamins and minerals, e.g. milk, egg, fish, liver.
2. Foods rich mainly in vitamins and minerals only, e.g. fruits and green leafy vegetables.

PLANNING OF A BALANCED DIET

A balanced diet is the one, which contains various groups of food stuffs such as energy yielding, bodybuilding and protective foods in the correct proportion and also make provision for extra nutrients to withstand short duration of leanness. The components of balanced diet will differ

Balanced Diet with High Cost

Balanced diet with high cost can include liberal amounts of costly foods such as milk, fish, fruits, meat, egg and moderate amounts of cereals and pulses.

Balanced Diet with Moderate Cost

Balanced diet with moderate cost includes moderate amounts of cereals, pulses, nuts and green leafy vegetables.

Balanced Diet with Low Cost

Balanced diets of low cost will include large amounts of cereals, pulses and vegetables, but small amounts of milk, eggs, fish and meat (Table 32.1).

A balanced diet has become an accepted means to safeguard the population from nutritional deficiencies. Its goals are:
1. The requirements of protein should be met, which amounts to 15%–20% of daily energy needs.

TABLE 32.1: The recommended composition of balanced diet for Indians (ICMR)

Food items	Adult (man)			Adult (woman)	
	Sedentary	Moderate	Heavy	Sedentary	Moderate
Cereals	460 g	520 g	670 g	410 g	440 g
Pulses	40 g	50 g	60 g	40 g	45 g
Leafy green vegetables	40 g	40 g	40 g	100 g	100 g
Other vegetables	60 g	70 g	80 g	40 g	40 g
Roots and tubers	50 g	60 g	80 g	50 g	50 g
Milk and milk products	150 g	200 g	250 g	100 g	150 g
Oils and fats	40 g	45 g	65 g	20 g	25 g
Fruits	60 g	60 g	60 g	60 g	60 g
Sugar and jaggery	30 g	35 g	55 g	20 g	20 g

2. Fat should be limited to 20%–30% daily energy needs.
3. Carbohydrates rich in natural fiber should constitute the remaining food energy.

For non-vegetarians, pulses should be reduced by 50% plus one egg or 30 g fish or meat. If no pulses, two eggs or 50 g fish or meat.

Refer to Table 32.1 for the ICMR recommended composition of balanced diet for Indians.

33 Assessment of Nutritional Status

The nutritional status of a community is the sum of nutritional status of individual who form that community. The aim of nutritional assessment of a community is to know the magnitude and geographic distribution of malnutrition as a public problem, to analyze the factors responsible for it and to effectively plan to control and eradicate them to maintain good nutrition. The nutritional status of a population is influenced profoundly by diet, infections and parasitic diseases. Malnutrition and under nutrition affect adversely the growth and health of children, and the health and physical efficiency of adults. The incidence of malnutrition is high among pregnant women, weaned infants and preschool children among low-income groups in developing countries.

NUTRITIONAL ASSESSMENT

The methods employed include:
1. Clinical examination.
2. Anthropometric measurement.
3. Laboratory and biochemical examination.
4. Dietary examination.
5. Study of vital statistics.
6. Assessment of ecological factors.

Clinical Examination

The goal is to assess the levels of health of individuals or by population groups in relation to the food they consume. The following drawbacks are possible in clinical examinations:
1. Malnutrition cannot be quantified on the basis of clinical signs.

2. Many deficiencies are unaccompanied by physical signs.
3. Lack of specific as well as subjective nature of most of the physical signs.

To minimize subjective and objective errors in clinical examination, standard schedules have been devised to cover all the areas of the body.

Anthropometric Measurements

Anthropometric measurements such as weight, height, median circumference, head circumference and skinfold thickness are valuable indicators of nutritional status. Anthropometric measurements recorded over a period of time would show the patterns of growth and development, when correctly interpreted.

If children do not get sufficient food, they fail to grow properly. Similarly, adults without enough food to eat loose weight and those who overeat gain weight. Measurements of adults and large groups of children at various ages have been used as an index of nutritional status. The weighing machine has also been widely used in school medical services and at child health clinics as a simple diagnostic tool for screening children who may be undernourished.

It is important to realize that there are other factors besides food intake that determine weight, notably constitutional or genetic makeup. There are tall, thin, light people and short, thick/fat heavy individuals who may each be equally healthy. Weighing machine alone cannot determine their relative nutritional status. Other physical measurements and particularly height are useful.

Height should be measured against a flat surface and the subject must stand as upright as possible without raising the heels from the ground.

Mid-upper Arm Circumference

The weight recording is a useful method, but at times it is not measured accurately by paramedical personnel. Height may give a fallacious impression in a genetically tall or short children.

The mid-arm circumference gives an assessment of muscle mass, subcutaneous tissue and hence indirectly to the nutritional status. It is relatively simpler to measure for a rapid community survey and varies very little between age 1 and 4 years. The upper arm is uniformly round and free from edema and does not vary with the height of the child. It can be measured quickly, requires no specific equipment and can be measured accurately by any trained paramedical personnel as following:

1. It is measured at the midpoint of the left upper arm.
2. Midpoint is marked by making central point of the distance between the olecranon of the ulna and the acromion of the scapula, when the arm is fixed at the elbow.
3. The left arm will be hanging loosely on the side. With a steel tape, the circumference of the arm is measured by passing it around the arm applying firmly, but without disturbing the contours of the arm.

Laboratory and Biochemical Examination

The laboratory and biochemical examination are as given below.

Laboratory Tests

Hemoglobin: The estimation of hemoglobin plays a vital role in health in nutritional surveys, as it acts as a major index for overall nutrition state.

Stool and urine: Stool examination would detect any intestinal parasites present. Urine can be examined for albumin and sugar.

Biochemical Tests

Biochemical tests are time consuming and expensive and hence they cannot be applied in large scale. Most of the biochemical tests would give information about the current nutritional status.

Dietary Examination

The value of nutrition assessment is greatly enhanced when it is supplemented by the food consumption assessment. A diet survey may be carried out by any of the following methods:
1. Weighing of raw foods.
2. Weighing of cooked foods.
3. Oral questionnaire methods.
4. Checking of stock inventory.

The data collected by any one of the above methods are analyzed for:
1. Mean intake of food in terms of cereals, pulses, vegetables, milk, meat, fish, etc.
2. Mean intake of calories, proteins, fats, vitamins, carbohydrates and minerals. The best guide for the analysis of the dietary questionnaire is the use of Indian Council of Medical Research (ICMR) publications.

Study of Vital Statistics

Vital statistics here involve mortality and morbidity data in a community, which enables one to identify high risk and extent of such risk to the community. Mortality data may not give a satisfactory picture, but morbidity (data from hospital or community health and morbidity surveys) would throw sufficient light on problems related to protein energy malnutrition, anemia, vitamin A deficiency and endemic goiter.

Assessment of Ecological Factors

In any nutritional survey, it is necessary to collect certain background information of the given community in order to make the assessment complete. The ecological factors related to malnutrition are:
1. Conditioning influence: Bacterial, viral and parasitic agents (amebiasis, ascariasis, etc).
2. Cultural influence: Food habits and practices. Cooking beliefs and taboos, child-rearing practices, feeding of pregnant or lactating mothers.
3. Socioeconomic factors: Family size, occupation, education, income, housing, expenditure on food.
4. Food production: Customs related to the methods of cultivation of food, storage and distribution.
5. Health and educational services: The number of hospitals and health personnel, preventive and curative services, mass media and communication.

Before initiating, steps for prevention and control of malnutrition, it is essential to make an ecological diagnosis of various causative factors, which coexist with other factors responsible for the malnutrition in the community.

NATIONAL AND INTERNATIONAL AGENCIES WORKING TOWARDS FOOD/NUTRITION

Food and Agriculture Organization

Food and Agriculture Organization (FAO) is one of the specialized agencies of the United Nations Organization, formed in 1945 with headquaters in Rome. The functions of FAO include:

1. To help nations raise their living standards.
2. To improve nutritional level of people of all countries.
3. To secure improvement in production and distribution of all food and agricultural products.
4. To improve the condition of rural masses.

The main activity of FAO is to promote production of food to meet the requirements of ever increasing world population. The joint WHO/FAO expert committee provides the base for many cooperative activities such as nutritional surveys, training courses, seminars and coordination of allied research programs.

Cooperative for Assistance and Relief Everywhere

Cooperative for Assistance and Relief Everywhere (CARE) was founded in North America in 1945. It is one of the world's largest independent non-profit, non-sectarian international relief and developmental organizations. CARE provides emergency aid and long-term development assistance.

CARE began its operation in India in 1950. Till the end of 1980s, the primary objective of CARE India was to provide food for children in the age group of 6–11 years. From mid 1980s CARE India focussed its food support in the Integraded Child Development Services (ICDS) program and in development programs in the areas of health and income supplementation.

CARE India has given help in the field of medicine, literacy, vocational training and agriculture. It also helps schools by providing garden tools, pumps and improved seeds to grow more food. It also provides mobile medical vans, X-ray machines, diagnostic equipments, eye glasses and frames, medical books, medicine and vitamins.

National Institute of Nutrition, Hyderabad

Setup under Indian Council of Medical Research (ICMR) is the premier research institution of the country. It has published many research publications including 'The nutritive value of Indian foods'. This handbook provides detailed information on the nutrients composition of a wide range of common Indian foods. Up-to-date information on nutritional requirement and recommended dietary allowances and guidelines for formulation of nutritionally rich diets are also provided by National Institute of Nutrition (NIN) for the benefit of health professionals and informed public.

The data on nutrient composition of foods given are based mainly on Indian research work carried out at the NIN, Hyderabad itself.

Central Food Technological Research Institute, Mysore

The Bengal famine of 1943 and the ravages of the second World War made the Government of India realize that the key to food security was in the right intervention of science and technology to conserve, preserve, process and distribute the available food resources. Central Food Technological Research Institute (CFTRI) was declared open on 21st October 1950 as the next step.

Through the decades since then, CFTRI has produced and provided scores of technology solutions that have given a powerful thrust to the development of indigenous food industries and played a notable role in the socioeconomic transformation of the nation.

Technology Milestones of CFTRI

1. Formation of infant food using buffalo milk.
2. Extraction of plant protein for the nutrition base for a new class of food supplements: energy food, Indian multipurpose food, miltone, bal-ahar and several weaning foods.
3. Improvement in the efficiency of process for handling, drying and milling of staple cereals.
4. Design and fabrication of energy efficient and cost-effective equipment for milling food grains and pulses.
5. Refinement of millets and production of diversified millet products with enhanced nutritive value.
6. Efficient methods for parboiling paddy.
7. Formulation of products for preparing traditional Indian snacks.
8. Production of spice and oil resins by indigenous technology.
9. Fermentation and drying of cocoa mass, cocoa butter and cocoa powder by indigenous technology.

Support Area Milestones

1. Establishment of the International Food Technology Training Center (IFTTC) in collaboration with FAO—the nucleus of an internationally referred center of excellence in advanced knowledge in foods.
2. Selection by the United Nations University (UNU) as an associated institution.

3. Recognition by the University of Mysore for postgraduate studies and research in food technology, food science and allied disciplines.
4. Adoption by the National Information System for Science and Technology (NISSAT) as a sectoral information center (NICFOS) for food science and technology in India.
5. Establishment of a state-of-the-art pilot plant.
6. Establishment of the International School of Milling Technology: An Indo-Swiss venture.
7. ISO 9001 certification.

34

CHAPTER

Role of a Nurse in Nutritional Programs

COMMUNITY NUTRITION PROGRAMS IN INDIA

The government of India, through various ministries have initiated large scale supplementary feeding programs and programs aimed at overcoming specific deficiency diseases as indicated in Table 34.1.

TABLE 34.1: Supplementary feeding programs

Program	Ministry
1. Vitamin A prophylaxis program	Ministry of Health and Family Welfare
2. Prophylaxis against nutritional anemia	Ministry of Health and Family Welfare
3. Iodine deficiency disorders control	Ministry of Health and Family Welfare
4. Special nutrition program	Ministry of Health and Social Welfare
5. Balwadi nutrition program	Ministry of Health and Social Welfare
6. Integrated Child Development Scheme (ICDS)	Ministry of Health and Social Welfare
7. Mid-day meal program	Ministry of Education
8. Supplementary nutrition program	Ministry of Women and Child Development

Vitamin A Prophylaxis Program

As part of the National Program for Prevention of Nutritional Blindness, the prophylaxis is to administer a single massive dose of an oily preparation of vitamin A containing 200,000 IU (110 mg of retinol palmitate) orally to all preschool children of 1–5 years of age in the community every 6 months through peripheral health workers. The scheme developed based on the technology by National Institute of Nutrition, Hyderabad and launched by the Ministry of Health and Family Welfare in 1970, is a remarkable success in preventing blindness.

Control of Iodine Deficiency Disorders

The National Goiter Control Program was launched by the Government of India in 1962, in the conventional goiter belt in the Himalayan region to supply iodized salt in place of common salt. But surveys showed that the deficiency disorder was more widespread with nearly 145 million people with iodine deficiency. As a result, a major national program—the IDD control program was initiated in 1986 with the objective to replace the entire edible common salt with iodized salt.

Integrated Child Development Program

Integrated Child Development Program (ICDP) was started in 1975, in pursuance of the National Policy on Children. The nutrition part of this program include supplementary nutrition, vitamin A prophylaxis, iron and folic acid distribution, immunization, health checkup, referral services, preshool education (3–6 years), nutrition and health educations.

Mid-day Meal Program

Mid-day meal program (MDMP) is also called the school lunch program with following principles:

1. The meal should be a supplement and not a substitute to the home diet.
2. The meal should supply at least one third of the total energy requirement and half of the protein used.
3. Cost of the meal should be reasonably low.
4. Cooking should be easy, no complicated cooking process should be involved.
5. As far as possible, locally available foods should be used to reduce its cost.
6. The menu should be frequently rotated to avoid monotony (Table 34.2).

TABLE 34.2: Model menu for a mid-day school meal

Food stuffs	Requirement (g/day/child)
Cereals and millets	75
Pulses	30
Oil and fats	8
Leafy vegetables	30
Non-leafy vegetables	30

OBJECTIVES OF NUTRITION EDUCATION

1. To develop nutrition advisory services and nutrition education programs for the public.
2. To participate and coordinate in community nutrition program with the cooperation of people working in other disciplines like social workers, village health workers and nurses, and also with the help of social welfare agencies.
3. To help in developing supplementary nutrition programs, wherever necessary.
4. To improve the nutritional levels of the community by available means.

MEANS FOR NUTRITION EDUCATION

1. The basic facts regarding the nutrition problems in a community can be gathered by nutrition survey and compiling the results of study of prevalent problems especially with reference to vulnerable groups like infants, preschoolers, pregnant and lactating mothers.
2. Studying the socioeconomic factors, religious beliefs, customs and traditions affecting dietary patterns and local prevalent problems.
3. Development of nutrition education material in local languages.
4. Supplementary feed programs in the mother and child activities.

METHODS FOR NUTRITION EDUCATION OF THE COMMUNITY

Important methods are:
1. Lectures and demonstration.
2. Workshops.

3. Films and slide shows.
4. Postures, charts and exhibitions.
5. Books, pamphlets, bulletins and newspaper.
6. Radio and television.

ROLE OF NURSES IN NUTRITIONAL ASSESSMENT AND NUTRITION EDUCATION

Nurses are concerned about the nutritional status of all their patients. What people eat affects their health from conception through old age. Chronic malnutrition affects physical and mental development. In industrialized societies, many diet-related diseases result from nutritional excess than undernourishment. For example, coronary heart disease is the result of excessive intake of saturated fats and cholesterol, cancer is linked to high fat, fiber and alcohol consumption, hypertension; a risk factor for strokes is associated with intake of excessive calories and salt; liver diseases are associated with heavy alcohol consumption and diabetes mellitus with excessive calorie intake and subsequent obesity.

Community health nurses are often the contact between community residents and healthcare system. Because of frequent and extended contact with patients in the community, nurses have excellent opportunities to provide information and counseling about the importance of nutrition in preventing illness and promoting health.

The role of the nurse has changed with the current preventive healthcare focus and emphasis upon wellness and with the expanding responsibilities, the nurses are assuring in the care of their patients in the hospitals as well as in primary healthcare centers. The nurse must follow an epidemiologic approach, while taking numerical histories and developing care plans for patients with nutritional inadequacies.

Nutritional problems are the result of multiple factors. All patients (hosts) have a genetic core and this together with the influence of past life experiences may make them more susceptible to problems. The factors influencing nutrition are biological, psychological, sociocultural and environmental factors.

The nurse within any healthcare setting should assume responsibility for provision of optimal nutrition and nutrition counseling for patients. Preventive health teaching should be initiated during first visit to patient or patient's first visit to the agency. Referral to appropriate community resources helps the patients to maintain a preventive approach to health care.

Role of Community Health Nurse in Nutrition

1. The community health nurse will have to study the food habits of people in her community, their views, etc.
2. She must impart the knowledge of the importance of good nutrition without hurting their cultural habits.
3. She must use all media of health education in nutrition education.
4. She needs to demonstrate simple recipes, which are affordable and locally available.
5. She will identify the malnutritioned children and refer them to appropriate nutrition programs.
6. She assists in nutrition rehabilitation programs.
7. She also takes part in nutrition research.

35 Nutrition in Pregnancy

Pregnancy and lactation are normal physiological processes. During pregnancy fetus draws its nourishments from the mother's diet. This increases the requirement of proteins, vitamins and minerals of the mother, as her body storages are used by the fetus.

During the first trimester of pregnancy, the food intake is generally lowered because of nausea and vomiting (morning sickness). During this period, frequent small easily digestible foods including fresh fruits, fruit juices and vegetables should be given.

ENERGY

The increase in calories trimester-wise is as follows:
Trimester I   : 10 kcal/day
Trimester II   : 90 kcal/day
Trimester III : 200 kcal/day

The increase in energy is to support the growth of the fetus, placenta and maternal tissue, and for the increase in basal metabolic rate (BMR) due to additional work of the growing fetus and the increase in maternal size.

PROTEINS

The normal protein requirement of an adult is 50 g/day. Indian Council of Medical Research (ICMR) has increased the requirement during pregnancy by 15 g/day. The additional protein is for:
1. The transfer of amino acids from the mother to fetus.
2. Rapid growth of the fetus.
3. Formation of amniotic fluid and storage reserves during delivery, labor and lactation.

4. The enlargement of the uterus, placenta and mammary glands.
5. For increase in maternal circulating blood volume and subsequent demand for increased plasma protein.

VITAMINS

Anemia due to B_{12} deficiency during pregnancy is not very common. Milk, fruits and vegetables can supply all necessary vitamins. Thus, when a good balanced diet is given, there is no need for vitamin supplements.

There is increased use for vitamin D to enhance the maternal calcium absorption and calcium metabolism in the fetus.

Vitamin K is of vital importance for the synthesis of prothrombin, which is necessary for normal coagulation of blood for preventing neonatal hemorrhage.

The water-soluble vitamins B complex and vitamin C must be supplied in adequate amounts. There is an increased requirement of folic acid for promoting fetal growth and to prevent macrocytic anemia during pregnancy. Deficiency of iron puts additional stress on folate metabolism.

MINERALS

An increased intake of calcium by mother is very essential not only for the calcification of fetal bones, but also for protection of calcium reserves of the mother to meet the large demands during lactation. Use of vitamin D and calcium supplements reduce muscular cramps during pregnancy.

IRON

During pregnancy, there is also an increased requirement of iron due to the following:
1. Iron is necessary for the growth of fetus and placenta.
2. It is necessary for the promotion of hemoglobin as there is 40%–50% increase in the maternal blood volume.
3. To replace the maternal iron losses.
4. To achieve high levels of hemoglobin in the infants, which is stored in the liver for 3–6 months. Iron must be transfused to uterus of the mother during gestation.

FATS

Fats must be provided according to the normal requirements.

NUTRITIONAL REQUIREMENTS DURING LACTATION

Milk is secreted by the mother for feeding the baby. Therefore, during lactation nutritional requirements are increased.

Calories

Mother requires total amount of about 13,000 kcal during lactation period of 6 months. Mother needs additional 700–750 kcal daily to convert food energy into milk.

Proteins

Daily milk produced is about 850–1,000 mL during lactation. Human milk contains about 1% protein and thus there is daily excretion of 8–10 g of protein. Therefore, lactating woman should take about 20–25 g of extra protein daily. In vegetarians 2–3 cups of milk and milk products will supply this need.

Non-vegetarians should take an average serving of either meat, chicken, egg or fish daily. In addition, two cups of milk should be taken. Balanced diet for pregnant women is given in Table 35.1.

TABLE 35.1: Menu plan for pregnancy

Time	Menu	Ingredient	Quantity	Energy (kcal/d)	Protein (g/d)	Fat (g/d)	CHO⁺ (mg/d)	Ca⁺ (mg/d)	Fe⁺ (mg/d)	P⁶ (mg/d)	Vit. A (µg/d)	Vit. B₁ (mg/d)	Vit. B₂ (mg/d)	Folic acid (mg/d)	Vit. C (mg/d)
7 AM	Bed coffee	Milk, sugar, coffee powder	1 cup	104	38	3.4	14.4	0.10	1.2	0.10	154	0.04	0.018	–	1.4
8.30 AM	Masala dosa	White rice, black gram	2 pcs	424	9.2	16.8	58.8	0.08	3.4	0.16	420	0.18	0.12	28.1	7.2
	Sambar	Dal, potato, tomato, beetroot, drumstick, lady's finger, pumpkin, cucumber, snake gourd, carrot, onion, chilli	1 serving	296.7	11.38	1.05	60.62	0.074	3.43	0.18	48.9	0.156	0.133	103.9	7.88
	Egg omelette	Egg, onion, pepper	1 cup	77	5.8	5.7	0.5	0.03	1	0.10	940	0.06	0.15	71.8	–
	Boiled banana	Banana	1 pc	153	1.3	0.2	36.4	0.01	0.4	0.05	80	0.05	0.08	–	7
	Tea	Milk, sugar, tea powder	1 cup	72	14	1.6	13	0.06	–	0.04	76	0.02	0.1	5.6	0.6
	Total			1,126.7	32.9	28.8	183.7	0.354	9.43	0.632	1,718.9	0.506	0.763	215	24.1
12.30 PM	Mutton pulav	Rice, mutton, onion, carrot, beans, peas	1 serving	343	10.2	19.5	31.8	0.05	1.75	0.11	50	0.10	3.10	7.5	0.56

Contd...

Contd...

Time	Menu	Ingredient	Quantity	Energy (kcal/d)	Protein (g/d)	Fat (g/d)	CHO* (mg/d)	Ca† (mg/d)	Fe‡ (mg/d)	P§ (mg/d)	Vit. A (μg/d)	Vit. B$_1$ (mg/d)	Vit. B$_2$ (mg/d)	Folic acid (mg/d)	Vit. C (mg/d)
	Vegetable salad	Tomato, cucumber, carrot, onion, curd, chilli		20.11	1.21	1.06	2.79	0.044	0.4	0.391	105.6	0.023	0.019	36.4	4.75
5 PM	Coffee	Milk, sugar, coffee powder	1 cup	104	3.8	3.4	14.4	0.10	1.2	0.10	154	0.04	0.18	5.6	1.4
	Ragi roti	Ragi flour, salt	2 pcs	460	8	9	87	0.40	6	0.30	255	0.50	0.13	5.2	–
	Total			927.1	23.12	32.9	135.9	0.594	9.35	0.901	564.6	0.663	3.43	54.7	6.7
8 PM	Chapati	Wheat flour, salt	2 pcs	193	5	5.5	30.8	0.02	3	0.13	128	0.20	0.05	12.1	–
	Amaranth curry	Amaranth, onion, salt, coconut oil	1 serving	47	1.4	2.3	5.1	0.04	6.6	0.04	1,942	0.03	0.03	54.2	51
	Fruit salad	Apple, banana, grape		101.8	0.925	0.023	24.1	0.083	0.725	0.035	43.8	0.065	0.055	–	4.4
10 PM	Milk	Milk, sugar	1 cup	130	7	7.4	9.8	0.24	0.8	0.2	280	0.06	0.34	5.6	4
	Total			471.8	14.33	15.22	69.8	0.323	11.13	0.405	293.8	0.355	0.645	71.9	9.4
	Grand total			2,525.5	70.3	76.9	389.5	0.913	29.91	1.36	4,678.2	1.52	4.84	341.6	90.18
	RDA			2,525	65	30	175	1,000	38	35	2,400	1.3	1.5	400	40

*CHO, carbohydrates; †Ca, calcium; ‡Fe, iron; §P, phosphorus.

36 Nutrition in Infancy

In early infancy most of the nutrient requirements are met by breast milk and weaning foods should start by 4–5 months.

ENERGY

The energy requirements of infants are much higher. Infants require 120 kcal/kg body weight.

PROTEINS

In infants, protein requirements are higher. In the initial months, the human milk provides the essential amino acids needed for growth.

The protein requirement of an infant is as follows:
1. 0–3 months: 2.3 g/kg body weight (a).
2. 3–6 months: 1.8 g/kg body weight (a).
3. 6–9 months: 1.8 g/kg body weight (b).
4. 9–12 months: 1.5 g/kg body weight (b).
   a. In terms of milk proteins.
   b. Partly vegetable proteins also.

If the protein and calorie requirements are not met adequately, it could lead to protein calorie malnutrition.

MINERALS

Rapid growth requires large quantities of minerals, especially calcium and phosphorus. Though mother's milk has less calcium, it is better absorbed from breast milk. The intake of cow's milk leads to hypokalemia due to its high phosphate content.

VITAMINS

Vitamins are essential for the rapid growth of infant. Breast milk provides sufficient vitamins. Cow's milk is deficient in vitamins C and D.

FAT

About 35%–45% of calories are provided by fat in the initial stages of infancy. Supplementary foods provide fat in the later stages.

CARBOHYDRATES

Lactose in human milk provides 25%–55% of calories.

FLUID

Water intake in full-term infants is 60 mL/kg body weight on day one. It increases to 150–170 mL/kg by day 3–4. As weaning starts, boiled and cooled water should be given along with fresh fruits and juices or porridges and gruels.

Table 36.1 shows the comparison of nutrient value of human and cow milk.

TABLE 36.1: Comparison of nutrient value of human and cow milk

Nutrient	Unit	Human milk	Cow milk
Water	mL	88.0	87.5
Fat	g	1.1	3.2
Protein	g	1.2	3.2
Energy	kcal	65.0	67.0
Calcium	mg	34.0	117.0
Sodium	mg/L	7.0	22.0
Zinc	mg/L	4.0	4.0
Iron	mg/L	0.5	0.5
Vitamin A	IU/L	1,898.0	1,025.0
Vitamin B	mg/L	46.0	11.0
Vitamin C	IU/L	22.0	14.0

BREASTFEEDING

Most infants start feeding by first few hours of birth. Early feeding helps to maintain normal metabolism and growth, promotes maternal-infant bonding and decreases risk of hypoglycemia, hyperkalemia, dehydration, fever and hyperbilirubinemia.

Advantages of Breastfeeding

1. Infant derives the sense of security and belongingness by the comfort of being held in the arms during the process of breastfeeding. There is an unbreakable bond created between the mother and infant.
2. It is economical to breastfeed the infant, as it is naturally available food, which is clean and hygienic.
3. Breastfeeding helps in birth control. The hormone prolactin, which stimulates milk production also decreases the synthesis of various hormones. It is a cost effective method of contraception. By breast-feeding, the uterus comes back to normal size and would stop bleeding by the secretion of oxytocin. It also helps to reduce weight in mothers.
4. Risk of breast cancer is higher in women who have not breastfed their babies.
5. There is proper development of jaws and teeth and they are not crowded as the infant must suckle hard to extract milk.
6. Reduced likelihood of child being allergic to milk as human milk proteins do not cause allergies.
7. There is less danger of the feed being contaminated, which could lead to gastrointestinal problems. Mortality rates are lower among breastfed infants.
8. Human milk contains bacterial and viral antibodies including high concentration of secretary IgA, which provide local gastrointestinal immunity.
9. It is available at correct temperature and needs no time for preparation.
10. It is convenient to feed the baby when it is in the mother's arms.
11. It protects the babies from obesity.
12. There is rapid maturation of the gastrointestinal tract due to the presence of growth factors and certain hormones.
13. The fats and proteins present are more easily digestible and there is less chance of child developing gastric and intestinal distress.

14. Milk has other anti-infective proteins due to the presence of microphages, complement, lysozyme and lactoferrin. All these provide protection against diarrhea and respiratory infections.
15. The breast milk also provides many biochemical advantages like prevention of neonatal hypoglycemia.

Conditions When Mothers are Advised not to Breastfeed

Septicemia, nephritis, active tuberculosis, typhoid fever, malaria, renal failure, grade IV cardiac failure, severe neurosis.

WEANING

Weaning is a stage in which supplementary foods are included along with the latest feed. It continues till the child is completely off the breastfeed up to 6 months. Breast milk alone is not sufficient to provide the required amounts of nutrients for expected growth rate and remain healthy. Therefore sufficient feed should be started from about 4–5 months of life.

Types of Supplementary Foods

For infants of 5–6 months—mashed banana, apple, sapota; for 7 months—boiled and mashed vegetables, soups and purees. Egg and starchy foods are introduced in the second 6 months of life. Egg yolk is given initially with hard cooking. Quality is gradually increased and egg white is introduced by 1 year. Boiled potatoes, carrot, rice, idly, bread are introduced from 7 months of age by which the baby is able to chew. Groundnut is introduced after 6 months. Homemade ragi/wheat ceri or commercially available cereal preparations are started from 4 months.

Factors to be Considerd while introducing Weaning

1. One food at a time should be introduced to check the tolerance of the child.
2. The infant should get familiarized with the food before getting a new food.
3. The food contains no fibrous material and the consistency should be very thin.
4. Make the child to eat all types of foods. Parents should not show personal prejudices and dislikes towards any food.

5. It is not necessary to cook separately for the child, as the family meals can be early modified in consistency, etc. Any new food should be initially offered once a day in small amounts (1–2 teaspoons). Food is frequently pushed out by the tongue rather than back as the baby cannot yet swallow well. This should not be mistaken as dislike to the food.

Problems of Weaning

1. Diarrhea: Acute diarrhea is the major cause of morbidity in infants during weaning. This may be due to indigestion when weaning food is introduced too early. Also there is lack of secretion in the digestive tract and this could cause diarrhea along with bottles and other unhygienic conditions.
2. Obesity: Diet containing too high fats or carbohydrates and too frequent feeds may produce overweight children.
3. Underweight: Ingestion of less quantity of feed could lead to underweight babies. Frequent illness and repeated diarrhea lead to weight loss. Symptoms are irritability, excessive crying, constipation and less sleep.
4. Allergy: Food generally found allergic to children are milk, certain fruit juices, wheat, egg, meat and fish.
5. Refusal to take new food: If the child does not like a particular food, it will refuse the same.
6. Chocking: Hard and big pieces of fruits like apple or vegetable may chock children to death. Such materials should not be given to children before 3 years.
7. Regurgitation and vomiting: Bringing out small quantity of swallowed food is called regurgitation. During the first 6 months, this is quite natural. It can be reduced by adequate burping during and after feeding. Vomiting is the complete emptying of stomach and may be due to a variety of disturbances and should be investigated.
8. Constipation: It is practically unknown in breastfed babies. It is due to insufficient feeds in artificially fed children. Increasing fluids or sugar may be a correct measure in older babies. Fruit juice, cereals and vegetables may be increased. Sometimes, the constipation may be due to any anal tissues and spastic colon.
9. Cholic: This is due to abdominal pain and associated with excessive crying in babies below 3 months. It usually occurs during afternoon or evening. Holding the baby upright or permitting the baby prone access the lap or giving mild sedative may be helpful.

ARTIFICIAL FEEDING

Though there is no substitute for mother's milk, but under certain circumstances artificial feeding is essential.
1. When pregnancy hinders with lactation.
2. When the infant is too weak to suckle due to cleft palate or hard lip.
3. When breast milk is less and eventually stops.
4. When mothers are not available for feeding especially when mother dies after childbirth.

For artificial feeding, bottles are used, which have to be sterilized to prevent infection.

Method of Sterilization of Feeding Bottle

1. Bottle should be sterilized every time before use.
2. Bottle should be rinsed with warm water to remove milk particles.
3. The bottle should be cleaned with brush.
4. No soap or detergents to be used.
5. The cap, nipple and bottle should be separated and kept in boiling water for 10 minutes.

PRETERM BABIES

Preterm babies are the babies born before the completion of the gestation period of 9 months. Most of these have low weight. Feeding these babies is difficult. The main aim of feeding preterm babies is to achieve the normal growth rate. The infant has poor sucking and swallowing reflexes.

Nutritional Management in Infants Suffering from Diarrhea

Usually parents try to withdraw food during diarrhea, which is harmful and leads to malnutrition. They should continue feeding during diarrhea and increase thereafter. Breastfeeding should continue without interruption. Other foods including undiluted cow's milk, cereals and vegetable extracts should be given to babies over 3 months. Food should be cooked, mashed/ground to make it easily digestible. Foods like banana, apple and tender coconut water are very beneficial. Frequent and small feeds every 3–4 hours 6–7 times a day are well tolerated than large ones.

Many hospital practices contribute to difficulties in breastfeeding by enforcing 4 hours feeding schedules, limiting nursing time, using only one breast at a feeding, washing with substances other than milk delaying the first feeding, providing formula supplementaries and using heavy intrapartum sedations.

Hospitals, which encourage breastfeeding are baby friendly. These include immediate postpartum mother-infant contact with sucking, rooming in demand feeding and support from experienced women. Prelacteal feeds like honey, sugar, water and milk should be strictly discouraged.

SUPPLEMENTARY FOODS FOR INFANTS AND TODDLERS

Infants

A menu plan for a 9-month-old infant is given in Table 36.2.

The first solid foods are introduced at 5–6 months of age. The foods given are cereals, cereal milk or cereal dal preparations such as suji halwa, rice milk, upma, rice dal, khichdi, pongal, bread, rice flakes/poha, etc. Fruits such as ripe banana, mango, papaya, which are soft and pulpy are also given. Well-cooked non-fibrous vegetables such as ash gourd, potato, pumpkin are fed along with rice.

Most of the problems of food acceptance begin in the toddler stage. The child will show a remarkable decrease in appetite in the 2nd year as compared to the 1st year. So, it is important to give small portion of food and let the child enjoy the food. Allow the child some freedom to decide when he is satisfied. Allow some flexibility in choices and help the child to form good food habits.

Toddlers

Children can share family meals, by the time they are 2 years old. A few alterations may be needed when the family makes spicy food. Toddler should not be given foods, which are too fatty or too sweet. Such foods may fill his limited space, without providing the nutrients needs. The child may be encouraged to eat sweets towards the end of the meal so that he may not eat these to the exclusion of other foods.

It is good to give appetizing beverages such as fruit juices and milk to the children. It is good to serve part of his milk needs in the form of soups, kheer, custard or ice cream. Fruits are ideal snacks. Crisp crackers or toasts are liked and children can eat these without help, which helps them feel independent.

Menu plan for toddlers (1–3 years) is given in Table 36.3.

Nutrition in Infancy

TABLE 36.2: Menu plan for a 9-month-old infant

Time	Menu	Ingredients	Amount (g)	Calorie (kcal/d)	Carbohydrates (g/d)	Protein (g/d)	Fat (g/d)	Calcium (g/d)	Iron (mg/d)	Vitamin A (µg/d)	Thiamine (mg/d)	Riboflavin (mg/d)	Niacin (mg/d)	Vitamin C (mg/d)
6 AM	Breast-feeding	–	–	–	–	–	–	–	–	–	–	–	–	–
8 AM	Carrot mashed	Carrot	25	12.711	2.675	0.225	0.05	0.02	0.375	472.5	0.01	0.0005	0.1	0.75
10 AM	Breast-feeding	–	–	–	–	–	–	–	–	–	–	–	–	–
12 PM	Banana mashed	Banana	25	39.55	9.1	0.325	0.05	0.0025	0.1	0.2	0.0125	0.02	0.075	1.75
3 PM	Breast-feeding	–	–	–	–	–	–	–	–	–	–	–	–	–
5 PM	Ragi porridge	Ragi, milk, jaggery	25	183.8	37.48	2.88	1.46	0.135	3.55	58.87	0.12	0.117	0.4	0
7 PM	Breast-feeding	–	–	–	–	–	–	–	–	–	–	–	–	–
9 PM	Breast-feeding	–	–	–	–	–	–	–	–	–	–	–	–	–
	Total			236.06	49.255	3.43	1.56	0.1575	4.025	531.57	0.1420	0.1425	0.575	2.5
	RDA			784	–	18	–	540	15	2,000	0.5	0.6	8	35

TABLE 36.3: Menu plan for toddler (1–3 years)

Time	Menu	Ingredients	Quantity	Calorie (kcal/d)	Protein (g/d)	Fat (g/d)	Carbo-hydrates (g/d)	Calc-ium (mg/d)	Iron (mg/d)	Vita-min A (µg/d)	Thiam-ine (mg/d)	Ribo-flavin (mg/d)	Niacin (mg/d)
7 AM	Milk	Milk, sugar	100 mL	65	3.5	3.7	4	0.12	0.4	140	0.03	0.17	0.1
10 AM	Pongal (hot)	Rice dal vegetables	1 cup	200	5.5	6	30.6	0.03	1.6	174	0.09	0.08	0.6
	Total			265	9	9.7	34.6	0.15	2	314	0.12	0.25	0.7
12 PM	Rice	Rice	½ cup	148.7	2.97	0.22	0.33	0.005	1.2	–	0.05	0.02	0.75
	Fish curry	Fish masala	½ serving	55	4.3	4.05	0.35	0.012	0.3	54	0.02	0.32	0.02
	Apple	Apple	1 pc	85.9	0.3	0.1	13.4	0.01	1.7	–	0.12	0.03	0.12
	Total			289.6	5.5	4.37	14.08	0.027	3.2	54	0.197	0.377	0.89
4 PM	Milk	Milk, sugar	50 mL	32.5	1.75	1.8	2	0.06	02	70	0.015	0.08	0.5
	Ragi roti	Ragi flour, salt	1 cup	249	4	4.9	47	0.22	3.2	137	0.27	0.07	0.70
8 PM	Masala dosa	Rice, potato peas	1 cup	212	4.6	8.4	20.4	0.04	1.7	210	0.09	0.06	3.6
	Milk	Milk, sugar	100 mL	65	3.5	3.7	4.0	0.12	0.4	140	0.03	0.17	0.1
	Total			558.5	13.85	18.8	73.4	0.54	5.7	557	0.405	0.385	4.9
	Grand total			1,112	28.4	32.87	122.0	0.617	10.9	925	0.722	1.01	6.4
	RDA			1,240	22	25	–	0.4	12	400	0.6	0.7	8

Menu for Preschool, School-age Children and Adolescents

DIET FOR A PRESCHOOL CHILD

Preschoolers have a very short span of attention and are easily distracted from eating. Their response to food is rather inconsistent. The muscle coordination is limited and eating behavior is generally messy. When opportunity is provided, the preschooler learn things faster by taking advantages of parents. Young children have extreme taste sensitivity and prefer mildly flavored foods.

Three times meal pattern along with mid-morning and mid-afternoon snacks are the best for extremely active children.

Types of Food Suitable for a Preschooler

1. Fresh fruit juices.
2. Milk and milk beverages, curd, cheese pieces.
3. Fruit pieces like slices of apple, papaya, mango, sapota.
4. Boiled/raw vegetables, carrots, cucumber, potato, cauliflower, beans.
5. Mixed cereals like ragi, cornflakes, puffed rice, idlis (Table 37.1).

DIET FOR SCHOOL CHILDREN

Calories and Proteins

The requirements of calories are increased steadily in this age group (Table 37.2). It increases further during adolescence. The increased requirements of proteins would meet demands of growth. Girls require more protein to meet the needs of approaching menarche.

Minerals

Children of 10–12 years old require more calcium than adults to meet skeletal growth. As the blood volume increases, there is an increased demand for iron.

ADOLESCENT

Adolescent (12–16 years) is an age of rapid growth and intense activity. Individual variation is marked in this age group. A number of physical, emotional and mental changes occur in this period of life. Girls mature between 11 and 13 years, whereas major changes occur in boys between 13 and 15 years.

It is normal for boys to eat a lot at this age, especially if they are fond of outdoor sports.

Dietary Consideration for Teenagers

The transition phase from childhood to adulthood is known as adolescence with speeded physical, biochemical and emotional development. It is during this period that the final growth occurs. There are many changes in the body due to hormones. Even boys and girls who had an excellent pattern of food intake are likely to succumb to strange in balanced diets during adolescence. They feel independent and seek own identity and freedom to make their own decisions. Emotional difficulties often stem from feelings of social inadequacy or pressure of school work.

Meeting Food Needs of Adolescents

Adolescence is the age of group activities. Therefore, if nutrition education is introduced as a group activity, it may help in improving eating habit.

Boys may need to consume a lot of energy-rich foods. Girls must give special attention to foods rich in protein, iron and other nutrients necessary for synthesis and regeneration of red blood cells. Girl's diet should include iron-rich foods such as dals, leafy green vegetables, dried fruits, egg, liver and red meat (if acceptable).

It is important for adolescents to gain appropriate weight for their height and body build. Any deviation from normal indicates some feeding problem, which must be identified and corrected with the help of a dietitian. Checking a 3-day food intake record, may help in identifying the specific lack or excess and thus form the basis or a plan of action.

Menu plans for preschool child, school-age children (6–12 years) and for an adolescent boy are given in Tables 37.1, 37.2 and 37.3, respectively.

Menu for Preschool, School-age Children and Adolescents

TABLE 37.1: Menu plan for preschool children

Time	Menu	Ingredient	Quantity	Calorie (kcal)	Protein (g/d)	Fats (g/d)	CHO (g/d)	Ca (mg/d)	P (mg/d)	Fe (mg/d)	Vit. A (µg/d)	Vit. B_1 (mg/d)	Vit. B_2 (mg/d)	Niacin (mg/d)	Vit. C (mg/d)
7 AM	Milk	Milk, sugar	1 cup	100	7.0	7.4	9.8	0.24	0.20	8	280	0.06	0.2	0.34	4.0
9 AM	Dosa	Rice, black gram	2 pcs	216	4.1	9.7	28.2	0.03	0.07	1.5	239	0.10	0.3	0.06	–
	Sambar	Vegetable, oil, chilli	½ serving	202.5	6.75	2.55	38.1	0.04	0.08	1.7	66	0.10	0.85	0.05	2.5
	Total			518.5	17.8	19.6	76.1	0.31	0.35	4	585	0.26	1.3	0.45	6.5
12:30 PM	Rice	Rice	½ serving	74.3	1.4	1.11	16.6	0.002	0.025	0.6	–	0.025	0.3	0.01	–
	Fish fry	Fish, oil		110	8.75	8.1	0.7	0.025	0.225	0.6	108	0.055	0.65	0.01	0.5
	Grapes juice	Grapes, sugar, water	1 cup	45	1	0.1	10	0.03	0.03	0.02	–	0.12	0.3	–	–
	Total			229.3	11.15	9.31	27.3	0.05	0.28	1.22	108	0.2	1.25	0.02	0.5
3:30 PM	Milk	Milk, sugar	1 cup	100	7.0	7.4	9.8	0.24	0.20	0.8	280	0.06	0.2	0.34	4.0
	Ragi roti	Ragi flour	1 pc	230	4	4.5	43.5	0.2	1.15	3	127.5	0.25	0.6	0.065	–
7 PM	Chapathi	Wheat flour, salt	2 pcs	193	5.0	5.5	30.8	0.02	0.13	3	128	0.20	2.0	0.05	–
	Green gram curry		½ serving	42.7	1.75	1.92	4.6	0.02	2.25	0.67	8.25	0.035	1.2	0.27	0.04
8 PM	Milk	Milk, sugar	1 cup	100	7.0	7.4	9.8	0.24	0.20	0.8	280	0.06	0.2	0.34	4
	Total			665.7	24.75	26.72	98.5	0.7	2.93	8.27	411.97	0.605	4.2	0.822	8.04
	Grand total			1,413.5	53.75	55.68	201.9	1.06	3.56	13.49	931.7	0.865	5.55	1.292	15.04
	RDA			1,690	30	25	240.4	4	40	18	400	0.9	1.0	11	40

TABLE 37.2: Menu plan for school-age children (6–12 years)

Time	Menu	Ingredient	Quantity	Calorie (kcal/d)	Protein (g/a)	Fats (g/d)	CHO* (g/d)	Ca† (mg/d)	Fe‡ (g/d)	Vit. A§ (µg/d)	Vit. B$_1$ ∥ (mg/d)	Vit. B$_2$ ¶ (mg/d)	Niacin (mg/d)	Vit. C** (mg/d)
6 AM	Coffee	Milk, sugar, coffee powder	1 cup (200 mL)	104	3.8	3.4	14.4	0.10	1.20	1.54	0.04	0.18	1.18	1.6
8 AM	Idli	Black gram, rice	2 pcs	130	4.6	0.02	27.6	0.03	0.8	8	0.10	0.05	1.2	–
	Radish sambar	Radish, tomato, potato, lady's finger, dal	1 serve (100 g)	52	1.2	1.8	67	0.02	1.1	37	0.04	0.02	0.026	1.6
	Banana	Banana	1 pc	153	1.3	0.2	36.4	0.01	0.04	80	0.05	0.08	0.3	7
	Milk	Milk, sugar	1 cup (100 mL)	65	3.5	3.7	4.9	0.12	0.64	140	0.03	0.17	0.1	2
	Total			504	25.3	9.3	150.3	0.28	3.64	419	0.26	0.5	1.806	11.9
1 PM	Rice	Rice	1 cup	118	2.4	0.2	26.8	0.004	1.0	–	0.04	0.02	0.60	–
	Curd	Milk	1 cup	51	2.9	2.9	3.3	0.1	0.3	3.9	0.05	0.06	0.1	1.2
	Papad	Wheat, salt	1 cup	288	18.8	0.3	52.4	0.08	17.2	–	–	–	–	–
	Potato curry	Potato, coconut, oil, chilli	1 cup	99	1.5	0.1	22.9	0.01	0.7	24	0.10	0.01	1.2	17.1
	Apple	Apple	1 pc	56	0.3	0.1	13.4	0.01	1.7	–	0.12	0.03	0.2	2.6
	Total			612	26	3.6	118.8	0.204	20.9	27.9	0.31	0.12	2.1	20.9

Contd...

Menu for Preschool, School-age Children and Adolescents

Contd...

Time	Menu	Ingredient	Quantity	Calorie (kcal/d)	Protein (g/d)	Fats (g/d)	CHO* (g/d)	Ca† (mg/d)	Fe‡ (g/d)	Vit. A§ (μg/d)	Vit. B₁‖ (mg/d)	Vit. B₂¶ (mg/d)	Niacin (mg/d)	Vit. C** (mg/d)
4 PM	Ragi porridge	Ragi, milk, coconut	1 cup	263	6.9	6.3	44.7	0.30	1.7	3.21	0.20	0.34	0.2	2
8 PM	Chappati	Wheat, salt	1 pc	193	5	5.5	30.8	0.02	3	128	0.20	0.05	2	–
	Egg curry	Egg, onion, chilli	1 cup	77	5.8	5.7	9.5	0.03	1.0	940	0.06	0.15	0.1	–
10 PM	Milk	Milk, sugar	1 cup (200 mL)	130	7	7.4	9.8	0.24	0.8	280	0.06	0.34	0.2	4
	Total			663	24.7	24.9	94.8	0.59	6.5	1,351.21	0.52	0.88	2.5	116
	Grand total			1,779	66	37.8	363.9	1.07	31.04	1,798.11	1.09	1.5	6.40	38.9
	RDA			1,690	40	25	350	1	26	1,600	1.0	1.2	13	40

*CHO, carbohydrate; †Ca, calcium; ‡Fe, iron; §Vit. A, vitamin A; ‖Vit. B₁, thiamine; ¶Vit. B₂, riboflavin; **Vit. C, vitamin C.

TABLE 37.3: Menu plan for adolescent boy

Time	Menu	Ingredient	Quantity	Weight serving	Calorie (kcal/d)	Protein (g/d)	Fats (g/d)	CHO* (g/d)	Ca† (mg/d)	P‡ (mg/d)	Fe§ (mg/d)	Vit. A‖ (μg/d)	Vit. B₁¶ (mg/d)	Vit. B₂** (mg/d)	Niacin (mg/d)	Vit. C†† (mg/d)
6 AM	Bed coffee	Milk, sugar	1 cup	100	52	1.9	1.7	7.2	0.05	0.05	0.10	0.77	0.02	0.90	0.90	0.7
8 AM	Idli	Rice, black gram	5 pcs	340	325	11.5	0.5	69	0.075	0.2	2	20	0.25	3	0.125	–
	Radish sambar	Radish, dal, potato, carrot, chillies, pumpkin	1½ cup	196	101	04.1	3.6	13.1	0.02	0.04	1.1	37	0.04	0.26	0.02	1.5
	Egg omelette	Egg, coconut, chilli, onion	½ cup	50	98.5	7.45	7.3	0.65	0.04	0.13	1.3	1,205	0.075	0.13	0.19	–
	Banana	Banana	1 serving	100	0.4	1.3	0.2	36.4	0.01	0.05	0.4	18	0.05	0.3	0.08	7
	Tea	Milk, sugar	1 cup	100	36	0.7	0.8	6.5	0.03	0.02	–	38	0.01	0.05	0.05	0.3
	Total			836	612.1	126.9	14.1	132.8	0.225	0.49	4.9	1,395	0.44	3.83	0.46	9.5
1 PM	Plain rice	Rice	2 serving	504	595	11.9	0.9	134.8	0.02	0.20	4.8	–	0.20	3.0	0.09	–
	Amaranth curry	Amaranth leaves, coconut, chillies, onion	½ plate	28	47	1.4	2.3	5.1	0.04	0.04	6.6	1,942	0.03	0.4	0.03	51

Contd...

Menu for Preschool, School-age Children and Adolescents

Contd...

Time	Menu	Ingredient	Quantity	Weight serving	Calorie (kcal/d)	Protein (g/d)	Fats (g/d)	CHO* (g/d)	Ca† (mg/d)	P‡ (mg/d)	Fe§ (mg/d)	Vit. A‖ (μg/d)	Vit. B₁¶ (mg/d)	Vit. B₂** (mg/d)	Niacin (mg/d)	Vit. C†† (mg/d)
	Fish fry	Fish, oil	1 serving	100	220	17.5	16.2	1.4	0.05	0.45	1.2	216	0.11	1.3	0.02	1.0
	Curd	Curd, salt, chilli	1 serving	50	51	2.9	2.9	3.3	0.12	0.19	0.3	39	0.05	0.1	0.06	1
	Total			682	913	33.7	22.3	144.6	0.23	0.88	12.9	1,197	0.39	4.8	0.2	53
4 PM	Tea	Milk, sugar	1 cup	100	36	0.7	0.8	6.5	0.03	0.02	–	38	0.01	0.05	0.05	0.3
	Ragi roti	Ragi, coconut	2 pcs	185	460	8	9	87	0.40	0.30	6.0	255	0.50	1.2	0.13	–
8.30 PM	Chapathi	Wheat flour, salt	3 pcs	85.5	289.5	7.5	8.25	46.2	0.03	0.19	4.5	192	0.3	3	0.75	–
	Bengal gram	Bengal gram, dal flour	1½ cup	151	284	9	16.4	25.2	0.07	0.13	3.8	366	0.14	2.4	0.10	2
10.30 PM	Milk	Milk, sugar	1 cup	100	65	3.5	3.7	4.9	0.12	0.10	0.4	140	0.03	0.1	0.17	20
	Total			621.5	1,134.5	28.7	29.1	169	0.65	0.74	14.3	861	0.98	6.7	0.5	22.3
	Grand total			2,139.5	2,660.4	89.35	65.5	447.71	1.105	2.57	32.1	3,443	1.81	15.3	1.185	84.8
	RDA				2,640	78	22	–	0.50	2.5	30	2,400	1.8	17	1.6	40

*CHO, carbohydrate; †Ca, calcium; ‡P, phosphorus; §Fe, iron; ‖Vit. A, vitamin A; ¶Vit. B₁, thiamine; **Vit. B₂, riboflavin; ††Vit. C, vitamin C.

38   Geriatric Nutrition

The process of aging brings about marked physiological changes in the body and these changes influence the nutritional requirements. Geriatric nutrition deals with the nutritional requirements of old people.

PHYSIOLOGICAL CHANGES IN AGING

1. Reduced BMR: Basal metabolic rate (BMR) is reduced in all tissues. BMR is highest in infants and then it goes on decreasing as age advances. Because of reduction of BMR in all organs, functions of all the organs are lowered to a certain extent.
2. Nervous system: There is decrease in memory, ability and rate of learning, reaction time and dimness of vision. Due to arteriosclerosis and lack of vitamins the mental faculty is depressed. This leads to lack of interest in living. Changes in behavior take place due to lack of work, isolation and loneliness.
3. Gastrointestinal tract (GIT): There is reduction in secretion of most of the digestive juices. Gastric acidity is also reduced. This leads to indigestion and affects absorptions. In addition, there are certain changes in the intestinal mucosa, which cause reduced absorption of nutrients. The motility of GIT is also reduced and there is tendency to develop constipation. Appetite is reduced due to lack of physical activity. Digestion is also affected because of improper mastication due to lack of teeth/artificial dentures.
4. Cardiovascular system: As the age advances cholesterol is deposited in the inner walls of arteries. This leads to atherosclerosis. Atherosclerosis occurring in the arteries supplying important organs (such as coronary arteries supplying the heart) causes decreased blood flow

to these organs thereby decreasing their efficiency. Atherosclerosis in the vessels also increases the tendency of clot formation (thrombosis) in the vessels leading to almost complete blockage of blood flow, e.g. cerebral thrombosis, coronary thrombosis, etc.
5. Renal system: Overall functioning of the kidney is reduced.
6. Skin: As age advances, elasticity of the skin is reduced. Wrinkles appear.
7. Endocrine system: Activities of the endocrine glands such as thyroid, adrenal cortex and islets of Langerhans (pancreas) are diminished. Hormones of these glands are responsible for different metabolic activities in the cells. So, overall cellular metabolism is influenced to a considerable extent.

NUTRITIONAL REQUIREMENTS

Diet of old people becomes imbalanced due to:
1. Often they live alone. They are reluctant to cook and also reluctant to go to a restaurant. The result is that they miss their meals.
2. In many, food intake is limited due to restriction in diet because of various diseases such as diabetes, hypertension and renal diseases. Therefore, certain foods are to be avoided.
3. There is constipation and worry about the failing health, which also reduces the appetite.
4. The teeth are lost due to decay. Many people use artificial teeth. Digestion is affected as there is improper mastication by artificial teeth.

Nutritional Requirements for Various Food Components

Calories

Because of reduction in BMR and restrictions in physical activity caloric requirement is reduced. Caloric intake is so adjusted that body weight remains constant preventing any tendency for obesity. But if there is loss of weight or emaciation, sufficient calories should be supplied to regain the normal weight.

Protein

Due to decreased appetite and poor digestion, the food intake is generally inadequate to meet the protein requirements of old people. Deficiency of proteins leads to anemia, edema and lowered resistance. The daily intake of protein should be increased. It should be about 70 g/kg body weight. For non-vegetarians, meat, fish and eggs can be given, but there may be problem of chewing or mastication. So, minced meat, half-boiled egg, milk and milk products should be given.

For vegetarians, pulses are rich sources of proteins. If the diet is not able to provide sufficient proteins it should be given in the form of food supplements such as skimmed milk powder.

Fats

Older people tend to have high cholesterol levels. Fats are also difficult to digest. So, in old age, daily intake above 40–50 g of fat is avoided. Half of this quantity should be in the form of vegetable oils rich in essential fatty acids to reduce serum cholesterol level.

Carbohydrates

Old people tend to take cheaper readily available food, which does not require cooking, e.g. bread, biscuits, cakes, etc. Diet containing larger quantities of these substances produces protein deficiency. It also causes constipation, loss of appetite resulting in further malnutrition.

Minerals

Osteomalacia and osteoporosis are common in old age. Though exact reason is not known, osteoporosis is partly due to diminished intake and absorption of calcium. Osteomalacia is due to diminished vitamin D because of limited exposure to sunlight. The daily calcium intake should be increased to 0.8–1.0 g and iron intake 30–40 mg. For calcium supply the person should take at least ½ liter milk and two eggs. Exposure to sunlight is essential for supply of vitamin D.

Vitamins

In old age, vitamin C deficiency is common in those who do not eat fruits and food is unbalanced. It is desirable that old people take one multivitamin tablet daily.

Fluids

Water intake should be liberal (more than 1.5 liters) to ensure that the volume of water excreted is not less than 1.5 liters per day. This will keep up the elimination of waste metabolic products such as urea, uric acid and creatine. Old people are reluctant to take liquid as they have to urinate frequently, especially old people with diabetes and enlarged prostate. They should be advised to take sufficient liquid during day and refrain from drinking at night so that sleep is not disturbed.

Roughage

Old people have a tendency to constipate. They should therefore take sufficient amount of fiber in the form of fruits and vegetables in the diet.

Meal Pattern

As far as possible, old people should take small frequent meals. They should take dinner early evening to prevent gaseous distribution and disturbance of sleep. Physical exertion after meals should be avoided especially in the people who have a poor coronary circulation.

Daily allowance of nutrients and balanced diet for adults and old people are given in Tables 38.1 and 38.2.

TABLE 38.1: Menu plan for adults

Time	Menu	Ingredients	Quantity	Calorie (kcal)	Protein (g/d)	Fats (g/d)	CHO* (g/d)	Ca† (mg/d)	P‡ (mg/d)	Iron (mg/d)	Vit. A (µg/d)	Vit. B_1 (mg/d)	Vit. B_2 (mg/d)	Vit. B_3 (mg/d)	Vit. C (mg/d)
6 AM	Coffee	Milk, sugar, coffee powder	1 cup	52	1.9	1.7	7.8	0.05	0.05	0.10	77	0.02	0.09	0.09	0.7
8 AM	Idli	Black gram, raw rice	4 pcs	260	9.2	0.4	44.2	0.06	0.16	1.6	16	0.2	2.4	0.10	–
	Radish sambar	Radish, onion, masala powder	1½ serving	101	4.1	3.6	13.1	0.04	0.07	2.2	73	0.07	0.6	0.03	3.0
	Tea	Milk, sugar, tea powder	1 cup	72	1.4	1.6	13	0.06	0.04	–	76	0.02	0.10	0.10	0.6
	Apple		1 pc	56	0.3	0.1	13.4	0.01	0.02	1.7	–	0.12	0.03	0.2	2
	Total			483	15	5.7	84.6	0.17	0.29	4.06	242	0.43	0.73	2.43	5.6
1 PM	Rice		2 serving	595	11.9	0.9	134.8	0.20	0.20	4.8	–	0.20	0.09	3.0	–
	Fish curry	Sardine fish, oil	100 g	101	21	1.9	–	0.09	0.06	2.5	–	–	–	2.6	–
	Dal rasam	Dal rasam mix, onion, garlic	1½ cup	29	1.6	0.9	3.8	0.03	0.03	0.9	72	0.03	0.2	0.2	1.5

Contd...

Contd...

Time	Menu	Ingredients	Quantity	Calorie (kcal)	Protein (g/d)	Fats (g/d)	CHO* (g/d)	Ca† (mg/d)	P‡ (mg/d)	Iron (mg/d)	Vit. A (μg/d)	Vit. B_1 (mg/d)	Vit. B_2 (mg/d)	Vit. B_3 (mg/d)	Vit. C (mg/d)
	Curd	Milk	1 cup	36	1.8	2.8	2.0	0.07	0.07	0.2	102	0.03	0.11	0.10	0.9
	Banana		1	153	1.3	0.2	36.4	0.01	0.05	0.4	80	0.05	0.08	0.3	7
	Total			914	37.6	6.7	177	0.22	0.71	8.8	254	0.31	0.48	6.2	9.4
4 PM	Coffee	Coffee powder, milk, sugar	1 cup	52	1.9	1.7	7.8	0.05	0.05	0.10	77	0.02	0.09	0.09	0.7
	Ragi roti	Ragi powder, salt	2 pcs	460	8	9	87	0.40	0.30	6	2.55	0.50	0.13	1.3	–
9 PM	Mutton pulav	Rice, salt, oil, mutton, spices	2 serving	402	12	22.8	37.4	0.06	0.12	2.06	58	0.12	0.12	3.6	0.64
	Vegetable salad	Cucumber, carrot, salt, onion	100 g	52.33	1.1	0.1	9.33	0.13	0.046	1.06	5	0.05	0.036	0.33	9.33
	Total			966.3	23	33.6	141.5	0.64	0.516	9.22	142.5	0.69	0.376	5.22	10.67
	Grand total			2,363.3	47.6	38.1	510.1	1.03	1.51	22.08	638.5	1.43	1.586	14.13	31.67
	RDA value			2,875	60	20	–	0.08	0.08	28	600	1.4	1.6	18	40

*CHO, carbohydrate; †Ca, calcium; ‡P, phosphorus.

TABLE 38.2: Menu plan for old age (above 65 years)

Time	Menu	Ingredients	Quantity	Weight	Calorie (kcal)	Protein (g/d)	Fats (g/d)	Carbohydrate (g/d)	Calcium (g/d)	Phosphorus (g/d)	Iron (mg/d)	Vitamin A (µg/d)	Thiamine (mg/d)	Nicotin (mg/d)	Riboflavin (mg/d)	Vitamin C (mg/d)
7 AM	Milk	Milk	1 cup	100	65	3.5	3.7	4.9	0.12	0.10	0.4	140	0.03	0.1	0.17	2
Breakfast 9 AM	Idli	Black gram, raw rice	3 pcs	204	195	6.9	0.3	41.4	0.45	0.12	1.2	12	0.15	1.8	0.045	–
	Green gram sundal	Green gram	1 plate	142	259	13.1	9.2	30.9	0.08	0.20	4.8	120	0.24	1.2	0.10	1.1
	Coffee	Milk, coffee powder, sugar	1 cup	200	104	3.8	3.4	14.4	0.10	0.10	1.20	154	0.04	0.18	0.18	1.4
11 AM	Ragi roti	Ragi powder, salt	1 pc	925	230	4	4.5	43.5	0.2	0.15	3	127.5	0.25	0.6	0.065	–
	Total			738.5	853	31.3	21.1	135	545	0.67	10.6	550.4	0.71	3.88	0.59	4.5
Lunch 12.30 PM	Rice	Rice	1 serving	252	297.5	5.95	.45	67.4	0.01	0.10	2.4	–	0.1	1.5	0.045	–
	Dal raita	Dal, salt, curd	¾ cup	98	14.5	0.75	.45	1.9	0.015	0.015	0.45	36	0.015	0.1	0.1	0.15

Contd...

Contd...

Time	Menu	Ingredients	Quantity	Weight	Calorie (kcal)	Protein (g/d)	Fats (g/d)	Carbohydrate (g/d)	Calcium (g/d)	Phosphorus (g/d)	Iron (mg/d)	Vitamin A (µg/d)	Thiamine (mg/d)	Nicotin (mg/d)	Riboflavin (mg/d)	Vitamin C (mg/d)
	Brinjal curry	Brinjal, onion, chilli	½ plate	45	122	1.4	10.7	4.9	0.02	0.05	0.9	9	0.03	0.5	0.06	10.1
	Meat curry	Meat, chilli powder, salt, onion	1 serving	128	220	11.6	18	2.7	0.10	0.10	2.1	277	0.10	0.9	0.20	2.4
4.30 PM	Tea	Milk, tea powder, sugar	1 cup	200	72	1.4	1.6	13	0.06	–	–	76	0.02	0.10	0.10	0.6
	Wheat upma	Wheat, onion, ginger, green chilli, salt	½ serving	64	81.5	1.9	2.7	12.35	0.005	0.02	0.35	70.5	0.025	0.2	0.005	0.6
	Total			787	807.5	23	33.9	102.5	0.21	0.235	6.2	468.5	0.29	3.3	0.51	14.45

Contd...

Contd...

Time	Menu	Ingredients	Quantity	Weight	Calorie (kcal)	Protein (g/d)	Fats (g/d)	Carbohydrate (g/d)	Calcium (g/d)	Phosphorus (g/d)	Iron (mg/d)	Vitamin A (µg/d)	Thiamine (mg/d)	Nicotin (mg/d)	Riboflavin (mg/d)	Vitamin C (mg/d)
8 PM	Ragi ball	Ragi powder, salt	½ pc	169	223	3	3.8	43.4	0.20	0.15	3	115	0.25	0.6	0.65	–
	Amaranth sambar	Amaranth, potato, onion, tomato	¼ cup	23.33	16.167	1.275	0.675	2.167	0.083	0.013	1.33	334.8	0.116	0.1166	0.005	8.83
	Banana	Banana	1 pc	93.2	142.59	12116	0.1864	33.925	0.0093	0.0466	0.3728	74.56	0466	0.2796	0.0746	6.524
10 PM	Milk	Milk	1 cup	100	65	3.5	3.7	4.9	0.12	0.10	0.4	140	0.03	0.1	0.17	2
	Total			384.56	446.786	8.9876	8.3614	84.392	0.4123	0.3096	5.102	664.36	0.3382	1.0962	0.3146	17.354
	Grand total			1,910	2,107.2	56.887	63.4	321.742	1.167	1.21	21.902	1,683.6	1.33	8.2762	1.415	36.304
	RDA value				2,100	55	50.70	7,500	0.5	0.6	20	750	1.2	16	1.3	50

39 CHAPTER

Naturopathic Medicine

CONCEPTS AND PRINCIPLES

Basic Concepts

In fact, 'nature cure' is a way of life of which we find a number of references in the Vedas and other ancient texts. The morbid matter theory, concept of vital force and other concepts upon which nature cure is based, are already available in old texts, which indicate that these methods were widely practiced in ancient India.

The whole practice of nature cure is based on the following three principles:
1. Accumulation of morbid matter.
2. Abnormal composition of blood and lymph.
3. Lowered vitality.

Nature cure believes that all the diseases arise due to accumulation of morbid matter in the body and if scope is given for its removal it provides cure or relief. It also believes that the human body possesses inherent self-constructing and self-healing powers. The fundamental difference in nature cure with other systems is that its theory and practice are based on holistic view point whereas the latter's approach is specific. Nature cure does not believe in the specific cause of disease and its specific treatment, but takes into account the totality of factors responsible for diseases such as one's unnatural habits in living, thinking, working, sleeping, relaxation, sexual indulgence, etc. It also considers the environmental factors involved, which on the whole disturb the normal functioning of the body and lead it to a morbid, weak and toxic state.

For treatment, it primarily stresses on correcting all the factors involved and allowing the body to recover itself.

Nature cure physician helps in nature's effort to overcome disease by applying correct natural modalities and controlling the natural forces to work within safe limits. The five main modalities of treatment are air, water, heat, mud and space.

Principles

1. All diseases, their cause and their treatment are one.
2. The basic cause of disease is not bacteria. Bacteria develops after the accumulation of morbid matter when a favorable atmosphere for their growth develops in body. Basic cause is morbid matter and not the bacteria.
3. Acute diseases are our friends and not enemies. Chronic diseases are the outcome of wrong treatment and suppression of the acute diseases.
4. Nature is the greatest healer. Body has the capacity to prevent itself from diseases and regain health if unhealthy.
5. In naturopathy, patient is treated and not the disease.
6. In naturopathy, diagnosis is easily possible. Ostentation is not required. Long waiting for diagnosis is not required for treatment.
7. Patients suffering from chronic ailments are also treated successfully in comparatively less time in naturopathy.
8. After emerging, suppressed diseases can be cured by naturopathy.
9. Nature cure treats all four aspects, i.e. physical, mental, social (moral) and spiritual at the same time.
10. Nature cure treats body as a whole instead of giving treatment to each organ separately.
11. Naturopathy does not use medicines. According to naturopathy 'food is medicine'.
12. According to Gandhiji, "Rama nama is the best natural treatment", means doing prayer according to one's spiritual faith is an important part of treatment.

In short, nature cure includes all the available non-invasive treatments and diagnostic modalities, which do not interfere with the body's natural functional capacity and healing process and are in affirmity with nature's constructive principles.

DEVELOPMENT AND ITS STATUS

Naturopathy is a system of healing science, stimulating the body's inherent power to regain health with the help of five great elements of nature—earth, water, air, fire and sky. Naturopathy is a call to 'return to nature' and to resort to simple way of living in harmony with the self, society and environment.

Naturopathy provides not only a simple practical approach to the management of diseases, but a firm theoretical basis, which is applicable to all the holistic medical care and by giving attention to the foundations of health. It also offers a more economical framework for the medicine of future generation.

Though the basic nature cure deals only with 'pancha mahabhootas', the recent developments advocate the practice of drugless therapies like massage, electrotherapy, physiotherapy, acupuncture and acupressure, magnetotherapy, etc. Diet plays a major role, above all.

History

Nature cure movement started in Germany and other Western countries with 'water cure' (hydrotherapy). Water cure was synonymous with nature cure in those early days. The credit of making water cure world famous goes to Vincent Priessnitz (1799–1851) who was a farmer. Dr Henry Lindlahr and others go to the extent of crediting him as 'Father of naturopathy'. The word 'naturopathy' has been coined by Dr John Scheel in the year 1895 and was propagated and popularized in the Western world by Dr Benedict Lust. A number of doctors of modern medicine and others became nature cure enthusiasts and gradually added a number of modalities within the fold of naturopathy and scientifically developed them. Nature cure movement gained momentum in India as Mahatma Gandhi, Father of the Nation became much interested in this system and included it in his programs. He has also established a Nature Cure Hospital in Uruli Kanchan, Pune district, Maharashtra, which is still functioning.

Background

Naturopathy adopts the following diagnostic methods:
- Full life case history covering all the facts of life, since birth
- Facial diagnosis—the science of facial expressions by studying the various characteristic features upon the body
- Iris diagnosis—study of iris indicating the condition of various visceral organs
- Modern clinical diagnosis to some extent.

METHODS OF NATURE CURE

The methods applied for cure in naturopathy are the following:
1. Water therapy: Water is the most ancient of all the remedial agents. It is employed in different forms in treatment and produces several types of physiological effects depending upon the temperature and duration. Hydrotherapy is employed in almost all types of disease conditions.
2. Air therapy: Fresh air is essential for good health. Air therapy is employed in different pressures and temperatures in variety of disease conditions.
3. Fire therapy: Existence of all the creatures and forms depends upon 'agni' (fire). In nature cure treatment, different temperatures are employed through different heating techniques to produce different specific effects.
4. Space therapy: Congestion causes disease. Fasting is the best therapy to relieve congestion of body and mind.
5. Mud therapy: Mud absorbs, dissolves and eliminates the toxins and rejuvenates the body. It is employed in treatment of various diseases like constipation, skin diseases, etc.
6. Food therapy: Most of the disease are amenable to food therapy. "As you eat so will you be physically as well as mentally fit." "Your food is your medicine." These are the main slogans of nature cure.
7. Massage therapy: Massage is generally employed for tonic, stimulant and sedative effects. It is an effective substitute for exercise.
8. Acupressure: There are different points on hands, feet and body, which are associated with different organs. By applying pressure on these selected points, related organs can be influenced for getting rid of their ailments.
9. Magnetotherapy: Magnets influence health. South and north poles of different powers and shapes are employed in treatment. By applying directly on different parts of the body or through charged up water or oil.
10. Chromotherapy: Sun rays have seven colors—violet, indigo, blue, green, yellow, orange and red. These colors are employed through irradiation of body or by administering charged water, oil and pills for treatment.

Natural Food Remedies

TABLE 39.1: Healthy food items in nature cure

Food items	Contents
Apple	Iron, vitamin C, good for nerves and brain
Amla	Contains maximum vitamin C (gooseberry) good for hair, bile, phlegm
Banana	Constipation and diarrhea
Bitter gourd	Diabetics, vitamin C, iron, copper, etc.
Carrots	Eye sight, teeth and bone weakness, vitamin A
Curd	Good for digestion, teeth and skin
Fig	Laxative, liver, asthma
Garlic	Blood pressure, arthritis, asthma, cough, cold and rheumatic pains, gout
Ginger	Gas trouble, indigestion, ginger tea for cold and cough
Grape and raisin	Rich in iron, copper, manganese and potassium
Honey	General debility, lungs, cough
Ispaghula (psyllium)	Piles, diarrhea and constipation
Lemon	Heart and skin diseases, vitamin C
Lettuce	Nervousness and palpitation
Neem leaves	Fresh and powder—good for skin, blood
Onion	Blood cholesterol
Papaya	Dsypeptic, laxative, digestive, vitamin C, A and iron
Pomegranate	Hemorrhage, diarrhea
Radish	Kidney stone, jaundice and scanty menses
Red tomatoes	Anemia, blood purifier, vitamin A, B, C
Soyabean	Diabetes, asthma, cough
Spinach	Constipation, vitamin A, E, iron and potassium
Triphala	Removes constipation, wind, increases appetite, memory
Tulasi tea	Fever, cold and cough

All sicknesses are caused by wrong eating, wrong drinking, wrong thinking and wrong living. Table 39.1 shows the natural food items and its contents used as part of natural food therapy.

Water Therapy

Every cell in our body depends upon water to function properly. Yet most of us do not understand the role of this vital nutrient.

It is a simple and good cure for new and old illnesses.

Benefits

Blood pressure, constipation, diabetes, headache, anemia, arthritis, asthma, bronchitis, hyperacidity, gastritis, dysentery, irregular menstruation, cough and/or pulmonary tuberculosis.

Dosage

Early morning before washing the face and brushing the teeth drink 1–3 large glasses of water (1½ liters). If this is not possible, start with one glass and go on increasing gradually.

Instructions

For 45 minutes nothing to be taken such as tea, coffee, milk. Avoid taking water for 1½–2 hours after breakfast, lunch and dinner. All persons, healthy or sick, should do the water therapy. Healthy persons will not fall sick and sick persons will restore good health.

Secret

Therapy by drinking water seems unbelievable and unconceivable, but proved reliable and commendable. Drinking sufficient quantity of water at a time, renders the colon for more effective function of mucosal folds, which inturn produces new/fresh blood. Water is an essential nutrient. Even shortage of water to a smaller extent can disrupt body's chemistry because adequate water dissolves and eliminates waste products, uric acid and urea through the body cells.

The process is curative and promotes better health. The treatment is simple, inexpensive, and a boon to the poor and the rich alike.

40 CHAPTER

Diet Therapy

PRINCIPLES OF DIET THERAPY

Diet therapy is concerned with the modification of the normal diet to meet the requirements of the sick individual. Its purposes are:
1. To maintain good nutritional status.
2. To correct deficiencies, which may have occurred.
3. To afford rest to the whole body or to ascertain body's ability to metabolize the nutrients.
4. To bring about changes in body weight whenever necessary.

Therapeutic nutrition begins with the normal diet. Advantages of using normal diet, as the basis for therapeutic diets are:
1. It emphasizes the similarity of psychologic and social needs of those who are ill and those who are well even though there is quantitative and qualitative differences in requirements.
2. Food preparation is simplified when the modified diet is based upon the family pattern and the number of items required in special preparation is reduced to a minimum.
3. The calculated values for the basic plan are useful in finding out the effects of addition or omission of certain foods, e.g. if vegetables are restricted, vitamin A and C deficiencies can occur.

FACTORS TO CONSIDER IN PLANNING THERAPEUTIC DIETS

The alteration of the normal diet require an appreciation of:
1. The underlying disease conditions, which require a change in the diet.
2. The possible duration of the disease.

3. The factors in the dietary, which must be observed.
4. The patients tolerance for food by mouth.

In planning meals for a patient, his/her economic status, food preferences, occupation and time of meals should also be considered.

MODIFICATION OF NUTRIENTS IN THERAPEUTIC DIETS

The normal diet may be modified:
1. To provide change in consistency as in fluid and soft diets.
2. To increase or decrease the energy value.
3. To include greater or lesser amounts of one or more nutrients, for example, high protein, low sodium, etc.
4. To increase or decrease bulk—high- and low-fiber diets.
5. To provide foods bland in flavor.

TYPES OF DIET USED IN HOSPITALS

1. Clear-fluid diet.
2. Full-fluid diet.
3. Soft diet.
4. Normal diet.

Clear-fluid Diet

Whenever an acute illness or surgery produces a marked intolerance for food as may be evident by nausea, vomiting, anorexia, distention and diarrhea, it is advisable to restrict the intake of food. In acute infection, in acute inflammatory conditions of the intestinal tract, following operations upon the colon or rectum when it is desirable to prevent evacuation from the bowel, clear-fluid diet is suggested. This diet is also given to relieve thirst, to supply the tissues with water, to aid in the removal of gas.

The diet is made up of clear liquids that leave no residue and it is non-gas forming action. This diet is entirely inadequate from a nutritional standpoint. Since it is deficient in protein, minerals, vitamins and calories. It should not be continued for more than 24–48 hours. The amount of fluid is usually restricted to 30–60 mL/hour at first, with gradually increasing amounts being given as the patients tolerance improves.

This diet can meet the requirement of fluids and some minerals and can be given in 1–2 hour intervals.

Full-fluid Diet

Full-fluid diet bridges the gap between the clear fluid and soft diet. It is used following operations in acute gastritis, acute infections and in diarrhea. This diet is also suggested when milk is permitted and for patients not requiring special diet, but too ill to eat solid or semisolid foods.

In this diet, foods which are liquid or which readily become liquid on reaching the stomach are given. This diet may be made entirely adequate and may be used over an extended time without fear of deficiencies developing, provided it is carefully planned. This diet is given at 2–4 hours interval.

Soft Diet

Soft diet bridges the gap between acute illness and convalescence. It may be used in acute infections, following surgery and for patients who are unable to chew. The soft diet is made up of simple, easily digestible food and contains no harsh fiber. Patients with dental problems are given mechanically soft diet. It is often modified further for certain pathologic conditions as bland and low residue diets. In this diet, three meals with intermediate feeding should be given.

Normal Diet

Normal diet is used for ambulatory and bed patients whose conditions do not necessitate a special diet as one of the routine diets. Many special diets progress ultimately to a regular diet.

The regular hospital diet is simple in character and preparation, easy of digestion and calculated to afford maximum nourishment with minimum effort to the body. The diet is well balanced, adequate in nutritional value and attractively served to stimulate a possible poor appetite.

SPECIAL FEEDING METHODS (MANAGEMENT OF SPECIAL DIETS)

Oral feeding is the best for the nourishment of a patient. But in the following conditions it is not possible to give the feeding orally:
1. Those who cannot swallow due to paralysis of the muscles of swallowing (diphtheria, poliomyelitis), etc. or cancer of the oral cavity or larynx.
2. Those who cannot be persuaded to eat.

3. Those with persistent anorexia requiring forced feeding.
4. Semiconscious or unconscious patients.
5. Severe malabsorption requiring administration of unpalatable formula.
6. Short bowel syndrome.
7. Those who are undernourished or at risk of becoming so.
8. Those who cannot digest and absorb.
9. After surgery.
10. Patients with neurological and renal disorders or have continued fevers or diabetes.
11. Babies of very low birth weight.

Tube Feeding

Tube feeding is done by passing a tube into the stomach or duodenum through the nose, which is called nasogastric feeding or directly by surgical operation known as gastrostomy and jejunostomy feeding.

A satisfactory tube feeding must be:
1. Nutritionally adequate.
2. Well tolerated by the patient, so that vomiting is not induced.
3. Easily digested with no unfavorable reactions such as distension, diarrhea or constipation.
4. Easily prepared.
5. Inexpensive.

Nutrition supplied through the tube may be:
- Natural liquid foods
- Blenderized to make liquid food
- Commercially supplied polymeric mixtures or elemental diet (pre-digested diet).

Feeding Requirements

A concentration of about 1 kcal/mL is satisfactory. Lesser concentration increases the volume, which must be given to meet the nutrient and energy needs and greater concentration are more likely to produce diarrhea and may be too thick to pass through a nasogastric tube.

The feeding is started through a continuous drip at a rate of 50 mL/hour. The rate is increased by 20 mL every 24 hours until the required volume is achieved. Usually with 100–120 mL/hour. The concentration or rate of flow may have to be reduced, if there is vomiting, abdominal cramps or diarrhea.

Feeding requirements are based on previous nutritional status and other feeds given to the patient.
- Fluids: 30 mL/kg
- Energy: 32 kcal/kg
- Protein: 1 g/kg body weight
- Sodium: 30–40 mmol/(provided there are no external losses)
- Potassium: 1 mmol/g of protein.

Vitamins and minerals supplementation should be given.

Care of the Solution

Feeding solutions have to be treated with full hygienic precautions during the preparation, storage and administration. Feeds should be stored in a refrigerator to avoid bacterial growth and taken out before administering in time to reach room temperature; very cold feeds are not tolerated. A feed should be discarded when it has been more than 2 hours out of storage.

Documentation

Nursing staff should accurately record:
1. The time when a feed is started and completed.
2. The volume administered.
3. Water used to irrigate the tubing.
4. The patients output of urine. Careful monitoring is needed to see that the patient is in fluid balance.

Parenteral Feeding

In parenteral feeding the nutrient preparations are given directly into a vein. This method may be used to supplement normal feeding by mouth, but can provide all the nutrients necessary to meet a patient's requirements. Then, it is known as total parenteral nutrition or TPN.

The same process is called hyperalimentation when at least 50% of the daily requirements are provided to produce a positive nitrogen balance for gain in weight.

Partial parenteral nutrition provides 30%–50% of daily requirements.

PRE- AND POSTOPERATIVE DIET

Good nutrition prior to and following surgery ensures fewer postoperative complications and better wound healing. Short convalescence, lower mortality and chronic diseases, increase the nutritional requirements.

Malnutrition can lead to weight loss, poor wound healing, decreased intestinal motility, anemia, edema or dehydration and ulcers. The circulating blood volume and the concentration of the serum proteins, hemoglobin and electrolytes may be reduced.

Preoperative Nutritional Assessment

The objectives in the dietary management of surgical conditions are:
1. To improve the preoperative nutrition whenever the operation is not of an emergency nature.
2. To maintain correct nutrition after operation or injury as far as possible.
3. To avoid harm from injudicious choice of foods.

Protein

A satisfactory state of protein nutrition ensures:
1. Rapid wound healing.
2. Increases the resistance to infection.
3. Exerts a protective action upon the liver against the toxic effects of anesthesia.
4. Reduces the possibility of edema at the site of the wound.

The level of protein to be used in preoperative and postoperative diets depends on the previous state of nutrition, the nature of the operation and the extent of the postoperative losses. Intake of 1.0–1.5/kg of body weight or about 100 g of protein are necessary as a rule.

Energy

With 2,500–3,000 kcal patients make progress. Obesity constitutes a hazard in surgery. Whenever possible it should be corrected. Rapid weight loss results in loss of lean body mass and should be avoided.

Minerals

A liberal intake of protein and ascorbic acid and administration of iron salt is necessary.

Fluid

A patient should not go to operation in a stage of dehydration, since the subsequent dangers of acidosis are great. If the patient is unable to ingest sufficient liquid by mouth, parenteral fluids are administered.

Vitamins

Vitamin C is important for wound healing. Loss of vitamin K results in bleeding. Hemorrhage is especially likely to occur in patients who have diseases of the liver.

Postoperative Diet

Following minor surgery, liquids are often tolerated within a few hours and rapid progression to a normal diet is made after major surgery, oral intake may be delayed for days. Complete nutritional support are provided by conventional intravenous feeding, catheter jejunostomy, TPN, tube feeding or semisynthetic fiber free diets.

FEVER

Fever is an elevation in body temperature above the normal, which may occur due to exogenous and endogenous factors. Types:
1. Short duration fever: Colds, tonsillitis and influenza.
2. Chronic fever: Tuberculosis.
3. Intermittent: Malaria.

General Dietary Considerations

Energy

The caloric requirement may be increased as much as 50%, if the temperature is high and the tissue destruction is great. The patient may be able to ingest only 600–1,200 kcal daily, but this should be increased as rapidly as possible.

Protein

About 100 g protein or more is prescribed for the adult when a fever is prolonged. High protein beverages may be used as supplements to the regular meals.

Carbohydrates

Glycogen stores are replenished by a liberal intake of carbohydrates. Glucose which is readily absorbed is preferred.

Fats

The energy intake may be rapidly increased through the judicious use of fats, but fried foods and rich pastries are to be avoided.

Minerals

A sufficient intake of NaCl is accomplished by the use of salty broth and soups and by liberal sprinklings of salt on food. Fruit juices and milk are relatively good sources of minerals.

Vitamins

Fevers apparently increase the requirement for vitamin A and C just as the B complex vitamins are needed at increased levels.

Fluids

Daily 2,500–5,000 mL is necessary including beverages, soups, fruit juices and water.

Ease of Digestion

Bland readily digested food should be used to facilitate digestion and rapid absorption. The food may be soft or of regular consistency. Fluid diets can be used initially.

Intervals of Feeding

Small quantities of food at interval of 2–3 hours will permit adequate nutrition without overtaking the digestive system at any time. During an acute fever the patient's appetite is often very poor and small feeding of soft or liquid foods as desired should be offered at frequent intervals. Sufficient intake of fluids and salt is essential. If the illness persists for more than a few days, high protein, high calorie foods will be needed.

TYPHOID

Typhoid is an infectious disease with an acute fever of short duration and occurs only in human. *Salmonella typhi* causes typhoid. Feces and urine of the patients or carriers of the disease are the source of infection. Drinking water or milk and food contaminated by intestinal contents of the patients or carriers or by flies often transmit the disease.

The disease is characterized by a continued and high inflammation of the intestine. Formation of intestinal ulcers, hemorrhage and enlargement of spleen can occur. The patient may complain of diarrhea or constipation and severe stomach ache. Abdominal absorption of nutrients can cause headache.

Principles of Diet

A high calorie, high protein, high carbohydrates, low fat, high fluid, low fiber and bland diet is suggested for typhoid patients.

At first clear-fluid diet is given followed by full fluid and soft diet is suggested because of the intestinal inflammation. Great care must be exercised to eliminate all irritating fibers and spices in the diet. Refined cereals, bread, eggs, boiled potato and simple desserts like custards, porridges can be given. Adequate nutrition reduces convalescence period.

Foods to be Included

Fruit juices with glucose, coconut water, barley water, milk and milkshakes. If there is no diarrhea custards, thin dal curries, eggs, baked fish, minced meat, curds, cottage cheese, cereals, gruels, steamed vegetable juices, milk puddings and vegetable puree can be included.

Foods to be Avoided

Butter, ghee, vegetable oil, non-irritating fibrous food, chillies and other spices, rich pastries, fried foods, heavy puddings and cream soups.

INFLUENZA

General principles of dietary treatment is followed for influenza patients.

TUBERCULOSIS

Tuberculosis is an infectious disease caused by the bacillus *Mycobacterium tuberculosis*. It affects the lungs most often, but may also be localized in other organs such as the lymph nodes or kidneys or it may be generalized.

Pulmonary tuberculosis is accompanied by wasting of tissue, exhaustion, cough, expectoration and fever. The acute phase resembles pneumonia with high fever and increased circulation and respiration.

As the disease progresses, the patient begins to exhibit loss of appetite, pain in the chest, worsening cough.

Principles of Diet

A high calorie, high protein, high vitaminized and mineralized, high fluid, soft diet is recommended.

Energy

Since the metabolic rate is not as high as in other fevers, satisfactory weight can be maintained with 2,500–3,000 kcals.

Protein

A protein intake, somewhat in excess of normal requirements is necessary in tuberculosis. The daily requirement may be from 80 to 120 g.

Minerals

Calcium, especially should be provided liberally, since, it is essential for the healing of tuberculosis lesion. At least 1 L of milk should be taken daily. The iron needs may also be increased, if there has been hemorrhage. Calcium, iron and phosphorus help in regeneration of cells, blood and fluids.

Vitamins

The metabolism of vitamin A is adversely affected in tuberculosis. Ascorbic acid deficiency is present with slight tuberculosis. Vitamin C is essential for many regenerative purposes.

Dietary Management

1. Many patients with tuberculosis have very active peristalsis so that the selection of food should be from those bland in flavor, non-stimulating and easily digested.
2. Since patients have poor appetite, food must be appetizing and patients likes and dislikes must be considered.
3. During the acute stage, a high calorie fluid and soft diet are prescribed followed by high calorie soft regular diet.

4. Initially small quantities of fluid diet should be given once in 3 hours when the fever comes down the interval can be increased to every 4 hours.
5. In meeting the protein requirement, good quality protein like eggs should be included.
6. Fatty foods, highly fibrous foods and very spicy foods, which are hard to digest should be avoided.

DIET IN RELATION TO CONDITIONS OF GASTROINTESTINAL TRACT

Diarrhea

Diarrhea is the passage of stools with increased frequency, fluidity or volume compared to the usual for a given individual. Diarrhea is a symptom of underlying functional or organic disease and is acute or chronic in nature.

Acute Type

1. Chemical toxins: Such as arsenic, lead, mercury or cadmium.
2. Bacterial toxins: Such as Salmonella or staphylococcal food poisoning.
3. Bacterial infections: Such as *Streptococcus, E. coli.*
4. Drugs: Such as quinidine, neomycin.
5. Psychogenic factors: Such as emotional instability.
6. Dietary factors: Such as food sensitivity or allergy.

Chronic Type

1. Malabsorptive lesions of anatomic, mucosal or enzymatic origin.
2. Metabolic diseases, such as diabetic neuropathy, uremia or Addison's disease.
3. Alcoholism.
4. Carcinoma of small bowel or colon.
5. Postirradiation to small bowel or colon.
6. Cirrhosis.
7. Laxative abuse.

Nutritional Considerations in Diarrhea

Fluid electrolyte and tissue protein losses are usually severe, if diarrhea is prolonged.

Fluids: Losses of fluids should be replaced by a liberal intake to prevent dehydration, especially in susceptible age groups.

Electrolytes

Losses of sodium, potassium and others with severe diarrhea. Potassium loss is detrimental as potassium is necessary for normal muscle tone of the gastrointestinal (GI) tract. Losses can be replaced by liberal fluids such as tender coconut water and fruit juices that are high in potassium.

Nutrient Malabsorption

Long continued diarrhea may result in depletion of tissue, proteins and decreased serum protein levels. Fat losses are considerable in certain disorders with consequent loss of calories and fat-soluble vitamins. Intake of calories as high as 3,000 with 100–150 g protein, 100–120 g fat and the remainder as carbohydrates.

Vitamin deficiencies frequently seen in chronic diarrhea are related to the decreased intake of vitamins and the increased requirements because of losses in the stools.

Iron deficiency owing to the increased losses of iron in the feces, the occasional blood losses and the reduced intake of iron rich foods because of fear that some foods might aggravate an existing lesion.

Dietary Considerations

In acute diarrhea, current recommendations include oral intake of glucose electrolyte solutions for those able to drink with progression to foods as tolerated in small frequent feeding as appetitive improves.

Many patients with chronic diarrhea do not tolerate milk or foods high in fat or fiber content. Generally speaking, however the need is for a diet high in protein and calories with adequate amounts of vitamin and minerals and liberal amounts of fluids.

Constipation

In this condition, there is the duodenum and intrevent or difficult evacuation of feces from the intestine.

Insufficient or infrequent emptying of the bowel may lead to malaise, headache, coated tongue, foul breath and lack of appetite. These symptoms usually disappear after satisfactory evacuation has taken place.

Correction of constipation depends in large measure on establishing regularity in habits, eating, rest, exercise and elimination.

Dietary Considerations

The diet should contain sufficient fiber to induce peristalsis and to contribute bulk to the intestine. A regular diet with an abundance of both raw and cooked fruits and vegetables is suitable for such patients. Whole grain cereals should be substituted for refined ones. Bran is useful, but excesses are to be avoided since it may act as an irritant to sensitive intestinal tracts. Fat containing foods are useful because of the stimulating effect of the fatty acids on the mucous membranes. Excesses may cause diarrhea and should be avoided. Mineral oil, if used should not be taken at mealtime because of its interference with the absorption of fat-soluble vitamins.

A fluid intake of 8–10 glasses a day is useful in keeping the intestinal contents in a semi-solid state for easier passage along the tract. Some individuals find that 1 or 2 glasses of hot or cold water plain or with lemon are helpful in initiating peristalsis when taken before breakfast.

Peptic Ulcer

The term peptic ulcer is used to describe any localized erosion of the mucosal lining of those portions of the alimentary tract that come in contact with gastric juice. The majority of ulcers are found in the stomach although they also occur in the duodenum, jejunum or any other part of the GI tract exposed to the gastric juice.

Dietary Management

It was customary to suggest bland diet for ulcer patients. Bland diet is a diet which is mechanically, chemically and thermally non-irritating.
Protein foods: Milk and protein foods do have some buffering effect, but they also evoke gastric secretions more than carbohydrates and fats. Milk should be included as a source of nutrients factor for healing purposes. Protein provides the necessary amino acids for synthesis of tissue proteins, which helps in healing ulcer.

Fat: Moderate amounts of the fat help to suppress gastric secretion and motility through the enterogastrone mechanism.

Foods believed to be 'chemically irritating' because of their stimulatory effect on gastric secretion include meat extractives, caffeine, alcohol, citrus fruits and juices and some spicy foods. 'Mechanically irritating' foods include those with indigestible carbohydrates such as whole grains and most raw fruits and vegetables. Foods believed to be 'thermally irritating' are those ordinarily served at extremes of temperatures such as very hot or iced liquids. In addition, certain foods traditionally forbidden include strongly flavored vegetables such as cabbage, cauliflower, onions and turnips and fried foods. Restriction of these foods is based on subjective evidence from patients who experience distress following ingestion of these items including good food.

Foods to be Included

Diary products like milk, cream, butter, mild cheese and eggs (not fried) steamed fish, rice, rice flakes, puffed rice, margarine, well-cooked cereal, semolina, cooked green leafy vegetables, custards, malted drinks.

Foods to be Avoided

Alcohol, strong tea, coffee, cola, beverages, gravies, soups, pickles, spices, curries, condiments, all fried foods, pastries, cakes, heavy sweets like halwa, barfi, raw unripe fruits, raw vegetables like cucumber, onions, radish and tomatoes.

Modificaton of Diet in Bleeding Ulcer

The degree of dietary modification in bleeding ulcer depends on the peculiarities of the individual case. The severe hemorrhage, it is customary to give no food until the bleeding has been controlled and the patients conditions is stabilized. If hemorrhage is not severe and if nausea and vomiting are not a problem, the patient may desire food and tolerate it well. Initial dietary treatment consists of mild alternated at 2 hours interval with small feeding of easily puddings toast and tender-cooked fruits and vegetables. Gradual progression in amounts and types of foods is made as the patient improves.

DIET IN RELATION TO DISEASE OF THE LIVER AND GALLBLADDER

Infective Hepatitis (Jaundice)

Infective hepatitis is otherwise known as viral hepatitis. This is the common cause of jaundice. The two viruses responsible are hepatitis A and B virus. The former enters the body through oral fecal route like through food or water, while the latter is passed through by using infected blood products from carriers, use of unsterilized needles and through sexual contact.

Symptoms

Anorexia, fever, headache, rapid weight loss, loss of muscle tone and abdominal discomfort.

Dietary Management

A high protein, high carbohydrate, moderate fat diet is recommended. Small attractive meals at regular intervals are better tolerated.

Energy: In nasogastric feeding stage about 1,000 kcal are supplied. In severe cases, 1,600–2,000 kcal are suggested.

Protein: For the liver cells to regenerate an adequate supply of proteins is needed. Protein requirements vary according to the severity of the disease, with severe jaundice 40 g, while in mild jaundice 60–80 g of protein is permitted with hepatic precoma and coma, protein containing foods are withheld and only high carbohydrate containing foods are given.

Fats: During hepatic precoma and coma due to severe liver failure, fats are not metabolized by the liver and so fat is restricted, in severe jaundice 30 g and in moderate jaundice 50–60 g.

Carbohydrates: High carbohydrate content in the diet is essential to supply enough calories, so that tissue proteins are not broken down for energy.

Vitamins: They are essential to regenerate liver cells—500 mg of vitamin C along with 10 mg vitamin K and supplements of vitamin B.

Minerals: Oral feeds of fruit juice, vegetable and meat soups with added salt, given orally or through a nasogastric tube help in maintaining the electrolyte balance.

Foods to be Included

Cereal porridge, soft chapati, bread, rice, skimmed milk, tapioca, potato, yam, fruit, fruit juices, sugar, jaggery, honey, biscuits, soft custards without butter cream and non-stimulant beverages.

Foods to be Avoided

Pulses, beans, meat, fish, chicken, egg, soups, sweet preparations where ghee, butter or oil are used, bakery products, dried fruits, nuts, spices, papads, chutney, alcoholic beverages, fried preparations, whole milk creams.

Cirrhosis of Liver

Cirrhosis is a condition in which there is destruction of the liver cell due to necrosis, fatty infiltration and fibrosis.

The cirrhotic process may commence many years before it becomes clinically obvious and usually the patient when first seen is at a very late stage with complications, such as ascites, ruptured esophageal varices or hepatic coma. Almost 85%–90% of liver damage also do not produce symptoms. The initial change in cirrhosis is wide spread liver cell necrosis due to viral hepatic, alcohol, etc.

Causes

1. Viral infection by hepatitis A and B viruses.
2. Alcohol.
3. Malnutrition.
4. Toxins of food, aflatoxin, bush tea.

Symptoms

The onset of cirrhosis may be gradual with GI disturbances such as anorexia, nausea, vomiting, pain and distension. As the disease progresses jaundice and other serious changes occur.

Ascites is the accumulation of abnormal amounts of fluids in the abdomen.

Principles of Diet

A high calorie, high protein, high carbohydrate, moderate or restricted fat, high vitamin diet helps in regeneration of liver and helps to prevent the formation of ascites. Low fat with supplements of fat-soluble vitamin and minerals should be given. Sodium should be restricted only when there is ascites.

When there is danger of esophageal varices or portal hypertension, fiber should be restricted.

Dietary Treatment

Energy: Consumption of food is difficult because of anorexia and ascites. The patients are usually emaciated and require highly nutritious food, i.e. high calorie diet is necessary because of prolonged undernourishment. The calorie requirement should be between 2,000–2,500 kcal.

Proteins: A high protein diet is helpful for regeneration of the liver. In the absence of hepatic coma a high intake of proteins about 1.2 g/kg of body weight can be given. If the patient is in precoma or coma, proteins should be withheld till the patient tides over the crisis. Vegetable proteins containing more valine is beneficial in preventing encephalopathy.

Fats: About 1 g of fat/kg of body weight is given. Even if fatty changes are present in the liver, fats should be given provided adequate amounts of protein is supplied. Medium chain triglycerides containing C8–C10 fatty acids can be given as these are digested and absorbed in the absence of bile salts. Coconut oil contains medium chain fatty acids.

Carbohydrates: Should be supplied liberally so that the liver may store glycogen. Liver function improves when an adequate store of glycogen is present in liver cells. 60% of the calories should come from carbohydrate so that liver damage is minimized.

Vitamins: The liver is the major site of storage and conversion of vitamins into their metabolically active form. In cirrhosis, the liver concentration of complex of folate, riboflavin, niacin, vitamin B_{12} and vitamin A are decreased. Vitamin supplementation especially of B vitamins is required to prevent anemia.

Minerals: Sodium is restricted in edema and ascites. Potassium salt is administered for ascites and edema to prevent hypokalemia. Anemia is common among cirrhosis patients, so iron supplementation is essential.

Foods to be Included

Cereals in a soft form, cooked rice, chapati, bread and idli, milk pudding, milk shakes, curds, puree, cooked vegetables, kichidi and porridge, pulses, beans, meat, fruit and fruit juices.

Hepatic Coma

Complex syndrome characterized by neurologic disturbances, which may develop as a complication of severe liver disease. It results from entrance of certain nitrogen containing substances such as ammonia into the cerebral circulation without being metabolized by the liver.

Precipitating Factors

Gastrointestinal bleeding, severe infections, surgical procedures and excessive dietary protein and sedatives may precipitate hepatic coma.

Symptoms

Confusion, restlessness, irritability, inappropriate behavior, delirium and drowsiness are present. There may be incoordination and a flapping tremor of the arms and legs when extended. Electrolyte imbalance occurs. The patient may go into coma and may have convulsions. Breath has a fecal odor. Prompt treatment is imperative or death occurs.

Dietary Modifications

Low-protein diet should be given. At the same time, catabolism of tissue proteins must be avoided.

Energy: About 1,500–2,000 kcals are needed to prevent breakdown of tissue proteins for energy and are provided chiefly in the form of carbohydrates and fats. Although anorexia may occur, attempts should be made to keep the calorie intake as high as is practical to minimize tissue breakdown.

Protein: First 2 or 3 days protein is completely omitted or 20–30 g/day are given. As the patient improves the protein intake is gradually increased to 1 g/kg of body weight. Nitrogen balance can be achieved on protein intake as low as 35 g/day, if high quality protein is used and calorie intake is adequate.

Dietary Management

These patients pose problems in feeding because of anorexia and behavioral patterns ranging from apathy, drowsiness and hyperexcitability. The protein free diet consisting of commercial sugar, fat emulsions, a butter sugar mixture or glucose in beverages or fruit juices may be used initially through oral or tube feeding. With improvements, the diets providing 20, 40 and 60 g protein may be gradually introduced.

Cholelithiasis

The function of the gallbladder and bile ducts is to concentrate, store and deliver bile into the duodenum at appropriate times to assist digestion. Hormonal and nervous factors play a part in this process. The stimulus for this activity is the entry of food into the small intestine. This causes the mucosa of the duodenum and jejunum to secrete a hormone, cholecystokinin, which is carried in the blood to the gallbladder and causes it to contract. Fats and foods rich in fats are especially effective for this purpose.

The bile is concentrated in the gallbladder and when it is super saturated gallstones are likely to form. Supersaturation arises when there is insufficient amount of solubilizing agents such as bile acids and to a lesser extent lecithin to keep cholesterol and bile pigments in solution. By far the most common gallstones are mixed stones composed of cholesterol, bile pigment and various calcium salts including calcium palmitate.

Gallstones are more common in women than in men. Advanced age, repeated pregnancies and sedentary life, and use of oral contraceptives are the contributing factors.

In man, it has been suggested that high cholesterol diets, lack of dietary fiber and an insufficiency of polyunsaturated fats predispose to gallstones.

Energy

Excess calorie intake appears to be risk for development of gallbladder disease. The disease is more common in obese persons.

Fat

The patient receives no food initially during attacks of cholecystitis. Progression to 20–30 g fat diet is made. If this is tolerated, the fat can then be increased to 50–60 g/day.

THERAPEUTIC DIET IN CONDITIONS OF ENDOCRINE GLANDS AND METABOLIC DISORDERS

Diabetes Mellitus

Diabetes mellitus is a chronic metabolic disorder that prevents the body to utilize glucose completely or partially. It is characterized by raised glucose concentration in the blood and alterations in carbohydrate, protein and fat metabolism. This can be due to failure in the formation of insulin or, its liberation or action.

Causes

1. Genetic factors—heredity.
2. Obesity.
3. Sugar intake.
4. Infections.
5. Acute stress—body releases adrenaline, noradrenaline and cortisol hormones that raise blood glucose levels.
6. Secondary diabetes—results from diseases which destroy the pancreas and lead to impaired secretion of insulin, e.g. pancreatitis, hemochromatosis, carcinoma of the pancreas and pancreatectomy.

Symptoms

1. Polydipsia—increased thirst.
2. Polyuria—increased urination.
3. Polyphagia—increased hunger.
4. Weight loss.

Other Possible Symptoms

1. Blurred vision.
2. Skin irritation or infection.
3. Weakness, loss of strength.
4. Decreased healing capacity.

Continued Symptoms

1. Fluid and electrolysis imbalance.
2. Acidosis (ketosis, ketonuria).
3. Coma.
4. Weight loss (Table 40.1).

Types

Type I: Insulin-dependent diabetes mellitus (IDDM) is also known as juvenile-onset diabetes and the patients depend on insulin. There is usually sudden onset and the occurrence of IDDM in the younger age group of

TABLE 40.1: Diabetic patients and weight loss on work

Patients type	Weight loss (kcal)
Bedridden patient	25
Light work	30
Medium work	35
Heavy work	40

10–12 years and there is an inability of pancreas to produce adequate amount of insulin.

Type II: Non-insulin-dependent diabetes mellitus (NIDDM) is also known as adult-onset diabetes. In this form diabetes develops slowly and is usually wilder and more stable. Insulin may be produced by pancreas, but action is impaired.

Diabetic Diet Prescription

The nutrition and diet prescription (Table 40.2) is based on:
1. History of both, the patient and the family.
2. Sex, age, weight, height and activity of the patient.
3. Type I or type II diabetes.
4. Type of insulin taken by the patient amount.

Food Exchange Lists

Food exchange lists are groups of measured foods of the same calorific value and similar protein, fat and carbohydrate can be substituted from one another in a meal plan.

TABLE 40.2: Insulin and meal distribution of calories and carbohydrates

Types of insulin	Breakfast	Noon	Mid-afternoon	Evening	Bedtime
1. None	1/3	1/3	–	1/3	–
2. Short acting (before breakfast and dinner)	2/5	1/5	–	2/5	–
3. Intermediate acting NPH*	1/7	2/7	1/7	2/7	1/7
4. Long acting	1/5	2/5	–	2/5	20–40 g of CHO[†]
5. Long acting with regular insulin at breakfast	1/3	1/3	–	1/3	20–40 g of CHO

*NPH, neutral protamine hagedorn; [†]CHO, carbohydrates.

Food exchange list helps to:
1. Restrict the food intake according to the insulin prescription.
2. Have variety in the diet.
3. Easy learning of the principles of diets.

Dietary Fiber

Dietary fiber and complex carbohydrates and restricted fat, benefit type I and type II diabetes. Such diets lower:
1. Insulin requirements.
2. Increase peripheral tissue insulin sensitivity.
3. Decrease serum cholesterol and triglyceride values.
4. Aid in weight control.
5. Lower BP.

Soluble fibers such as pectin, gums, hemicellulose (in fruits) increase intestinal transit time, delay gastric, slow glucose absorption and lower serum cholesterol.

Insoluble fibers such as cellulose and lignin (vegetables, grains) decrease intestinal transit time, increase fecal bulk, delay glucose absorption and slow starch hydrolysis.

Fiber Content of Foods

Fiber content of foods includes:

Maize, whole wheat, coriander, mint, carrot, brinjal, cauliflower, French beans, lady's finger, green mango 1%–3%.

Ragi, whole legumes, groundnut, cluster beans, double beans, peas, guava 3.5%.

Nutritional Requirements

The nutritional requirements (Box 40.1) are calories 1,700–1,800, CHO 180 g, fats 60 g and protein 90 g.

A minimum amount of 100 g of CHO should be given to prevent ketosis. Suggested calories from protein is 15%–20%, from carbohydrate 55%–60%, 20%–25% as fat, cholesterol 100 mg/100 kcal and 50 g of fiber.

This diet reduces insulin requirements, improves glycemic control, lower fasting serum cholesterol and triglyceride values and promote weight loss.

BOX 40.1: Daily nutrition evaluation sheet

Physicians details:			Patients details:	Date:
Name of the Doctor:			Name of the Patient:	
Hospital/Nursing Home:		Age: Year	Sex: M/F	
Address:				
Phone No:				

Physical evaluation:

Height:	(m)	Weight:	(kg)	BMI:
Waist:	(cm)	Hip:	(cm)	Waist/Hip ratio:

Lifestyle evaluation: **Nutrition prescription:**

Sedentary: ☐   Moderate: ☐   Strenuous: ☐   Calories/day

Dear Sir/Madam,

You have been diagnosed for diabetes and are advised a diet plan to keep a check on your sugar levels. The good news is that our traditional Indian diet with a slight modification is quite close to what is considered 'diabetic diet'.

Basic advice

Avoid simple carbohydrate like:

Jaggery	Soft drinks	Jelly
Honey	Pastries	Candy
Glucose	Cakes	Beer
Sweets	Ice creams	Sweet wines
Oily pickles	Jams	Drinking chocolate, etc.

The above tend to cause a sharp rise in the blood glucose levels

A diet high in protein is good for the health of diabetic patient. It supplies essential amino acids. It does not raise blood sugar during absorption as carbohydrate.

Excess fat is avoided, as diabetic patients are prone to suffer from atherosclerosis. Ketone bodies, the intermediary product of fats are accumulated when carbohydrate is deficient.

Foods to be Included

Clear soups, lemons, salted pickle, pepper water, plain coffee or tea (without sugar), skimmed buttermilk, unsweetened lime juice, tomato juice, soda water, raw vegetables, salads, soup cubes, salt seasonings like onion, mint, pepper, garlic, curry leaf, coriander, vinegar, mustard and spices.

Foods to be Avoided

Sugar, glucose, honey, jaggery, sweets, halwas, burfies, nuts, jam, jellies, preserved fruits, dried fruits, aerated drinks, cake, pastries, candy, fried foods, alcohol.

VARIOUS METABOLIC DISORDERS

Hyperthyroidism

Hyperthyroidism is a disturbance in which there is an excessive secretion of the thyroid hormone with a consequent increase in the metabolic rate. It is believed to be an autoimmune disease occurring in genetically predisposed persons. The disease is also known as exophthalmic goiter, thyrotoxicosis, Graves' disease or Basedow's disease.

The chief symptoms are weight loss, sometimes to the point of emaciation, excessive nervousness, prominence of the eyes and a generally enlarged thyroid gland. Increased appetite, weakness and signs of cardiac failure are also present.

The increased level of energy metabolism increases the requirement of vitamin B. The excretion of calcium and phosphorus is greatly increased in hyperthyroidism.

Frequent feedings (125 g protein) will help satisfy hunger. A liberal calcium intake is desirable and may be provided in addition to the liberal use of milk.

Hypothyroidism

Decreased production or activity of the thyroid hormone or hypothyroidia is a relatively common problem.

Obesity is a problem for some patients with hypothyroidism, since they may continue in their earlier patterns of eating, even though the energy metabolism has been significantly reduced. In other patients, the appetite may be so poor that undernutrition results. For overweight persons, reduction of calories is necessary. Reduction of dietary cholesterol may be indicated. Adequate fluids and foods high in dietary fiber are needed to overcome constipation.

JOINT DISEASES

The term *arthritis* and *rheumatism* are applied to many joint diseases.

The most common form of arthritis is *osteoarthritis* or *degenerative arthritis*. Joint stiffness is characteristic. Pain is confined to joints. Joints of the fingers, knees, hip and spine are involved.

Rheumatoid Arthritis

Rheumatoid arthritis is a highly inflammatory and very painful condition having its onset in young women. This is characterized by fatigue, pain, stiffness, deformity, which may be severe and limited function.

DIETARY COUNSELING

Arthritic patients require the same amount of calories as other persons need.

Obesity is a common problem in osteoarthritis. Weight loss should be brought about in order to bring down the added stress on weight bearing joints.

Many patients with rheumatoid arthritis have lost weight and are in poor nutritional status. A high-calorie diet, high-protein diet is given.

Gout

Gout is a disorder of purine metabolism occurring principally in middle-aged and older men, women are susceptible after menopause.

Low-purine diet with moderate calories for obese individuals. The calories can be reduced up to 1,200–1,600 kcals.

Protein

Because the nitrogen of the protein nucleus is supplied by protein, the intake is restricted to 0.9 g/kg body weight. Fat is often restricted to about 60 g/day.

Fluids

The daily intake of fluids should be at least 3 L.

THERAPEUTIC DIET IN CONDITIONS OF THE URINARY SYSTEM

Glomerulonephritis

Glomerulonephritis is an inflammatory process affecting the glomeruli, the small blood vessels in the head of the nephron, most common in its acute form in children 3–10 years of age.

Symptoms

Hematuria, proteinuria, edema, shortness of breath, tachycardia, elevated BP and anorexia. There may be *oliguria* or *anuria*.

Principles of the Diet

Fluids: The fluid intake will be adjusted to output including losses in vomiting or diarrhea. Daily fluid replacement should be 1,000 mL plus daily amount excreted in the urine.

Insensible water loss is:
- 30 mL/kg body weight for infants
- 20 mL/kg body weight for older children
- 10 mL/kg body weight for adults.

Energy: Sufficient calories is given without increasing the protein intake by means of sugar, honey, glucose.

Protein: Usually the diet contains 0.5 g of protein/kg body weight for older children and 1–1.5 g/kg/day for younger children. A low-protein diet is recommended so as to give rest to the kidney. An intake of 20–40 g/day is considered sufficient. Out of the recommended protein 50 g should be from animal protein.

Sodium: The restriction of sodium varies with the degree of oliguria and hypertension. If renal function is impaired, the sodium (Na) will be restricted to 500–1,000 mg/day. If edema is present, Na is restricted.

Potassium: When the kidneys do not work properly, potassium (K) builds up in the body and causes heart to beat uneven and stop suddenly.

Phosphorus: Eating foods high in phosphorus (P), will raise the phosphorus in the blood and this can cause calcium (Ca) to be pulled from the bones. This will make bones weak and cause them to break easily.

Nephrosis (Degenerative Bright's Disease)

Symptoms

Heavy proteinuria, hypoalbuminemia and peripheral edema.

Principles of Diet

High protein, high calorie, high carbohydrate, salt restricted moderate fat with restricted fluid are recommended. Vitamin supplements especially vitamin C are given.

Dietary Treatment

To ensure protein use for tissue synthesis, sufficient kilocalories must always be provided. 200 kcal is suggested.

About 100–120 g of protein should be provided. A high-protein diet is required to meet the heavy loss of albumin and protein depletion of the tissues.

Sodium is restricted to prevent accumulation of edema fluid and prevent hypertension.

Special Instructions

Since Ca and K deficiency may accompany severe proteinuria, bone refraction and hypokalemia are common and hence:
1. The diet has to be soft.
2. Low quality proteins like pulses should be mixed with cereals or milk to improve quality of protein. High quantity proteins like egg, meat are preferred.
3. Vitamin supplements especially vitamin C are essential.

Acute Renal Failure

There is a sudden shut down of renal function following metabolic or traumatic injury to normal kidneys.

Symptoms

Anuria or oliguria—low urine volume, i.e. 20–200 mL/day. Due to accumulation of waste products of protein metabolism in blood, excretion of K is diminished. There is also increased phosphate and sulfate with decreased sodium, calcium and base bicarbonate. Lethargy, anorexia, nausea, vomiting, blood pressure, uremia.

Dietary Management

Energy: A minimum of 600–1,000 kcal is necessary. A high calorie intake is desired mainly from carbohydrates and fats.

Protein: All foods containing protein is stopped if the patient is under conservative treatment and blood urea nitrogen is rising. However, 40 g is allowed when the patient is on hemodialysis or peritoneal dialysis.

Carbohydrates: A minimum of 100 g/day is essential to minimize tissue protein breakdown.

Fluids: The total fluid permitted is 500 mL plus losses through urine and gastrointestinal tract with visible perspiration, an additional 500 mL may be necessary.

Sodium: Sodium loss through urine is measured and replaced. Na restriction is also judged based on Na loss in the urine.

Potassium: Hyperkalemia occurs with a daily rise of 0.7 mEq, in serum potassium. It has deleterious effects on heart.

Chronic Renal Failure

Chronic renal failure is also known as uremia. When the level of urea in the blood is very high, i.e. when 90%, the function of renal tissue is destroyed, and uremia occurs. It may be the end result of acute glomerulonephritis, pyelonephritis and nephritic syndrome.

Dietary Management

Diet should be palatable, must have varieties, adjusted according to altered biochemistry and physiology (hyperphosphatemia and hypertension) and adequate enough for growth in children.

Energy: Adequate kilocalories are mandatory. Carbohydrate and fat must supply sufficient non-protein in kilocalories to spare protein for tissue protein synthesis and to supply energy.

Requirements: The energy requirements are:
Infancy: 100–120 k/kg/day.
Childhood: 80–110 kcal.
Adults: 35–50 kcal.

Protein: Failing kidney needs to be given rest. Protein intake can be reduced to 0.5 g/kg of body weight per day.

Fluid: The usual fluid permitted is volume of daily urine plus 500 mL.

Sodium: Strict restriction is necessary, only if hypertension and edema are present.

- 1–2 mmol/kg of body weight for infants
- 40–60 mmol/day for older children.

Potassium: This has to be restricted to 1 mmol/kg of body weight. Double boiling and draining excess water reduces potassium content.

Urolithiasis or Urinary Calculi

Urolithiasis or urinary calculi are found to be lodged in the urinary system namely kidneys, ureters, bladder or urethra.

Small foci are formed and supersaturated urinary salts are precipitated around the foci of mucoid structures.

Causes

1. Climate: In warm climate, the urine volume is low.
2. Occupation: People working under the sun and perspire a lot pass concentrated urine.
3. Infection of urinary tract: Frequent infection of urinary tract may be contributory to the formation of pus cells and epithelial cells may form a focus around which the stone may be formed.
4. Dietary habits: Foods rich in oxalates, calcium, purines and phosphate may predispose to form renal calculi.
5. Heredity.
6. Vitamin A and B complex deficiency.
7. Hyperthyroidism.

Types of Calculi

1. Calcium phosphate.
2. Calcium oxalate–mostly found in India.
3. Uric acid.
4. Magnesium ammonium phosphate.

Dietary Management

a. Planning acid-ash diet.
   A liberal fluid intake
   - Salt in moderation
   - The fruits and vegetables so selected should not contribute more than 25 mL of base daily.

b. **Planning alkaline-ash diet:** If stones of uric acid or cystine type occur, the diet should be alkaline ash. Alkaline producing foods such as fruits, vegetables and milk, while acid producing foods like meat, eggs and cereals are restricted.
c. **Planning low-oxalate diets:** An acid or alkaline reaction of the diet is of little value for oxalate urolithiasis. Sources of oxalates should be omitted which include beans, beet greens, chocolate, cocoa, dried figs, plums, potatoes, spinach, tea and tomatoes.

Fluid: About 0.2–2.5 L should be given. Coconut water, barley water and fruits.

DIET THERAPY IN CONDITIONS OF THE CIRCULATORY SYSTEM

Cardiovascular Diseases

Cardiovascular diseases are characterized by the thickening of the arterial valves and their loss of elasticity.

Types

1. **Atherosclerosis:** It is a degenerative disease of the arteries and consists of focal accumulation in the intimal lining of arteries of a variable combination of lipids, complex carbohydrates, blood and blood products, fibrous tissue and Ca deposits.
2. **Coronary heart disease:** It is syndrome arising from failure of the coronary arteries to supply sufficient blood to the myocardium. Also known as ischemic heart disease (IHD).
3. **Myocardial infarction:** Necrosis or destruction of part of the heart muscle due to failure of blood supply and may lead to sudden death.
4. **Angina pectoris:** Pain in the chest, exercise or excitement provokes severe chest pain and so limits patients physical activities.

Objectives of Dietary Management

1. Maximum rest for the heart.
2. Prevention or elimination of edema.
3. Maintenance of good nutrition.
4. Acceptability of the program.

Principles of Diet

Low calories, low fat particularly low-saturated fat, low cholesterol, high in polyunsaturated fatty acids (PUFA), low carbohydrate and normal protein. Minerals, vitamins and high-fiber diet is also recommended.

Energy

Usually a 1,000–1,200 calorie diet is suitable for an obese patient in bed. Those patients with desirable level are permitted a maintenance level of calories, during convalescence and their return to activity.

Fat

The first step involves restriction of fats to not more than 30% of the total calories consumed. Levels as low as 20% are tolerated without side effects. Total fat from 30% met by saturated 10% and monounsaturated vegetable oil.

Proteins, Vitamins and Minerals

Normal allowances.
Duration of meal: Three or four smaller meals are suggested instead of two big meals. The evening meals must be 2 hours before retiring to bed.
Sodium: It is restricted when there is hypertension.
Fluid: The restriction of fluid is not required as long as Na is not restricted.
High-fiber diet: Increasing fiber will serve to reduce cholesterol.

Hypertension

Elevation of the blood pressure (BP) above normal is a symptom, which accompanies many cardiovascular and renal diseases.

High BP of unknown cause is known as essential hypertension.

Causes

Cardiovascular diseases, renal diseases, tumors of the brain or adrenal glands, hyperthyroidism or diseases of ovaries and pituitary may cause hypertension.

Types

1. Mild hypertension: Diastolic pressure is 90–104 mm Hg.
2. Moderate hypertension: Diastolic pressure is 105–119 mm Hg.
3. Severe hypertension: Diastolic pressure is 120–130 mm Hg.

Symptoms

Headache, dizziness, impaired vision, failing memory, shortness of breath, pain over the heart and gastrointestinal disturbance, unexplained tiredness.

Principles of Diet

Low calorie, low fat, low-sodium diet with normal protein intake is prescribed.

Energy: Obese patient must be reduced to normal body weight with low-calorie diet.

Protein: A diet of 50 g protein is necessary to maintain proper nutrition.

Fats: About 40 g fat, partly as vegetable oil is permitted.

Sodium: Restrictions for a moderate low-sodium diet (1,000 mg).

  Do not use:
1. Salt in cooking or at the table.
2. Salt preserved foods, pickles, canned foods.
3. Highly salted foods such as potato chips.
4. Spices and condiments such as ketchup, sauce.
5. Cheese, peanut butter, salted butter.
6. Frozen peas.
7. Shellfish.
8. Regular baking powder, sodium metabisulfite, ajinomoto.
9. Prepared mixture.

Appendices

Appendix I: Normal Values of Important Tests
Appendix II: University Examination Question Papers

Appendices

APPENDIX I: NORMAL VALUES OF IMPORTANT TESTS

Test	Normal values	Test	Normal values
◆ FBS	70–100 mg%	Calcium	8.5–10.5 mg%
◆ RBS	80–120 mg%	◆ Phosphorus	2.5–5 mg%
◆ PPBS	100–140 mg%	◆ **Lipid profile**	
◆ Urine sugar	Nil	◆ Cholesterol	150–250 mg%*
◆ Glycosylated hemoglobin	4.5–8%	◆ HDL cholesterol	30–70 mg%*
◆ Urea	10–45 mg%	◆ Triglyceride	10–160 mg%
◆ Creatinine	0.7–1.5 mg%	◆ VLDL	6–40 mg%
		◆ LDL	180 mg%
◆ Uric acid	3–7 mg%	◆ Acid phosphatase	0–3 KAU/dL
◆ Sodium	133–143 mEq/L	◆ Amylase	25–125 U/dL
◆ Potassium	3.9–5.3 mEq/L		
◆ Chloride	98–108 mEq/L		
◆ Blood non-protein nitrogen (NPN)	20–40 mg%	*Better to keep serum cholesterol level below 200 mg%	
◆ **Liver function tests**		◆ **Iron profile**	
◆ Total protein	6–8 g/dL	◆ Iron	60–150 µg/dL
◆ Albumin	3.4–5 g/dL	◆ TIBC	230–380 µg/dL
◆ A/G ratio	1.2–1.7	◆ Transferrin	1.2–2 g/dL
◆ Total bilirubin	0.2–1.2 mg%	◆ Transferrin saturation	20–50%
◆ Conjugated bilirubin	0.1–0.4 mg%	◆ **Urine**	
◆ SGOT (AST)	5–50 IU/L	◆ Creatinine	1.0–1.8
◆ SGPT (ALT)	5–50 IU/L	◆ Reducing sugars	100 mg/day
◆ Alkaline phosphatase	100–250 IU/L	◆ Urea	30 g/day
◆ Gamma GT (GGT)	10–45 IU/L	◆ Uric acid	0.8 g/day
◆ CPK	0–192 IU/L	◆ Chloride as NaCl	10–15 g/day
◆ CPK-B	0–13 IU/L	◆ Urobilinogen	0.4 g/day
◆ CPK-MB	0–25 IU/L	◆ Ketone bodies	1 mg/day
◆ LDH	200–400 IU/L	◆ Phosphorus	10 g/day
		◆ Titrable acidity	200–400 mL 10N acid

APPENDIX II: UNIVERSITY EXAMINATION QUESTION PAPERS

RAJIV GANDHI UNIVERSITY OF HEALTH SCIENCES KARNATAKA

First Year BSc Nursing Degree Examination
April 2014

Biochemistry

I. Long Essays (Answer any one)   1 × 10 = 10 Marks

1. Describe the sources, biochemical functions, requirement and deficiency manifestations of Vitamin D.
2. What are ketone bodies? How are they formed and utilized in the body?

II. Short Essays (Answer any two)   2 × 5 = 10 Marks

3. Denaturation of proteins.
4. Essential fatty acids.
5. Why is sucrose a nonreducing sugar?

III. Short Answers   5 × 2 = 10 Marks

6. Anomers.
7. Ketone bodies.
8. Name the bile alts and their functions.
9. Benedict's test.
10. Give the normal levels of serum calcium and blood urea.

RAJIV GANDHI UNIVERSITY OF HEALTH SCIENCES KARNATAKA

First Year BSc Nursing Degree Examination
April 2014

Nutrition

I. Long Essays (Answer any one)   1 × 10 = 10 Marks

1. Explain the methods of cooking. Write briefly on the effect of heat on food constituents.
2. Classify the vitamins. Explain about the functions, sources and deficiencies of fat-soluble vitamins.

II. Short Essays (Answer any five)   5 × 5 = 25 Marks

3. Explain the methods of assessment of nutritional status.
4. Define food preservation and write its principles.
5. Write the absorption and metabolism of iron.
6. Define balanced diet. Write the role of nutrition in maintaining health.
7. Functions of proteins.
8. Determine the basal metabolic rate.

III. Short Answers   5 × 2 = 10 Marks

9. Expand: CARE, FAO.
10. Explain steaming.
11. List out the macro- and microminerals.
12. Define Nutrition and Health.
13. Give good sources of Vitamin C.

RAJIV GANDHI UNIVERSITY OF HEALTH SCIENCES, KARNATAKA

First Year BSc Nursing Degree Examination
August 2013

Nutrition

I. Long Essays (Answer any one) 1 × 10 = 10 Marks

1. a. Define Nutrition
   b. Role of nutrition in maintaining health
   c. Factors affecting food and nutrition
2. a. Explain the nutritional problems in India
   b. Discuss the nutritional programmes in detail.

II. Short Essays (Answer any five) 5 × 5 = 25 Marks

3. Food standards
4. Functions, sources and classification of lipids
5. Diet in Pregnancy
6. Weaning
7. NIN
8. Principles and methods of cooking

III. Short Answers 5 × 2 = 10 Marks

9. Rickets
10. Food preservation
11. BMR
12. Oral rehydration therapy
13. Scurvy

Biochemistry

I. Long Essays (Answer any one) 1 × 10 = 10 Marks

1. Give the IUB classification of enzymes with two examples for each class.
2. Give the sources, functions, deficiency manifestation and RDA of Vitamin C.

II. Short Essays (Answer any two) 2 × 5 = 10 Marks

3. Deficiency manifestations of vitamin A.
4. Urea cycle.
5. Functions of plasma proteins.

III. Short Answers 5 × 2 = 10 Marks

6. Essential amino acids
7. Rothera's test
8. Mention two proteolytic enzymes
9. Name the coenzyme form the Thiamine and Pyridoxine
10. Normal blood levels of cholesterol and urea.

RAJIV GANDHI UNIVERSITY OF HEALTH SCIENCES, KARNATAKA

First Year BSc Nursing (PC) Degree Examination
August 2013

Biochemistry

I. Long Essays (Answer any one)   1 × 10 = 10 Marks

1. Define oxidative phosphorylation. Describe the components of electron transport chain.
2. Describe the regulation of blood sugar level.

II. Short Essays (Answer any four)   4 × 5 = 20 Marks

3. Give an account of digestion and absorption of lipids
4. Glycogenolysis
5. Functions of plasma proteins
6. Urea cycle
7. What are isoenzymes? Give two examples with their clinical importance

III. Short Answers   4 × 2 = 8 Marks

8. Write the normal range of; (a) Blood urea, (b) Serum creatinine
9. Mitochondria
10. Name ketone bodies and test for detection of ketone bodies
11. Define Gluconeogenesis.

RAJIV GANDHI UNIVERSITY OF HEALTH SCIENCES, KARNATAKA

First Year BSc Nursing (PC) Degree Examination
August 2013

Nutrition and Dietetics

I. Long Essays (Answer any one)   1 × 10 = 10 Marks

1. a. Discuss the importance of breast feeding. b. Explain the role of nurse in promoting and implementing BFHT policy in a hospital/community setting.
2. a. What are vitamins. b. Explain the sources, functions and deficiency of Vit. B complex.

II. Short Essays (Answer any three)   3 × 5 = 15 Marks

3. Growth chart
4. Pasteurization
5. Complementary feeding
6. Rickets

III. Short Answers   5 × 2 = 10 Marks

7. Food poisoning
8. Goiter
9. Colostrum
10. Baking
11. Vit K

APPENDIX II: UNIVERSITY EXAMINATION QUESTION PAPERS

RAJIV GANDHI UNIVERSITY OF HEALTH SCIENCES, KARNATAKA

**First Year BSc Nursing (Basic) Degree Examination
March 2013 (Revised Scheme)**

Nutrition

I. Long Essays (any one)   1 × 10 = 10 Marks

1. Define nutrition. Explain the factors affecting food and nutrition.
2. Define proteins. Explain in detail the digestion, absorption, metabolism and storage of proteins.

II. Short Essays (any five)   5 × 5 = 25 Marks

3. Nutritional problems in India.
4. Food standards.
5. Function of carbohydrates.
6. Menu plan for school-going child.
7. ICDS program.
8. Vitamin A deficiency disorders.

III. Short Answers   5 × 2 = 10 Marks

9. Food Adulteration Act (PFA).
10. Scurvy.
11. Basal metabolic rate (BMR).
12. Dehydration.
13. Dietary sources of fats.

RAJIV GANDHI UNIVERSITY OF HEALTH SCIENCES, KARNATAKA

First Year BSc Nursing (Basic) Degree Examination
March 2013 (Revised Scheme)

Biochemistry

I. Long Essays (any one)   1 × 10 = 10 Marks

1. Describe the reactions of gluconeogenesis. Mention its significance.
2. What are the different types of enzyme inhibition? Explain with suitable examples.

II. Short Essays (any two)   2 × 5 = 10 Marks

3. Primary structure of proteins.
4. Isoenzymes and their clinical significance.
5. Biological role of pyridoxal phosphate.

III. Short Answers   5 × 2 = 10 Marks

6. What is the daily requirement of vitamin A and D?
7. Glucose tolerance test.
8. Active transport.
9. Define Km value. What is its significance?
10. Give the normal levels of serum cholesterol and triglycerides.

RAJIV GANDHI UNIVERSITY OF HEALTH SCIENCES, KARNATAKA

First Year BSc Nursing (Basic) Degree Examination
(Revised Scheme)

Biochemistry

I. Long Essays (any one)   1 × 10 = 10 Marks

1. Explain factors affecting enzymes activity.
2. Write a note on glucose tolerance test. Explain how blood glucose is regulated.

II. Short Essays (any four)   4 × 5 = 20 Marks

3. Clinical applications of serum enzymes.
4. Secondary structures of proteins.
5. Gout.
6. Urea cycle.
7. Classification and functions of lipoproteins.

III. Short Answers   5 × 2 = 10 Marks

8. Name any three electrolytes and their normal values.
9. Coenzymes.
10. Any four functions of plasma proteins.
11. Hyperglycemia.

RAJIV GANDHI UNIVERSITY OF HEALTH SCIENCES, KARNATAKA

First Year BSc Nursing (Basic) Degree Examination
March 2013 (Revised Scheme)

Nutrition and Dietetics

I. Long Essays (any one)   1 × 10 = 10 Marks

1. Explain in detail the method of cooking keeping in mind the preservation of nutrition.
2. Plan a therapeutic diet for a patient suffering from diabetes mellitus.

II. Short Essays (any three)   3 × 5 = 15 Marks

3. Diet in postoperative care.
4. Principles of nutrition.
5. Diet for a sick child.
6. Methods of assessing nutritional status of a child below 5 years.

III. Short Answers   5 × 2 = 10 Marks

7. Nutritive values of milk.
8. Low-cost nutritious food.
9. Proteins.
10. Food hygiene.
11. Substitutes for non-vegetarian foods.

RAJIV GANDHI UNIVERSITY OF HEALTH SCIENCES, KARNATAKA

First Year BSc Nursing (Basic) Degree Examination
March 2009 (Revised Scheme)

Biochemistry

I. Long Essays (any one)   1 × 10 = 10 Marks

1. Krebs citric acid cycle is the final common pathway of metabolism. Justify the statement, describe the cycle.
2. Give the sources, functions, deficiency manifestations and requirement of vitamin C.

II. Short Essays (any four)   4 × 5 = 20 Marks

3. Name the ketone bodies. Give their formation and fate.
4. Describe the digestion of proteins. How are the amino acids absorbed?
5. Outline the β-oxidation of fatty acids. Give the energy formed from oxidation of palmitic acid.
6. What are transaminases? Give the reactions and clinical applications.
7. Role of kidney in acid-base balance.

III. Short Answers   5 × 2 = 10 Marks

8. Name and indicate the role of two hormones that regulate blood glucose levels.
9. Coenzyme forms of vitamin B_6 and nicotinic acid.
10. Tests for detection of glucose and fructose in urine.
11. Normal serum levels of cholesterol and calcium.
12. Rickets: Cause and prevention.

RAJIV GANDHI UNIVERSITY OF HEALTH SCIENCES, KARNATAKA

First Year BSc Nursing Degree Examination
March 2009 (Revised Scheme—2)

Biochemistry

I. Long Essays (any one)   1 × 10 = 10 Marks

1. Give an account of the citric acid cycle and explain why it is called the common renal metabolic pathway. Write a short note on its energetics.
2. Discuss the sources, daily requirements and biochemical functions of vitamin A.

II. Short Essays (any three)   3 × 5 = 15 Marks

3. Classify lipoproteins. Explain their biological significance.
4. Give the sources and fate of acetyl-CoA.
5. Functions and deficiency symptoms of pyridoxine.
6. Renal regulations of blood pH.

III. Short Answers   5 × 3 = 15 Marks

7. Antioxidants.
8. Significance of isoenzymes in diagnosis of myocardial infarction.
9. Invert sugar.
10. Functions of vitamin E.
11. Normal levels of
    a. Calcium.
    b. Urea.
    c. Sodium in blood.

RAJIV GANDHI UNIVERSITY OF HEALTH SCIENCES, KARNATAKA

First Year BSc Nursing Degree Examination
March 2009 (Revised Scheme—2)

Nutrition

I. Long Essays (any two) 2 × 10 = 20 Marks

1. Discuss the various methods of food preservation. Write a note on food adulteration and its prevention.
2. Discuss the dietary management in diabetes mellitus.
3. Define balanced diet. What factors do you consider while planning?

II. Short Essays (any five) 5 × 5 = 25 Marks

4. Special nutrition program.
5. Dietary sources, functions, requirements and deficiency of calcium.
6. Steps to be taken to prevent food contamination.
7. List the nutrients which supply energy and basic factors influencing the energy needs of the body.
8. Digestion of fat in the GI tract.
9. Xerophthalmia.
10. Protein-energy malnutrition.

III. Short Answers 5 × 3 = 15 Marks

11. Pasteurization.
12. Bland diets.
13. Megaloblastic anemia.
14. Egg flip and whey water.
15. Weaning.

RAJIV GANDHI UNIVERSITY OF HEALTH SCIENCES, KARNATAKA

First Year BSc Nursing Degree Examination
September/October 2008
Nutrition and Biochemistry (Revised Scheme—2)

Nutrition

I. Long Essays 2 × 10 = 20 Marks

1. Discuss the various methods of cooking and its effects on nutrients. How can you preserve the nutrients while cooking the food?
2. Discuss proteins under the following heading:
    a. Classification.
    b. Dietary sources and requirements.
    c. Functions.
    d. Deficiency.

II. Short Essays 5 × 5 = 25 Marks

3. Define food adulteration. What are the various food adulterants commonly found in foods and how can it be prevented?
4. Discuss the digestion and absorption of carbohydrates.
5. CFTRI.
6. Short notes on pressure cooking and simmering.
7. Write the functions and imbalance of sodium in the body.

III. Short Answers 5 × 3 = 15 Marks

8. Various food standards used to ensure food quality.
9. Rickets.
10. What are macronutrients? Write its calorific value.
11. Clear liquid diets.
12. Functions of fat in the body.

RAJIV GANDHI UNIVERSITY OF HEALTH SCIENCES, KARNATAKA

First Year BSc Nursing Degree Examination
September/October 2008
Nutrition and Biochemistry (Revised Scheme—2)

Biochemistry

I. Long Essays   1 × 10 = 10 Marks

1. Describe the sources, biochemical functions, normal requirements and deficiency manifestations of thiamine.

II. Short Essays   3 × 5 = 15 Marks

2. Classify enzymes, give examples of each class.
3. Homeostasis of blood calcium.
4. Hexose monophosphate shunt and its significance.

III. Short Answers   5 × 3 = 15 Marks

5. Bile salts in urine.
6. Polysaccharides.
7. Metabolic role of zinc.
8. Pyruvate dehydrogenase enzyme complex.
9. Normal levels of:
   a. Glucose.
   b. Uric acid.
   c. Creatinine in blood.

RAJIV GANDHI UNIVERSITY OF HEALTH SCIENCES, KARNATAKA

First Year BSc Nursing Degree Examination
April 2005

Biochemistry

I. Long Essays (any one) $1 \times 10 = 10$ Marks

1. Describe citric acid cycle.
2. Explain sources, biochemical functions and deficiency of ascorbic acid.

II. Short Essays $4 \times 5 = 20$ Marks

3. Name essential fatty acids. Write its importance.
4. Define buffers. Name blood buffers and explain its role in acid-base balance.
5. Classify proteins on the basis of functions giving examples.
6. Renal function tests.

III. Short Answers $5 \times 2 = 10$ Marks

7. Glutamine formation and its importance.
8. Coenzymes of thiamine and niacin.
9. Benedict's test.
10. Night blindness.
11. Normal blood levels of calcium and phosphorus.

RAJIV GANDHI UNIVERSITY OF HEALTH SCIENCES, KARNATAKA

First Year BSc Nursing (Basic) Degree Examination
2004

Biochemistry

I. Long Essays (any one)   1 × 10 = 10 Marks

1. Describe various mechanisms of acid-base balance.
2. Describe beta-oxidation of fatty acids.

II. Short Essays   4 × 5 = 20 Marks

3. Digestion of proteins and absorption of amino acids.
4. Functions of vitamin D and its deficiency manifestations.
5. Name abnormal constituents of urine. Give their significance. How are they detected?
6. Glucose tolerance test (GTT).

III. Short Answers   5 × 2 = 10 Marks

7. Functions of nucleic acids.
8. Coenzymes of pyridoxine and riboflavin.
9. Normal blood urea and creatinine level.
10. Rickets.
11. Renal glycosuria.

RAJIV GANDHI UNIVERSITY OF HEALTH SCIENCES, KARNATAKA

First Year BSc Nursing Degree Examination
September 2003

Biochemistry

I. Long Essays (any one)   1 × 10 = 10 Marks

1. Describe the digestion and absorption of proteins.
2. What are the normal physical characteristics of urine? Mention the pathological components of urine, how are they detected?

II. Short Essays (any four)   4 × 5 = 20 Marks

3. Explain in detail the significance of the pentose phosphate pathway.
4. Write briefly on phenyl ketonuria.
5. Explain in brief alkalosis and acidosis.
6. Outline the transamination reaction with a suitable example. Give its clinical significance.
7. Describe GTT.

III. Short Answers   5 × 2 = 10 Marks

8. Name two biologically important compounds derived from cholesterol.
9. Give four hormones formed from tyrosine.
10. Beriberi.
11. RDA of vitamin D and vitamin C.
12. Name the renal function tests based on glomerular filtration.

RAJIV GANDHI UNIVERSITY OF HEALTH SCIENCES, KARNATAKA

First Year BSc Nursing Degree Examination
April 2003

Biochemistry

I. Long Essays (any one)   1 × 10 = 10 Marks

1. Explain metabolism of glycine and state its metabolic importance.
2. Explain sources, daily requirements, functions and deficiency diseases of vitamin A.

II. Short Essays   4 × 5 = 20 Marks

3. Diagnostic importance of enzymes.
4. Mucopolysaccharides.
5. Fatty liver and lipotropic factors.
6. Liver function tests.

III. Short Answers   5 × 2 = 10 Marks

7. Blood glucose level and renal threshold value.
8. Nucleotides of biological importance.
9. Functions of vitamin K.
10. Test for urinary ketone bodies.
11. Sodium and potassium levels in plasma.

RAJIV GANDHI UNIVERSITY OF HEALTH SCIENCES, KARNATAKA

First Year BSc Nursing Degree Examination
May 2002 (New Scheme)

Biochemistry

I. Long Essays (any one) $1 \times 10 = 10$ Marks

1. How are carbohydrates digested and absorbed?
2. Name the renal function tests. Indicate their significance. How is creatinine clearance test performed?

II. Short Essays $4 \times 5 = 20$ Marks

3. Oral glucose tolerance test.
4. Ketone bodies.
5. Classification of proteins.
6. Ascorbic acid.

III. Short Answers $5 \times 2 = 10$ Marks

7. Sources and daily requirements of vitamin A.
8. What are essential fatty acids? Name them.
9. Name the major plasma lipoproteins.
10. What is the normal pH of blood? Name two plasma buffers.
11. What is the function of 1,25-dihydroxycholecalciferol?

RAJIV GANDHI UNIVERSITY OF HEALTH SCIENCES, KARNATAKA

First Year BSc Nursing Degree Examination
April 2002

Nutrition

I. Long Essays (any one)   1× 10 = 10 Marks

1. What is balanced diet? Name essential nutrients. Mention basic functions of this nutrients.
2. Enumerate kidney function tests. Describe any one test which will help for the assessment of kidney function.

II. Short Essays (any four)   4 × 5 = 20 Marks

3. Physical characteristics of urine.
4. Serum electrolyte levels.
5. Acidosis and alkalosis.
6. Digestion of carbohydrates.
7. Homeostasis of blood.

III. Short Answers   5 × 2 = 10 Marks

8. Mention the normal range of fasting and postprandial blood sugar, serum cholesterol and total protein.
9. Enumerate the kidney function tests.
10. Name two fat soluble vitamins and their food sources.
11. Name two water soluble vitamins and their requirements.
12. Name the tests which detect carbohydrates and protein in urine. Explain one test for the detection of protein in urine.

RAJIV GANDHI UNIVERSITY OF HEALTH SCIENCES, KARNATAKA

First Year BSc Nursing Degree Examination
October 2001 (New Scheme)

Biochemistry

I. Long Essays (any one)   1 × 10 = 10 Marks

1. Describe glycogen metabolism.
2. Describe the sources, daily requirements, functions and deficiency diseases of vitamin A.

II. Short Essays   4 × 5 = 20 Marks

3. Digestion and absorption of lipids.
4. Functions of plasma proteins.
5. Urea cycle.
6. Classification of amino acids.

III. Short Answers   5 × 2 = 10 Marks

7. Benedict's test.
8. Dietary sources and RDA of vitamin C.
9. Protein digesting enzymes secreted by pancreas.
10. Bile salts.
11. Milk sugar.

RAJIV GANDHI UNIVERSITY OF HEALTH SCIENCES, KARNATAKA

First Year BSc Nursing Degree Examination
October 2001 (Old Scheme)

Biochemistry

I. Long Essays (any one)   1 × 10 = 10 Marks

1. Write about the dietary sources, daily requirements and functions of vitamin A.
2. How is oral glucose tolerance test performed? How is blood glucose level maintained?

II. Short Essays (any four)   4 × 5 = 20 Marks

3. Essential amino acids.
4. Digestion and absorption of carbohydrates.
5. Name bile acids and mention about the functions of bile salts.
6. Metabolic acidosis.
7. Benedict's qualitative test.

III. Short Answers   5 × 2 = 10 Marks

8. What is a simple protein? Give two examples.
9. What is lecithin?
10. van den Bergh test.
11. What is normal sodium and potassium level?
12. Give two important functions of insulin.

RAJIV GANDHI UNIVERSITY OF HEALTH SCIENCES, KARNATAKA

First Year BSc Nursing Degree Examination
September 2001

Biochemistry

I. Long Essays (any one)   1 × 10 = 10 Marks

1. Describe digestion and absorption of proteins.
2. Mention the normal pH of blood. Explain how is it maintained?

II. Short Essays (any four)   4 × 5 = 20 Marks

3. Describe the pathway of fatty acid oxidation.
4. Regulation of plasma calcium level.
5. Role of insulin in regulation of blood glucose level.
6. Sources and functions of vitamin A.
7. Structure and functions of glycogen.

III. Short Answers   5 × 2 = 10 Marks

8. Ketogenesis.
9. Test for detection of proteins in urine.
10. Essential fatty acids.
11. Glycosuria.
12. van den Bergh test.

RAJIV GANDHI UNIVERSITY OF HEALTH SCIENCES, KARNATAKA

First Year BSc Nursing Degree Examination
May 2001 (New Scheme)

Biochemistry

I. Long Essays (any one) 1 × 10 = 10 Marks

1. Write an essay on digestion and absorption of proteins.
2. Name B complex vitamins with an essay on the biochemical functions of any one of them.

II. Short Essays 4 × 5 = 20 Marks

3. Polysaccharides.
4. Classification of lipids.
5. Clearance tests.
6. Vitamin K.

III. Short Answers 5 × 2 = 10 Marks

7. Sources of vitamin D.
8. Test for ketone bodies.
9. Calorific value of proteins and fats.
10. Xerophthalmia.
11. Insulin effect on carbohydrate metabolism.

RAJIV GANDHI UNIVERSITY OF HEALTH SCIENCES, KARNATAKA

First Year BSc Nursing Degree Examination
May 2001 (Old Scheme)

Biochemistry

I. Long Essays (any one)   1 × 10 = 10 Marks

1. Describe glycogen metabolism in the liver in the fed and fasting state.
2. Write an essay on essential nutrients.

II. Short Essays (any four)   4 × 5 = 20 Marks

3. Name the dietary essential amino acids and classify them.
4. Name the plasma lipoproteins and give their functions.
5. Discuss the water balance.
6. Describe the renal tubular mechanism operating for the reabsorption of sodium.
7. What are the functions of vitamin C.

III. Short Answers   5 × 2 = 10 Marks

8. Name the enzymes catalyzing the following reactions:
   a. Arginine → Ornithine + urea.
   b. $CO_2 + H_2O \rightarrow H_2CO_3$.
9. What is the percentage of NaCl in isotonic saline?
10. How is glutamine synthesized in the brain?
11. What is the clinical significance of plasma HDL cholesterol.
12. Give the normal range of values in blood of:
    a. Fasting glucose.
    b. Serum creatinine.
    c. Blood urea.
    d. Serum total cholesterol.

RAJIV GANDHI UNIVERSITY OF HEALTH SCIENCES, KARNATAKA

First Year BSc Nursing Degree Examination
April 2001

Biochemistry

I. Long Essays (any one) $1 \times 10 = 10$ **Marks**

1. Discuss about the digestion and absorption of lipids.
2. What is the normal fasting blood glucose level? Discuss in detail about blood glucose homeostasis.

II. Short Essays $4 \times 5 = 20$ **Marks**

3. Structure of starch.
4. Respiratory acidosis.
5. Ketosis.
6. Primary structure of proteins.

III. Short Answers $5 \times 2 = 10$ **Marks**

7. Name any four enzymes of diagnostic importance.
8. Write the normal serum levels of:
   a. Total bilirubin.
   b. Total cholesterol.
   c. Bicarbonate.
   d. Uric acid.
9. What is uronic acid? Mention the functions of glucuronic acid.
10. Name the key enzymes of gluconeogenesis.
11. Pellagra.

RAJIV GANDHI UNIVERSITY OF HEALTH SCIENCES, KARNATAKA

First Year BSc Nursing Degree Examination
October 2000 (New Scheme)

Biochemistry

I. Long Essays (any one)   1 × 10 = 10 Marks

1. Discuss glycolysis in liver.
2. Write the dietary sources of proteins, requirements, functions and deficiency disorders.

II. Short Essays   4 × 5 = 20 Marks

3. Discuss the sources, requirements and functions of vitamin C.
4. What is the normal biochemical composition of CSF? How do they vary in disease?
5. How are proteins digested?
6. Give the significance of breastfeeding.

III. Short Answers   5 × 2 = 10 Marks

7. NPN substances excreted in urine.
8. Isotonic saline, its preparation and uses.
9. Normal levels of total cholesterol and HDL cholesterol in serum.
10. Creatinine clearance test.
11. Gout.

RAJIV GANDHI UNIVERSITY OF HEALTH SCIENCES, KARNATAKA

First Year BSc Nursing Degree Examination
October 2000 (Old Scheme)

Nutrition

I. Long Essays (any one)   1 × 10 = 10 Marks

1. Define homeostasis. How do hormones maintain blood glucose homeostasis?
2. Give the dietary sources, requirements, functions and deficiency manifestations of vitamin A.

II. Short Essays   4 × 5 = 20 Marks

3. How is a 5% dextrose solution preferred and sterilized? What are its uses?
4. Why should an uncontrolled diabetes mellitus patient develop metabolic acidosis?
5. Explain the functions of bile in digestion.
6. Name the digestive enzymes of pancreas. Brief out their functions.

III. Short Answers   5 × 2 = 10 Marks

7. Give the significance of blood urea estimation.
8. What is the normal color of urine? What do you infer when the urine of a patient is deep yellow?
9. A sample of urine reduces Benedict's reagent. Give two reasons for the reduction.
10. What is the nutritional value of ripe papaya fruit?
11. How is parboiled rice nutritionally superior to raw rice?

KERALA UNIVERSITY

First Year BSc Nursing Degree Examination
September/October 2008

Paper II—Physiology Including Biochemistry Response Sheet for MCQs

Time: 10 Minutes **Maximum: 5 Marks**

Directions

1. Write the name of examination, month and year, subject of the day's examination and register number in the space provided.
2. Select the one most appropriate response and encircle the corresponding alphabet against each Question Number in the Response Sheet.
3. Enter the total number of your responses in the appropriate box provided at the end.

Question No.

1.	A	B	C	D
2.	A	B	C	D
3.	A	B	C	D
4.	A	B	C	D
5.	A	B	C	D
6.	A	B	C	D
7.	A	B	C	D
8.	A	B	C	D
9.	A	B	C	D
10.	A	B	C	D

Total Number of Responses

Name of Examination…..……………....………………….….2008
Subject…………………………………….....……………………
Register Number….....….

Nutrition and Biochemistry for Nurses

Note: 1. Do not write anything on the question paper.
2. Write your register number on the answer sheet provided.
3. Select the appropriate answer and encircle the alphabet against each question in the answer sheet provided.
4. In the answer sheet enter the total number of your answers in the appropriate box provided.
5. Each question carries ½ mark.

1. **Hypermetropia is corrected by:** (10 × ½ = 5 Marks)
   A. Biconvex lens B. Biconcave lens
   C. Cylindrical lens D. None of the above
2. **Hormone which increases blood calcium level is:**
   A. Insulin B. Parathormone
   C. Glucagon D. Calcitonin
3. **Hormone responsible for secretion of milk is:**
   A. Oxytocin B. Prolactin
   C. Estrogen D. FSH
4. **Intrinsic factor is secreted by:**
   A. Chief cells B. Mucus neck cells
   C. Parietal cells D. Peptic cells
5. **Renal threshold for glucose in a normal individual is:**
   A. 0 mg/100 mL B. 300 mg/100 mL
   C. 180 mg/100 mL D. 325 mg/100 mL
6. **Lateral geniculate body receives:**
   A. Auditory fibers B. Touch fibers
   C. Olfactory fibers D. Visual fibers
7. **Hyperbaric oxygen therapy is useful in following condition:**
   A. High attitude B. Severe anemia
   C. Cyanide poisoning D. Congestive cardiac failure
8. **Gastric acid secretion is inhibited by:**
   A. Acetylcholine B. Histamine
   C. Gastrin D. Somatostatin
9. **Pacinian corpuscle is:**
   A. Pain receptor B. Taste receptor
   C. Temperature receptor D. Pressure receptor
10. **In conduction deafness:**
    A. Air conduction is better than bone conduction
    B. Bone conduction is better than air conduction
    C. There is no relationship between air conduction and bone conduction
    D. Both air conduction and bone conduction are equal.

KERALA UNIVERSITY

(Pages : 1 + 2 = 3)

Name.....................
Reg. No..................

First Year BSc Nursing Degree Examination
September/October 2008
Part I—Biological Sciences
Paper II—Physiology Including Biochemistry

Time: 2 Hours Maximum: 50 Marks

1. Answer Sections A and B in separate answer books.
2. Draw diagrams wherever necessary.
3. Question I should be answered first in the response sheet provided.

SECTION A (PHYSIOLOGY)

I. Multiple choice questions (on attached separate sheet).
   (5 Marks)
II. Enumerate the clotting factors. Explain the intrinsic mechanism of coagulation. **(3 + 5 = 8 Marks)**
III. Write briefly on any four questions: **(4 × 2 = 8 Marks)**
   a. Vital capacity.
   b. Juxtaglomerular apparatus.
   c. Reflex arc.
   d. Normal ECG as in lead II.
   e. Tests for ovulation.
IV. Explain the mechanism of skeletal muscle contraction. **(4 Marks)**

SECTION B (BIOCHEMISTRY)

V. a. Write an essay on liver function tests. **(6 Marks)**
   b. Write briefly the regulation of blood glucose level. **(4 Marks)**
VI. Write briefly on: **(2 × 3 = 6 Marks)**
   a. Phenyl ketonuria.
   b. Metabolic acidosis.
VII. Write briefly on: **(3 × 3 = 9 Marks)**
   a. Plasma proteins.
   b. Hypocalcemia.
   c. Lysosomes.

KERALA UNIVERSITY

Name......................
Reg. No..................

First Year BSc Nursing Degree Examination, January 2008

Part III—Community Health
Paper II—Nutrition (New Scheme)

Time: 2 Hours   Maximum: 50 Marks

SECTION A

(5 + 10 = 15 Marks)

I. a. Bring out the importance of protein in human body.
   b. Discuss protein under the following headings:
   i. Metabolism.
   ii. Sources.
   iii. Requirements.

II. Write briefly on any two of the follwing: (2 × 5 = 10 Marks)

   a. Anemia.
   b. Kwashiorkor.
   c. Food spoilage.

SECTION B

(5 + 10 = 15 Marks)

III. a. Explain the principles of food preservation.
   b. Enumerate the various methods adopted in home situation for food preservation and storage.

IV. a. Write any two short notes given below or answer the essay:
(2 × 5 = 10 Marks)

   i. Nutritional needs of infants.
   ii. Rickets.
   iii. Ariboflavinosis.

Or

(10 Marks)

   b. Give an account of functions and deficiencies of thiamine.

KERALA UNIVERSITY
First Year BSc Nursing Degree Examination
Nutrition and Biochemistry

I. Short Notes (any five)   **5 × 4 = 20 Marks**

1. Nutritional problems in India.
2. Classification of foods.
3. Food standards in India.
4. Better methods of cooking.
5. Food Adulteration Act.
6. Food additives and its principles.
7. Methods to retain nutrients in food.

II. Multiple Choice Questions   **10 × ½ = 5 Marks**

1. Optimum of nutrition means:
   a. Lack of nutrition
   b. Correct amount of nutrition
   c. Imbalance of nutrition
   d. Correct amount and proportion of nutrition
2. All enzymes are:
   a. Protein
   b. Carbohydrate
   c. Vitamin
   d. Mineral
3. One of the most important function of vitamin is:
   a. Energy giving
   b. Protection from infection
   c. Body building
   d. Production of enzymes
4. The maximum energy source in ones diet should be from:
   a. Fat
   b. Protein
   c. Carbohydrate
   d. Water
5. The energy contribution from protein is:
   a. 4 kcal
   b. 6 kcal
   c. 7 kcal
   d. 9 kcal

6. Nutrients needed in amounts of a gram or more per day are categorized as:
    a. Micronutrients
    b. Macronutrients
    c. Essential nutrients
    d. Mineral nutrients
7. The source of cellulose is:
    a. Liver
    b. Meat
    c. Plant food
    d. Sugar
8. Storage form of carbohydrate in the body:
    a. Glycerol
    b. Glycogen
    c. Fatty acid
    d. Fiber
9. Malnutrition means:
    a. Lack of nutrition leading to ill health
    b. Undesirable kind of nutrition leading to ill health
    c. Correct amount of nutrition
    d. Correct proportion of nutrition
10. Scurvy is a deficiency disease of:
    a. Vitamin A
    b. Vitamin D
    c. Vitamin C
    d. Iodine

CALICUT UNIVERSITY

First Year BSc Nursing Degree Examination 2008
(Revised Syllabus—2007)

Nutrition and Biochemistry
(Pattern of Questions)

Time: 2 Hours 30 Minutes   Maximum: 75 Marks

(SECTION A Nutrition—50 Marks
and
SECTION B Biochemistry—25 Marks)

TEST DESIGN—Details of weightage. For Nutrition
(50 Marks)

I. Objective Type (20%)	
a. MCQs	5 Marks
b. Matching type	5 Marks
II. Very Short Answer Type (40%)	
a. Definitions/List	5 Marks
b. Give reasons/Differentiate between	5 Marks
III. Short Answers (20%)	
To answer 3 questions out of 4	$3 \times 5 = 15$ Marks
IV. Essay Type (20%)	
One essay question	$1 \times 15 = 15$ Marks
Total	50 Marks

TEST DESIGN—Details of weightage. For Biochemistry
(25 Marks)

I. MCQs	5 Marks
II. Short Answers	10 Marks
III. Essay	10 Marks

DIFFICULTY INDEX

Sl No	Difficulty Index	Percentage
1.	Average	60
2.	Difficult	20
3.	Easy	20

Index

Page numbers followed by *f* refer to figure and *t* refer to table respectively.

A

Acetoacetic acid, Gerhardt's test 249
Acetone bodies 249
Acetyl-CoA synthesis 177*f*
Acid-base
  balance, measurement 235
  imbalance 235
  regulation 310
Acidosis 235
Acquired immunity 202
Acrolein formation 40
Actin 208
Active transport of glucose 133
Acupressure 410
Acute
  renal failure 439, 440
    dietary management 440
    symptoms 439
  type diarrhea 423
Addison's disease 423
Adenosine
  diphosphate 140
  triphosphate 7, 52, 140
Adipose tissue, metabolism 178
Adolescent 392
  boy, menu plan 396*t*
ADP See Adenosine diphosphate
Adrenal
  cortex 221
  medulla 220
Adrenaline 216
Adrenocorticotropic hormone 165, 167, 223
Adult gastric juice 128
Adult-onset diabetes 433

Adults, menu plan 402*t*
Aerobic glycolysis 151
Agmark standard 347
Air therapy 410
Alanine 53
  transaminase 191
Albumin 231
Albumin See Plasma proteins
Albumin See Proteins, test
Albumin water 353
Aldehyde 23
Alkalosis 235
Allergy 386
Alpha-hydroxy ketone See also
    Aldehyde
Amine hormones 216
Amino acids 13, 52, 60, 192, 299
Amino acids See Proteins, absorption
Amino acids
  chemical properties 55
  classification 54
  functions 55
  metabolism 146
  occurrence 55
  physical properties 55
  properties 55
  structure 54
Amino group, properties 60
Amla 360
Ammonia 70
  test 247
Ammonium sulfate 112
Amylopectin 30
Amylose 30
Anabolism, features 190*t*

Anaerobic glycolysis 151
Androgens 214
Anemia 399
  causes 321
  deficiency of iron 321
  hemochromatosis 322
  hemosiderosis 322
Animal
  foods 361
  starch See Glycogen
Anthropometric measurements 366
"Antibody-mediated immune response" 203
Anticoagulants 226
Antioxidants 206
Antioxidants, action 206
Antithyroid agents 218
Anuria 439
Arginine to form ornithine and urea, cleavage 194
Argininosuccinic acid
  synthesis 194
  to produce arginine, cleavage 194
Arrowroot conjee 356
Arthritis 437
Artificial feeding 387
Ascorbic acid 41
Ascorbic acid See also Vitamin C
Aspartate transaminase 191
Aspartic acid 53, 194
Asymmetric carbon atoms 19
Atherosclerosis 442
ATP See Adenosine triphosphate
ATP
  generated in TCA cycle 157
  "molecules gain in aerobic glycolysis" 153t
  synthetase complexes 7
Autoradiography 10
"Average water balances in normal adult" 329t

B

B complex group of vitamins 85
B complex vitamins 359
BMR See Basal metabolic rate
Balanced diet 18
  budgeting 357
  planning 362
  with high cost 363
  with low cost 363
  with moderate cost 363
Barfoed's test 24
Barley water, beverages 353
Basal metabolic rate 217, 285
  definition 285
  measurement 285
  normal value 286
Basedow's disease 436
Benedict's
  qualitative 247
  test 23, 247
  for reducing sugar 247t
Benzidine test for blood in urine 248
Benzoic acid 341
β-hydroxybutyric acid 180
β-oxidation of fatty acids 175
Bicarbonate buffers 233
Bile
  pigments 136, 248
  salts 137, 248
Bilirubin 136, 258
  level, abnormalities 260t
  metabolism, abnormalities 258
Biliverdin 136
Biochemistry
  scope 3
  to nursing, importance 4
Biological oxidation 141
Biosynthesis 217
Biotin 89
Biuret test 73
Black coffee, beverages 352
Blood
  buffers 233
  chemistry 226
  clotting 226
  constituents 226, 227t
  functions 228
  glucose
    in postabsorptive state 164
  level 165
    abnormalities 159
    homeostasis 163
    regulation 163
  urea 253
Body
  building foods 362
  mass index 289

Body's defence system 303
Boiling food 340
Bones, calcification 310
Brain cells 16
Breast milk 382
Breastfeeding 384
    advantages 384
Bright's disease 439
Bromsulfalein excretion test 264
Buttered egg See also Scrambled

C

Calcium
    absorption 308
    dietary
        allowance 308
        sources 308
    distribution 308
    functions 308
    hypercalcemia 309
    hypocalcemia 309
        causes 309
        osteoporosis 309
        symptoms 309
        tetany 309
    product 307, 309
    source 359
Calories 379, 391, 399
    and carbohydrates, insulin and meal distribution 433t
Calorigenic effect 218
Canning food 340
Carbohydrates 143, 144, 146, 284, 290, 383, 400, 419, 429, 440, 433t,
    absorption 132
    changes 337
    characteristics 18
    chemistry 16
    digestion 130
    excess 293
    foods 361
    functions 290
    in mouth, digestion 130
    in small intestine, digestion 130
    in stomach, digestion 130
    metabolism 145, 217, 218
        effects 220
    reactions 22
    requirements 291
    sources 17, 290

    test 23
    tolerance 161
Carbon
    dioxide 229
    tetrachloride 259
Carboxylic
    acid group 65
    group, properties 55
Cardiovascular diseases 442
    causes 443
    energy 443
    fat 443
    hypertension 443
    minerals 443
    of diet 443, 444
    of dietary management 442
    proteins 443
    symptoms 444
    types 442, 444
    vitamins 443
Cardiovascular system 398
Catabolism, features 190t
Catachrome system 141
Cell
    composition 5
    functions 5
    mediated immune response 203
    structure 5
    ultrastructure 5f
Cellular enzymes 6
Cellulose 17, 31
"Central nervous system, depression" 236
Cephalins 43
Cereals 359
Cerebral thrombosis 399
Cerebrosides 18, 37, 44
Child development
    program 373
    services 273
Chloride 314
    dietary sources 314
    functions 315
    hypochloremia 315
    normal level 314
    recommended dietary allowance 314
    test 246
Chloroform 259
Cholecystokinin 222
Cholelithiasis
    energy 431
    fat 431

Cholestatic syndrome 266
Cholesterol
　absorption 135
　biosynthesis 181
　biosynthetic pathway 183f
　functions 46, 296
Cholic 386
　acid 137
Chromium 322
　requirements 323
　sources 322
Chromotherapy 410
Chronic
　renal failure 440
　　dietary management 440
　type diarrhea 423
Chyme 128
Cirrhosis of liver hepatic coma
　precipitating factors 430
Citric acid cycle 153, 155f
　common pathway 157, 157f
　steps 156
　summary 156
Citrulline, synthesis 193
Classification and structure of amino
　acids 54
Clear-fluid diets 351
Climate 286
Clonal selection theory 204
Clostridium botulinum 342
Coagulation
　factors 264
　vitamin See Vitamin K
Cobalamin 94
Cobalt 323
　deficiency manifestation 323
　dietary
　　allowance 323
　　sources 323
Coenzymes 105, 120
　classification 121
　in metabolism 142f
　with groups 121t
Cold
　storage and freezing 339
　test 247
Collagen 207
Colloidal nature 71
Color reactions of proteins 73
Colors, changes 337

Community
　health nurse in nutrition 376
　Nutrition Programs in India 372
Competitive inhibition 119f
Complete proteins 53
Compound lipids 37
Conjugated proteins 69
　based 70
Constituent of bones and teeth 310
Contractile
　muscle 70
　proteins 208
Cookery rules 332
Cooking
　baking 335
　boiling 336
　changes 337
　food
　　aims 332
　　objectives 332
　frying 335
　grilling 336
　in air 334
　in water 334
　media 334
　methods 333
　microwave cooking 336
　poaching 336
　pressure cooking 337
　purpose 332
　roasting 334
　steaming 336
Copper 316
　dietary
　　requirement 316
　　sources 316
　function 316
Coronary
　heart disease 442
　thrombosis 399
Corticosteroids, effects 221
Corticotropin See also
　Adrenocorticotropic hormone
Cow's milk 382, 387
Creatine synthesis 245
Creatinine 244
　clearance test 254
Crohn's disease 206
Cushing's syndrome 314
Cytoplasm 6, 7
Cytosol 7

D

Daily nutrition evaluation sheet 435*t*
Daily recommended protein intake 301*t*
Dal soup 354
D-amino acid-oxidase acts 114
Dark field microscopy 10
Decarboxylation 192
Deep fat frying 335
Deficiency manifestations of
   macrominerals 326*t*
   microminerals 326t
Degenerative arthritis 437
Dental caries 293
Deoxyribonucleic acid 102
Derived
   lipids 37
   proteins 69
Dextran 31
D-glucuronic acid 32
Diabetes 167
   mellitus 160, 216, 431
      causes 160, 432
      continued symptoms 432
      dietary fiber 434
      fiber 434
      food exchange lists 433
      foods 436
      nutritional requirements 434
      oral glucose tolerance test 161
      other possible symptoms 432
      symptoms 432
      types 432
   types 161
Diabetic
   diet prescription 433
   "patients and weight loss on work" 433*t*
   type of GTC 163
"Diagnostic value of plasma enzymes" 121
Dialysis 73
Diarrhea 274, 386, 423
   constipation 424
   dietary
      considerations 424, 425
      management 425
   electrolytes 424
   foods to
      avoided 426
      included 426
   "modificaton of diet in bleeding ulcer" 426
   nutrient malabsorption 424
   peptic ulcer 425
Diazotized sulfanilic acid 259
Diet 270
   for preschool child 391
   for school children 391
   in hospitals, types 414
   in relation to
      "conditions of gastrointestinal tract" 423
      disease of liver and gallbladder 427
   therapy 413
      in conditions of circulatory system 442
      principles 413
Dietary
   consideration for teenagers 392
   counseling 437
   examination 367
   fibers 291, 292
   "management, precipitating factors" 430
   "modifications, precipitating factors" 430
   sources 310
   of proteins 302
Dietetics 270
Digestive fluids 127
Dihydroxyacetone phosphate, isomerization 151
Dilution test 255
Dioxygen See Oxygen, supply
Diphtheria, poliomyelitis 415
Disaccharides 26, 27*t*
Disturbances in homeostasis 235
DNA See Deoxyribonucleic acid
DNA
   "molecule, double helix structure" 104*f*
   structure 102
Drugs 286
Duration of meal 443

E

Ease of digestion 420
Edema 399
EFA See Essential fatty acids
EFA
   contents of vegetable sources 297
   deficiency 297

effects 297
Egg 361
　flip 353
　preparation 352, 353
Eggnog See Egg flip
Ehrlich test 261
"Ehrlich's aldehyde test for
　　urobilinogen" 249
Elastin 207
Electrolyte sodium 330
Electrolytes 329
　content of ECF and ICF 330*t*
　distribution 329
Electron
　carriers 143
　microscopy 10
　transport 142
　　chain 144*f*, 156
Electrophoresis 231
　principle 231
Elevated serum lipoproteins 173
Embden-Meyerhof pathway 150
Endocrinal 286
Endocrine
　factors 222
　"glands, therapeutic diet in
　　conditions" 431
　system 399
Endoplasmic reticulum 6
Energetics 157, 176
"Energy" 377, 382, 418, 419, 429, 438,
　440
　expenditure, factors affecting 284
　"from metabolic fuels, extraction" 144
　production in glycolysis 153
　　and TCA cycle 157
　source 140
　yielding foods 362
Enforcement 346
Enteropeptidase 128
Environmental temperature 286, 289
Enzyme 7, 70, 112
　action 310
　　mechanism 115
　activity 117*f*
　　and pH 118*f*
　　and substrate concentration 116*f*
　　and temperature 118*f*
　　factors affecting 115
　regulation 310

aminopeptidases 188
carboxypeptidases 188
chymotrypsin 188
classification 113
concentration 117*f*
　effect 117
differences 211
dipeptidases 188
in diseases, increase of different 122*t*
inhibition 119
isomerases 114
ligases 114
lyases 113
non-specific inhibition 120
oxidoreductases 113
pepsin 188
properties 112
proteins 65
"reactions with free radicals
　byproducts" 205
role 188
similarities with 210
specific inhibition 119
specificity 114
transferases 113
trypsin 188
Enzymology 112
Epinephrine 166, 220
Erythrocytes See Red blood cells
Essential
　amino acids 53
　fatty acids 297
　hypertension 443
Ethanolamine cephalin See
　Phosphatidyl ethanolamine
Ethereal sulfate, test 246
Ethylenediaminetetraacetic acid 228
Eukaryotes 9
Eukaryotic cells 9
Exophthalmic goiter 436
Extracellular fluid 329
Extraction of energy from metabolic
　fuels 144*f*

F

Factors
　affecting BMR 285
　influencing nutrition 276*f*
　regulating hormone action 212

FAD See Flavin adenine dinucleotide
Fasciculata cells 223
Fat 291, 383
  requirements of individuals 295
Fate of glucose after absorption 149
Fats 294, 297, 361, 379, 400, 420, 429
  "types iodine numbers, different" 41*t*
  biological significance 36
  characteristics 41
  chemical
    composition 38
    properties 40
  digestion 131
  important sources 294*t*
  in mouth, digestion 131
  in small intestine, digestion 131
  in stomach, digestion 131
  physical properties 39
  properties 39
  sources 359
Fat-soluble
  and water-soluble vitamins,
    differences between 77
  "vitamins See also Vitamins not
    acting as coenzymes"
Fatty
  acids 36, 38
  contents in blood 42*t*
  liver
    and lipotropic factors 179
    causes 180
    physiological 180
Feeding
  bottle, method of sterilization 387
  requirements 416, 417
Fever 419
  general dietary considerations 419
Fiber 290
Fibrous proteins 68
  collagens 68
  elastins 68
  fibrin 68
  keratins 68
  myosins 68
Fire therapy 410
Fish 361
Five food group system 281
Flavin
  adenine dinucleotide 107, 142
  mononucleotide 86, 107

nucleotide coenzymes 107
Fluid 383, 400, 418, 420, 438, 440
  diets 352
  mosaic model of cell membrane 11
Fluorine 323
  absorption and excretion 323
  deficiency syndromes 324
  dietary sources 323
  functions 323
  recommended dietary allowance 323
  toxicity 324
FMN See Flavin mononucleotide
Folacin 88
Folic acid See also Folacin
Food 269, 270
  and agricultural organization 368
  budget, plans 357
  calorie 283
    value 283
  choice 282
  classification 281
  content 434
  convection 333
  different types 352
  functional classification 362
  functions 278
  "groups and guidelines for selection"
    358
  guide pyramid for older adults 283*f*
  habits and selection of foodstuffs,
    factors influencing 276
  intoxication 342
  laws 345
  medicinal value, role 279
  methods 338
  needs of adolescents 392
  chemical composition 281
  function 281
  nutrition value 281
  origin 281
  preparation 357
  preservation 338
    methods 339
    principles 339
  principles 338
  radiation 334
  selection 357
  spoilage, causes 338
  standards 345
  storage 357

suitable for preschooler, types 391
therapy 410
Foodborne
  diseases 342
    types 342
  infections 343
Forbidden clones 204
Fouchet's
  reagent 249
  test 258, 261
    for bile pigments 249
Free nucleotides 104
Free radicals 205
Fruit juice, beverages 353
Fruits 360
Full fat milk powder 360
Full-fluid diet 351, 415
Functions manifestations of
  macrominerals 326*t*
  microminerals 326*t*
Furanose ring 21

G

Galactose by intestinal epithelial cells
    See also Active transport of glucose
Galactosemia 167
Gallbladder, function 431
Gamma-glutamyltransferase 266
Gastric juice, digestive fluids 127
Gastrin 221
Gastrointestinal
  bleeding 430
  hormones 221
  tract 398
Gastrostomy 416
Gelatin 68
Gender 286
Geriatric nutrition 398
Globular proteins 69
  albumins 69
  globulins 69
Globulin 230, 231
  ratio See albumin
  ratio See Plasma proteins
Glomerular
  filtration rate 253
  function, tests 253
Glomerulonephritis 438
  principles of diet 438
  symptoms 438
Glucagon 166, 216
Glucocorticoids 166
Gluconeogenesis 165
Glucose 13
  active transport 132*f*
  plus
    fructose 28
    galactose See Lactose
  to cells, transport 150
  tolerance test 162*f*
Glucosis 149
Glutamate
  oxaloacetate transaminase 191
  pyruvate transaminase 191
Glycogen 31
  synthesis See Glycogenesis
Glycogenesis 149
Glycogenic amino acids 165
Glycogenolysis 149, 164
Glycogenolytic hormone 216
Glycolipids 37
Glycolipids See Cerebrosides
Glycolysis 151, 154*f*
  "Embden-Meyerhof pathway" 150, 152*f*
  reactions 150
Glycoproteins 70
Glycosuria 160
Gmelin's test 258
  for bile pigments 248
Goiter 219
Gout 437
  fluids 437
  protein 437
Graves' disease 436
Green leafy vegetables 360
Growth hormone 167, 222

H

Hard-cooked egg 354
Haworth projections 21
Hay's test for bile salts 248
Health 269, 271
Healthy food items in nature cure 411*t*
Heart ailment 297
Heat and acetic acid test 247
Heller's nitric acid test 247
Heme 228
Hemoglobin 233, 367

Index

buffers 234
Hemolytic 258
  jaundice 259, 261
    types obstructive jaundice,
      difference between 261
Hemoproteins 70
Heparin 227
Hepatic
  jaundice 258, 259
  transport function, test 264
Hepatitis virus 259
Heteropolysaccharides 29
Hexose 25
  monophosphate 145
    shunt 150, 159
High infant-mortality rate 281
High-calorie diet 437
High-protein diet 437
Histocompatibility complex 204
Homeostasis 163f
Homopolysaccharides 29
Hormonal state See also Endocrinal
Hormones 70
  chemistry 210
  classification 211
  functions 210
  in homeostasis of blood sugar level,
    role 165
  introduction 210
  mode of action 212
  of anterior pituitary 222
  secreting glands 211
  secretion 211
Hospital diets 351
  types 351
Human leukocyte antigens 204
  complex 204
Humoral response 203
Hydrochloric acid 128, 240
Hydrogenation 40
Hydrolysis of starch 30, 30f
Hydroxyl radical 206
Hydroxyproline 208
Hyperbilirubinemia 258
Hyperglycemia
  causes 160
  in diabetes mellitus 215
Hyperthyroidism 219, 436
Hypervitaminosis
  A 81
  B_2 87

B_3 88
B_6 87
C 85
D 82
E 83
K 84
Hypocalcemia, cause 82
Hypoglycemia, causes 160
Hypoglycemic in nature see Blood
  glucose levels
Hypophosphatemia, cause 82
"Hypothalamic hormones and pituitary"
  222
Hypothyroidism 219, 436

I

ICF See Intracellular fluid
Icterus 258
Immune response 202
Immunity 202
  types 202
Immunochemistry 202
Immunocompetent cell 203
Indian gooseberry See Amla
Infection, resistance 279
Infective hepatitis 427
  cholelithiasis 431
  cirrhosis of liver symptoms 428
  dietary management 427
  foods to
    avoided 428
    included 428
  symptoms 427
Influenza 421
Innate immunity 202
Inorganic
  ions 243
  sulfates, test 246
Insulin 165, 215
  antagonism 161
  deficiency 216
  dependent diabetes mellitus 216, 432
Intestinal juice
  digestive fluids 129
  disaccharidase 129
  enterokinase 129
  lecithinase 129
  nucleosidase 129
  peptidase 129
  phosphatase 129
  polynucleotidase 129

Intracellular fluid 329
Inulin 32
   clearance test 254
Invert sugar See Mutarotation
Iodine 318
   deficiency
      disorders, control 373
      manifestation 319
         goiter 319
   dietary sources 319
   functions 319
   number 41
Iron 319, 360, 378, 395t
   absorption
      decreases 321
      factors influencing 320
      promote 320
   deficiency 321
   dietary
      allowance 320
      sources 320
   excretion 321
   storage 321
   utilization 320
Ischemic heart disease 442
ISI standards 347
Isoleucine 54
Isomerism of glucose 6-phosphate 151

J

Jaffe's test 246
Jams 340
Jaundice 258
Jaundice See also Icterus
Jaundice
   common cause 427
   diagnosis 260
   different types 260t
   types 259
Jejunostomy feeding 416
Joint diseases 437
Juvenile-onset diabetes 432

K

Keratin 208
Kesari dal 343
Ketogenesis 180
Ketone
   bodies 36
   body metabolism 180

Ketosis 181
Khichdi 388
Kidney
   function 252
   stones 244
Krebs cycle 153
Krebs-Henseleit cycle 192
Kwashiorkor 230, 304, 305t

L

Lactoflavin 86 See also Riboflavin
Lactose 28
   of milk 17
Lathyrism 343
Lathyrus sativus 343
Lathyrus sativus See Kesari dal
Lecithins See Phosphatidyl cholines
Legumes See Pulses
Leucine 54
Leukocytes See White blood cells
Levulose 18
Liebermann-burchard reaction 49
Light
   cereal preparations 355
   diets 355
   microscopy 9
Linoleic acid 295
Lipids 143, 146
   absorption 134
   changes in 337
   chemistry 36
   classification 37
   digestion and absorption 174
   functions 295
   layer, diffusion 13
   metabolism 145, 175, 218
      effects 220
Lipolysis 175
Lipoproteins 47, 70
   functions 48, 48t
   type 47t
Lipotropic agents 180
Liver 291
   "causes, infective hepatitis cirrhosis" 428
   dietary treatment, infective hepatitis cirrhosis 429
   "fat, factors influencing accumulation" 179f
   function tests 263

infective hepatitis cirrhosis 428
principles of diet, infective hepatitis cirrhosis 428
Lower blood cholesterol levels 298
Lower jejunum 133
Lysine 54
L-α-amino acids found in protein 56*t*

M

Macrominerals 307
Magnesium 316
  dietary sources 316
  function 316
Magnetotherapy 410
Maintenance of acid-base balance 232
Malnutrition 280
  causes 280
  for deficiencies 18
  in India, causes 274
  mortality and morbidity 281
Maltose 26
Manganese 322
  sources 322
Marasmic kwashiorkor 304
Marasmus 304, 305*t*
Marmalades 340
Massage therapy 410
Meat 361
  products order 346
Medicine, biochemical perspective 3
Melanin 55
Membrane lipids See Structural lipids
Metabolic
  acidosis 236
    symptoms 237
  actions of insulin 215
  alkalosis 237
  disorders 436
    of urea cycle 195
    therapeutic diet in conditions 431
  pool 188
    of amino acids 189, 189*f*
Metabolism 303
  biomedical importance 145
  concepts 140
  definition 140
  of amino acids 189
  of carbohydrates 149
  of glutamic acid 195
  of lipids 173
  of proteins 188

Metalloproteins 70
Methionine 53
Microminerals 316
Mid-day meal program 373
Milk
  and milk products 360
  preparations 352, 353
    whey 353
  protein 68
Millets 359
Minerals 359, 378, 382, 392, 400, 418, 420, 429
  changes 337
  metabolism 307
  required in human nutrition 307*t*
Minor nutrients 271
Misbranding 347
Mitochondria 7
Mitochondrion, structure 7, 8*f*
Mixed diets 284
Molisch's test See Carbohydrates, test for
Molybdenum 324
  absorption and excretion 324
  deficiency manifestation 324
  dietary sources 324
  functions 324
  recommended dietary allowance 324
Monosaccharides 18*t*, 25
Mucopolysaccharides 32
Mud therapy 410
Mutarotation 19, 20
Mycobacterium tuberculosis 421
Myosin 208

N

Na^+-K^+ pump 313
N-acetyl glucosaminidase 121
Nasogastric feeding 416
National Institute of Nutrition 369
National Nutritional Policy 274
Natural food remedies 411
Nature cure, methods 410
Naturopathic medicine 407
Naturopathy 408
Negative ions, addition 72
Nephrosis 439
  dietary treatment 439
  principles of diet 439
  symptoms 439

Nervous system 398
Net protein utilization 300
Neurotransmitters 70
Neutral
　fat See Triglycerides, functions of
　fats 173
　mucopolysaccharides 32
　protamine hagedorn 433
　salt solution, addition 72
NH_3, detoxification 195
Niacin 87
Nicotinamide adenine dinucleotide 106, 107, 142
Nicotinic acid 87
Night blindness 80
Ninhydrin
　reactions 60, 70
　test 73
Nitrogen
　balance 189
　base + sugar 101
　＋ phosphate 101
Non-essential amino acids 53
Non-insulin-dependent diabetes mellitus 216
Non-protein nitrogen 243
　containing compounds 52
Norepinephrine 220
　functions 220
Normal diet 415
Normal urine
　analysis 246
　constituents 242
Normal value of
　blood sugar 159
　important tests 447
Nucin 127
Nucleic acids 17, 99, 101
　functions 104
　purines 100
　size 103
　types 102
Nucleoproteins 70
　components 100*f*
Nucleosides 101
Nucleotides 99, 101
　of biological importance 104
Nucleus 6
Nurse in nutritional programs, role 372

Nurses in nutritional assessment 375
Nutrients 270, 271
　classification 271
　in therapeutic diets, modification 414
　preservation 332
　value of human and cow milk, comparison 383*t*
Nutrition 269, 306
　education 375
　　of community, methods 374
　　means 374
　education, objectives 374
　history 269
　in infancy 382
　in pregnancy 377
Nutritional
　aspects of fats 294
　assessment 365
　considerations in diarrhea 424
　problems in India 272, 272*t*
　requirements for various food components 399
　state 286
　status 279
　　assessment 365
Nuts 359
Nyctalopia 80

O

O_2 See Superoxide anion
Obesity 293, 386, 437
Oil seeds 359
Oils 361
Old age, menu plan 404*t*
Oligosaccharides 29
Oliguria See also Anuria
Optical isomerism 19, 61
Optimum temperature 118
Organelles 6
Ornithine cycle See also Krebs-Henseleit cycle
Osazone formation 24
Osmosis 14
Osteoarthritis 437
Osteomalacia 82
Ovarian hormones 214
Oven roasting 334
Overhydration 331
　symptoms 331

Oxidation 24
  of fatty acids 175
  of glyceraldehyde 3-phosphate 151
  of pyruvate to acetyl-coA 150
  reduction nucleotides 106
Oxidative deamination 192
Oxygen
  species, formation of reactive 205
  supply 205
  transport 228
Oxyhemoglobin 233

P

Pancha mahabhootas 409
Pancreatic
  islet cells 221
  juice 128
Pantothenic acid 89
Pantothenic acid See Vitamin B_5
Parasitic infections 274
Parathyroid
  glands and hormones 219
  hormone 219
Parenteral feeding 417
Pathological
  fatty liver 180
  urine, analysis 247
Pentoses 25
  examples 26t
Pepsin catalyzes 131
Peptide
  bonds 64
  hormones 215
Pernicious anemia 94
pH 232
  effect 117
  of blood
    homeostasis 232
    regulation 232
Phase contrast microscopy 10
Phenol red excretion test for kidney function See Phenolsulfonphthalein test
Phenolsulfonphthalein 255
  test 255
Phosphate
  buffers 233
  product 309
  test 246

Phosphatidyl
  cholines 42
  ethanolamine 43
Phosphoglycerides 42
Phospholipids 37, 42
  functions 296
Phosphoproteins 70
Phosphorus 259, 310, 438
  functions 310
Phosphorylation of
  fructose 6-phosphate 151
  glucose 151
Phrynoderma 297
Pigment metabolism 258
Plasma
  flow, measurement 256
  lipids 173
    estimation 49
    transportation 174
  proteins 229, 264, 303
    albumin 229
    during electrophoresis, distribution 231f
    separation 231
  sodium level alteration 312
  transport 321
Plasmalogens 44
Platelets 226
Poached egg 354
Poisoning by other organisms 343
Poisonous
  animals 343
  plants 343
Polyhydric alcohols 16
Polysaccharides 29
Polyunsaturated fatty acids 443
Pooled urine 240
Poor man's milk 359
Population growth 274
Porridge 356
Positive ions, addition 72
Posthepatic jaundice 259
Postoperative diet 419
Postprandial thermogenesis 287
Pot roasting 335
Potassium 313, 438, 440
  bicarbonate 233
  dietary
    allowance 313
    sources 313

hyperkalemia 314
hypokalemia 314
metabolic functions 313
oxalate 227
Pre- and postoperative diet 417
Precipitating factors 430
Prehepatic jaundice 259
Preoperative nutritional assessment 418
Preparation of simple beverages 352
Preschool children, menu plan 393t
Preterm babies 387
Prevention of Food Adulteration
    Act, 1954 345
Primary tissue building 303
Procollagen 207
Progesterone 215
Prokaryotes 9
Prokaryotic
    and eukaryotic cells, differentiation 9t
    cells 9
Proline 53
Proopiomelanocortin 223
Protective foods 282, 362
Protein 143, 144, 291, 299, 382, 391,
    399, 418, 419, 429, 438, 440
    absorption 54, 135
    aids metabolic functions 303
    and amino acid metabolism,
        pathway 190f
    animal sources 302
    biomedical importance 65
    by enzymes, digestion 188
    calorie malnutrition in children 305
    changes 337
    channels, diffusion 13
    chemistry 64
    classification 68
    composition 64
    content of some foodstuffs 302t
    deficiency 304
    denaturation 68, 71
    digestion 131
    efficiency ratio 300
    electrophoresis 264
    excess 306
    foods 305, 425
        deficiency 305
    functions 303
    in mouth, digestion 131

in small intestine, digestion 132
in stomach, digestion 131
inter-relationship in metabolism 146
metabolism 52, 218
    pathway 189
on biological function 70
on composition 69
on nutritional level 69
on solubility 68
plant sources 302
primary
    structure 66
    tissue building 303
properties 70
quality 299
quaternary structure 67
secondary structure 66
structure 66
tertiary structure 67
test for 274
transport 12, 70
    carrier 12
    channel 12
    utilization 52
Prothrombin time See Coagulation
    factors
Provitamin A See β-carotene
Ptyalin 127
Ptyalin See Salivary amylase
Pulses 359
Pyranose ring 21
Pyridoxine 87
Pyridoxine See Vitamin B_6
Pyrimidines of nucleic acids 100
Pyruvate, formation 152

Q

Quetelet's index 289

R

Ragi conjee 355
Rancidity 40
Raw tomato juice, beverages 353
RBCs See Red blood cells
Recommended dietary allowance 278,
    301
Red blood cells 16, 228
Reducing sugar, test 247

Reduction of pyruvate to lactate 153
Refusal to take new food 386
Religious belief 276
Renal
  blood, measurement 256
  function tests 252
  mechanism 234
  system 399
Reserve fuel supply 291
Respiratory
  acidosis 236
  alkalosis 236
  chain 142
  quotient 284
Rheumatism 437
Rheumatoid arthritis 437
Riboflavin 86
Riboflavin See Vitamin B_2
Riboflavin
  deficiency 87
  function 87
  sources 87
Ribonucleic acid 6, 102
Ribosomes 6, 102
Rice
  dal 388
  milk 388
Rickets 82, 310
RNA See Ribonucleic acid
RNA, secondary structure 102
Roasting of bread 337
Rothera's test 180
  for acetone and acetoacetic acid 249

S

Sago porridge 356
Salivary
  amylase 130
  digestion, digestive fluids 127
Salmonella typhi 420
Salt, addition 340
Saponification 40
  number 41
Scavenger enzymes 206
Schiff's test 244
School-age children, menu plan 394*t*
Scrambled 354
SDA See Specific dynamic action
Secretin 221

Secretion 217
Selenium 318
  deficiency 318
  dietary
    allowance 318
    sources 318
  excess 318
  functions 318
Semi-essential amino acids 52
Serine 53
Serum
  bilirubin, van den Bergh test 259
  glutamic
    oxaloacetic transaminase 263
    pyruvic transaminase 263
  potassium 313
  proteins, tests for detecting changes 265
Severe
  infections 430
  protein deficiency disease 230
Sex See also Gender
Sex hormones 213
Shallow fat frying 335
Simple
  lipids 37
  proteins 69
  tests to detect adulteration in items of
    daily use 348*t*
Skimmed milk powder 360
Smooth muscle, action 220
Sodium 311, 438, 440
  bicarbonate 233
  carbonate 23
  citrate 23, 227
  dietary
    allowance 313
    sources 312
  fluoride 228
  functions 311
  hypernatremia 312
    symptoms 312
  hypobromide test 243
  hyponatremia 312
    symptoms 312
Soft diet 352, 415
Soft-cooked egg 354
Solar vitamin 81
Somatotropin See also Growth
  hormone
Soups 354

Space therapy 410
Special diets, management 415
Special feeding methods 415
Special tissue function 290
Sphingomyelins 42, 44
Spit roasting 334
Standard urea clearance 253
Staphylococcus 342
   aureus 342
Starch 16, 17, 29, 290
   test 30
Steamed fish 355
Stereoisomerism 61
Stereoisomers 19
Stereospecificity 114
Steroid 45
   hormones 213
Sterol 213
Stool and urine 367
Storage proteins 70
Structural
   and contractile proteins 207
   lipids 42
   proteins 207
Substances associated with lipids 38
Sucrose 17, 28
Sugar 17, 290, 361
   cyclic forms 20
   non-reducing 23
   reducing 23
   See also Salt, addition
   See also Starch
   substitutes 293
Suji halwa 388
Sulfa drugs 218
Sulfolipids 37
Sulfosalicylic acid test 248
Sulfur 315
   containing amino acids 53
   dietary sources 315
   excretion 315
   functions 315
Superoxide anion 206
Supplementary
   feeding programs 372t
   foods, types 385
Synthesis, site 48t

T

Tea, beverages 352
Temperature
   correction 242
   effect 118
Tertiary structure 67f
Tetrahydrofolic acid 119
Tetroses 25
Thermogenic effect of food 287
Thiamine 85
   deficiency 86
   dry beriberi: 86
   function 86
   sources 86
   wet beriberi 86
Thiocarbamide 218
Thiocyanate 218
Threonine 53
Thymol 240
Thyroid hormones 167, 217
Thyroid-stimulating hormone 223
Thyrotoxicosis 436
Thyrotropic hormone See also
   Thyroid-stimulating hormone
Thyroxine 218
Thyroxine See Thyroid hormone
Thyroxine-binding
   globulin 217
   prealbumin 217
TMV See Tobacco mosaic virus
Toad skin 297
Tobacco mosaic virus 103
Toluene 240
Toxicity See Selenium excess
Toxins 259
Transamination 190
Transport mechanism 13
   across cell membrane 12
   active 13
   passive 13
Treponema pallidum 10
Triacylglycerols 36, 173
Tricarboxylic acid
   cycle 153
Trichloroacetic acid See also
   Ammonium sulfate

Index

Triglycerides, functions 295
Trioses 25
Tryptophan 53
Tube feeding 416
Tuberculosis 421
  dietary management 422
  energy 422
  minerals 422
  principles of diet 422
  protein 422
  vitamins 422
Typhoid 420
  foods to be
    avoided 421
    included 421
  principles of diet 421

U

Unconjugated bilirubin 259
Underweight 386
United Nations Children's Emergency Fund 273
Upma 388
Urea 243
  clearance 253
  clearance test 253
    procedure 254
  cycle 192, 196f
    significance 195
  synthesis 192
Urease
  catalyzes 114
  test 243
Uremia See also Chronic renal failure
Uric acid 244
Urinalysis 240
Urinary
  calculi See also Urolithiasis
  elevation 121
  system, therapeutic diet in conditions 438
Urine
  appearance 241
  collection 240
  color 241
  composition 241
  concentration test 254
  odor 241
  preservative 240
  specific gravity 241
  volume 241
Urolithiasis 441
  causes 441
  dietary management 441
  types of calculi 441
Uronic acid 24, 32
  pathway 159

V

Valine 54
Vegetable 360
  soup 355
Very low-density lipoproteins 174
Viral
  hepatitis 427
Vital statistics, study 368
Vitamin 77, 378, 383, 400, 419, 420, 429
  A 77, 78
    aldehyde 78
    and vision 80
    conversion of beta-carotene to retinal 78
    deficiency 280
      diseases 80
    functions 79
    prophylaxis program 372
    requirements 78
    sources 78
    toxin 81
  absorption 135
  B complex 344
  B_1 See Thiamine
  B_2 269
  B_{12} See Cobalamin
  B_{12}
    deficiency 94
      manifestations 94
    functions 94
    sources 94
  B_2 86
  B_3 106
  B_3 See Niacin
    deficiency 88
    functions 88
    source 88

B_5 89
  deficiency 89
  functions 89
  sources 89
B_6 269
B_6 See Pyridoxine
  deficiency 87
  function 87
  sources 87
B_7 See Biotin
  deficiency 94
  functions 89
  sources 89
B_7 functions 89
B_9 See Folacin
  deficiency 88
  functions 88
  sources 88
C 41, 84, 207, 360
  deficiency 85
  function 85
  sources 85
changes 337
classification 77
D 77, 81, 360
  deficiency 82
  physiological action 82
  sources 81
deficiency diseases 90t
definition 77
E 77, 83, 206, 359
  deficiency 83
  function 83
  source 83
functions 90t
K 77, 83
  deficiency 84
  function 84
  sources 84
  not acting as coenzymes 78
  sources 90t
Vomiting 386

W

Wald's visual cycle 80
Water 328
  and electrolyte balances,
    disorders 330
  balance 329
  dehydration 330
  functions 328
  importance 328
  intoxication 331
  metabolism 328
  soluble vitamins 77, 84
    B complex 378
    coenzymes 121
    relationship among 122t
    vitamin C 378
  therapy 410, 412
Weaning 385
  problems 386
White blood cells 226
Xanthinuria, causes 324
Xanthoproteic test 73
Zinc 317
  absorption 317
  dietary
    requirement 317
    sources 317
  excretion 317
  function 317
Zwitterion formation 60